Cognitive Impairment and Dementia in Parkinson's Disease

Cognitive Impairment and Dementia in Parkinson's Disease

Edited by

Prof. Dr. Murat Emre

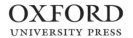

OXFORD

UNIVERSITY PRESS

OXFORD

UNIVERSITY PRESS

Great Clarendon Street, Oxford OX2 6DP

Oxford University Press is a department of the University of Oxford.
It furthers the University's objective of excellence in research, scholarship,
and education by publishing worldwide in

Oxford New York

Auckland Cape Town Dar es Salaam Hong Kong Karachi
Kuala Lumpur Madrid Melbourne Mexico City Nairobi
New Delhi Shanghai Taipei Toronto

With offices in

Argentina Austria Brazil Chile Czech Republic France Greece
Guatemala Hungary Italy Japan Poland Portugal Singapore
South Korea Switzerland Thailand Turkey Ukraine Vietnam

Oxford is a registered trade mark of Oxford University Press
in the UK and in certain other countries

Published in the United States
by Oxford University Press Inc., New York

© Oxford University Press, 2010

British Library Cataloguing in Publication Data

Data available

Library of Congress Cataloging in Publication Data

Data available

Typeset in Minion by Glyph International, Banglore, India
Printed in Great Britain
on acid-free paper by
CPI Antony Rowe, Chippenham, Wiltshire

ISBN 978-0-19-956411-8

10 9 8 7 6 5 4 3 2 1

Foreword

The realization that cognitive impairment is more frequent in Parkinson's disease than one would expect by chance has been slow to achieve universal acceptance amongst neurologists. The age of the patient rather than the duration of disease is the major risk factor for dementia, frontal executive functions and visuospatial impairment are often more prominent than amnesia. Young onset patients rarely develop severe memory loss before the seventh decade of life and when it occurs it is ushered in by daytime somnolence and visual hallucinations. On the other hand patients presenting in their late sixties may have bradyphrenia and difficulties drawing overlapping pentagons from the outset of their illness, raising the possibility of distinct subtypes of Parkinson's disease. Dementia with Lewy bodies (DLB) was claimed to be the second commonest neurodegenerative cause of dementia, but it seems likely that if current operational criteria are adhered to it is rare and extremely uncommon in the absence of any signs of Parkinsonism. Most but not all cases of both Parkinson's disease dementia and DLB are associated with neocortical Lewy bodies, but they are unlikely to be the primary pathological substrate for cognitive impairment.

Although cholinomimetics are efficacious in Parkinson's disease dementia the effect on an individual patient cannot be predicted with some patients improving strikingly while others not at all. This may reflect different underlying pathological substrates for the cognitive impairment or pharamaco-genetic differences. Cholinomimetics also seem to be helpful for daytime somnolence, reduced vigilance and visual hallucinations in some patients.

Professor Emre and his contributors have done a scholarly job in reviewing the complexities of a subject which remains the major challenge to effective management of Parkinson's disease and yet remains taboo. He is to be congratulated for publishing a book which will inform practicing clinicians and will hopefully stimulate the young generation of neurologists to intensify their research efforts into unravellling the enigma of neurodegenerative disease and the aging brain.

Andrew Lees
Reta Lila Weston Institute of Neurological Studies
University College London
UK

Contents

Contributors

Dag Aarsland
Psychiatric Division,
Section for Geriatric Psychiatry
Stavanger University Hospital
Department of Clinical Medicine
University of Bergen
Bergen, Norway

Clive Ballard
Wolfson Centre for Age-Related Diseases
Guy's Campus
King's College London
London, UK

Paolo Barone
Department of Neurological Sciences
University of Napoli Federico II and IDC
Hermitage-Capodimonte
Napoli, Italy

Kolbjørn Brønnick
Norwegian Centre for Movement
Disorders
Stavanger University Hospital
Stavanger, Norway

David J. Burn
Institute for Ageing and Health
Newcastle University
Newcastle upon Tyne, UK

Elise Caccappolo
Division of Aging and Dementia
Department of Neurology
Columbia University
New York, New York, USA

Murat Emre
İstanbul Faculty of Medicine
Department of Neurology
Behavioral Neurology and Movement
Disorders Unit
İstanbul University
İstanbul, Turkey

Michael Firbank
Institute for Ageing and Health
Newcastle University
Newcastle upon Tyne
UK

Nir Giladi
Department of Neurology
Faculty of Medicine
Tel Aviv Sourasky Medical Center
Tel-Aviv University
Tel-Aviv, Israel

Rita Guerreiro
Laboratory of Neurogenetics
National Institute on Aging
Bethesda
Maryland, USA

John Hardy
Institute of Neurology
Reta Lila Weston Institute of
Neurological Studies
University College London
London, UK

Jeffrey M. Hausdorff
Department of Neurology
Tel Aviv Sourasky Medical Center
Department of Physical Therapy
Faculty of Medicine
Tel-Aviv University
Tel-Aviv, Israel
and
Department of Medicine
Harvard Medical School

Alex Iranzo
Neurology Service
Institut Clínic de Neurociències
Hospital Clínic de Barcelona
Centro de Investigación Biomédica en
Red sobre Enfermedades
Neurodegenerativas (CIBERNED)
University of Barcelona
Barcelona, Spain

Jaime Kulisevsky
Movement Disorders Unit
Neurology Department
Sant Pau Hospital
Autonomous University of
Barcelona and CIBERNED
(Centro de Investigación en red
Enfermedades Neurodegenerativas)
Barcelona, Spain

Carol Lippa
Department of Neurology
Drexel University College of Medicine
Philadelphia
Pennsylvania, USA

Eugenia Mamikonyan
Department of Psychiatry
University of Pennsylvania
Philadelphia
Pennsylvania, USA

Karen Marder
Division of Aging and Dementia
Department of Neurology
Columbia University
New York, New York, USA

Ian McKeith
Wolfson Research Centre
Institute for Ageing and Health
Newcastle University

Anat Mirelman
Department of Neurology
Tel Aviv Sourasky Medical Center
Tel-Aviv, Israel

Yoshikuni Mizuno
Juntendo University Koshigaya Hospital
Koshigaya, Japan

John T. O'Brien
Institute for Ageing and Health
Newcastle University
Newcastle upon Tyne, UK

Yasuyuki Okuma
Department of Neurology
Juntendo University Shizuoka Hospital
Izunokuni, Japan

Javier Pagonabarraga
Movement Disorders Unit
Neurology Department
Sant Pau Hospital
Autonomous University of Barcelona
and CIBERNED (Centro de
Investigación en red Enfermedades
Neurodegenerativas)
Barcelona, Spain

Meir Plotnik
Department of Neurology
Tel Aviv Sourasky Medical Center
Tel-Aviv, Israel

Gonzalo J. Revuelta
Department of Neurology
Emory University School of Medicine
Atlanta
Georgia, USA

Gabriella Santangelo
Department of Neurological Sciences
University of Napoli Federico II and IDC
Hermitage-Capodimonte
Napoli, Italy

Galit Yogev-Seligman
Department of Neurology
Tel Aviv Sourasky Medical Center
Tel-Aviv, Israel

Andrew Singleton
Laboratory of Neurogenetics
National Institute on Aging
Bethesda
Maryland, USA

Eduardo Tolosa
Neurology Service
Institut Clínic de Neurociències
Hospital Clínic de Barcelona
Centro de Investigación Biomédica en
Red sobre Enfermedades
Neurodegenerativas (CIBERNED)
University of Barcelona
Barcelona, Spain

Daniel Weintraub
University of Pennsylvania
Philadelphia
Pennsylvania, USA

Chapter 1

Introduction

Murat Emre

James Parkinson was more than a physician. One of his biographers records that 'Like many of his contemporaries he had absorbing and overwhelming interests which ranged successively, and successfully, through politics, the church, medicine and geology' and that 'James was a careful, perhaps obsessional, man.' [1] He had many intellectual skills; above all he was a sharp and succint observer, which enabled him to find associations not described before, resulting in discoveries and descriptions in medicine, geology and palaeontology, which still bear his name. Yet Parkinson's 'An essay on the shaking palsy', which otherwise so succintly described the features of the disease that was later named after him, almost completely dismissed the mental aspects. He desribed the characteristic features of the disease as 'Involuntary tremulous motion with lessened muscular power, in parts not in action and even when supported, with a propensity to bend the trunk forwards and to pass from a walking to a running pace: the senses and intellects being uninjured.' [2] This statement, 'senses and intellects being uninjured', was probably one of the main reasons that mental dysfunction in PD was ignored for a long time to come, although his general descripton of the final stages of the disease ends with the statement that 'The urine and faeces are passed involuntarily; and at the last, constant sleepiness, with slight delirium, and other marks of extreme exhaustion, announce the wished-for release.' This brief statement on likely mental dysfunction caught less attention as it was less unequivocal. Parkinson was honest about the potential shortcomings of his descriptions as he admits in the opening remarks in the Preface that 'it therefore is necessary, that some conciliatory explanation should be offered for the present publication: in which, it is acknowledged, that mere conjecture takes the place of experiment; and, that analogy is the substitute for anatomical examination, the only sure foundation for pathological knowledge.' He realized that early and late stage symptoms may be different as he states that 'The disease is of long duration: to connect, therefore, the symptoms, which occur in its later stages with those which mark its commencement, requires a continuance of observation of the same case, or at least a correct history of its symptoms, even for several years. Of both these advantages the writer has had the opportunities of availing himself; and has hence been led particularly to observe several other cases in which the disease existed in different stages of its progress.' Parkinson was a modest and unassuming man; true to form, he ended his opening remarks as follows: 'Should the necessary information be thus obtained, the writer will repine at no censure which the precipitate publication of mere conjectural suggestions may incur; but shall think himself fully rewarded by having excited the attention of those, who may point out the most appropriate means of relieving a tedious and most distressing malady.' He did excite attention for decades to come, for which he received the well-deserved credit and recognition. His concluding remarks were examplary and constitute a timely reminder for all contemporary clinical scientists: 'Before concluding these pages, it may be proper to observe once more, that an important object proposed to be obtained by them is, the leading of the attention of those who humanely employ anatomical examination in detecting the causes and nature of diseases, particularly to this malady. By their benevolent labors its real nature may be ascertained, and appropriate modes of relief, or even cure, pointed out.'

Why would such an excellent observer miss or ignore the mental aspects of the disease? The reasons are probably rather simple: James Parkinson did not observe a large number of patients – his essay was based on the study of only six. Two of them were 'casually met with in the street' (one 62 and the other about 65 years of age), questioned and observed once, a third case 'the particulars of which could not be obtained, and the gentleman, the lamented subject of which was only seen at a distance.' He personally attended to the other three patients, two of them in their fifties, and the third was examined at the age of 72 years, with a disease duration ranging from about 5–12 years. One of these patients was lost to follow-up after the first examination, and probably only one was followed to his terminal stages. Of particular note is that five of his six cases were seen at a relatively young age. We now know that age is the most important risk factor for dementia and that it rarely occurs in patients below the age of 60 years.

In fact, the occurrence of cognitive dysfunction and dementia in some patients with what came to be known as Parkinson's disease was recognized shortly after the description by Parkinson himself. Charcot, who called the disease 'Maladie de Parkinson' in 1877 in his 'Lectures on Diseases of the Nervous System', stated during these that 'at a given point, the mind becomes clouded and the memory is lost.' He had already referred to these aspects of the disease during 1861–62, together with Vulpian that 'in general, psychic faculties are definitely impaired.' Nevertheless these statements drew less attention and for many years PD was perceived to be a pure motor disorder.

As survival time of PD patients became substantially longer with modern dopaminergic treatment, cognitive dysfunction and dementia became more apparent. Descriptions from the 1960s onwards pointed out that dementia may accompany PD. Even then, it was assumed that dementia in PD (PD-D) may be a consequence of the ageing process, as ageing was recognized to be the main risk factor for PD-D. The observation that Alzheimer's disease (AD)-type pathology, in particular plaques, frequently accompanies PD-D subsequently led to the contention that dementia in PD simply represents coincident AD. This perception delayed the recognition of PD-D as a separate entity. Subsequently, however, prospective epidemiological studies clearly demonstrated that both prevalence and incidence of dementia in PD is substantially increased as compared with age-matched controls, indicating that dementia was related to the disease pathology itself. With refining of neuropscyhological methods and understanding of circuits subserving discrete mental processes, the clinical profile of PD dementia was better worked out in comparative studies, demonstrating the differences between this disorder and AD. In parallel, comprehensive clinico-pathological studies were conducted, which gained particular momentum after the discovery that the main component of Lewy bodies (LB) is α-synuclein. Development of immunohistochemistry using antibodies against this protein, which turned out to be more sensitive to detect LB-type pathology than the conventional ubiquitin staining, was crucial in dissecting out the underlying pathology. All these developments were instrumental for the recognition of PD-D as a separate entity and dementia as an integral part of the disease spectrum of PD.

The consequences of considering dementia as part of the pathological substrate of PD are not only academic. As PD patients survive longer due to more efficient treatment for their motor symptoms, cognitive deficits and dementia occur more often and constitute one of the main reasons for severe disability in the later stages of the disease. These deficits are not responsive to dopaminergic substitution and often worsen under such treatment. Hence, understanding and managing all aspects of dementia in PD have practical relevance for patients and their families. Full recognition of its clinical features would allow accurate diagnosis as well as development of assessment measures to evauate the natural course of the disease and the potential benefits of future treatments. Understanding associated biochemical deficits, pathophysiology and pathology would allow such potential treatments to be developed.

Much has already been achieved. Major epidemiological studies produced valuable data as to the point prevelance, cumulative incidence and risk factors associated with PD-D. A number of clinical studies were able to discern the profile of cognitive deficits and the frequency as well as the spectrum of accompanying behavioural symptoms. Comprehensive clinical–pathological correlation studies successfully described the type and topography of the underlying pathology, and genetic findings provided data supporting the role of α-synuclein. Finally specific clinical diagnostic criteria were published and the first specific treatment became available.

The purpose of this book is to compile in one volume the data that have accumulated over the course of the last few decades. Physicians treating patients with PD will be able to find information on all aspects of the disease without need for time-consuming searches. It is also hoped that this book might invoke more interest on PD-D, giving rise to new ideas and initiatives. It would be appropriate to echo James Parkinson's concluding remarks: the editor and the authors of this book would feel fulfilled and satisfied if this latter purpose is served.

References

1 Gardner-Thorpe C. James Parkinson, 1755–1824. Exeter: A Wheaton & Co. Ltd, 1988.
2 Parkinson J. An essay on the shaking palsy. London: Whittingham & Rowland, 1817.

Chapter 2

Epidemiology of dementia associated with Parkinson's disease

Dag Aarsland

Introduction

Studies of the frequency of dementia in Parkinson's disease (PD) have used a variety of methods and designs, which may affect the outcome. Important methodological features include tests to assess cognition, definitions of dementia, and the criteria for selecting patients. For example, results vary according to whether attempts were made to identify all patients in a defined region or whether the study was based on convenience samples from hospital clinics. The optimal case identification method is door-to-door survey, but few studies have used this method to report the prevalence or incidence of Parkinson's disease with dementia (PD-D) in the general population. Most studies have been cross-sectional, providing an estimate of the proportion of PD patients who are demented (point prevalence). For several reasons, including the higher mortality rate in PD-D versus non-demented PD subjects [1], more accurate information regarding the true frequency of dementia in PD can be drawn from longitudinal studies. Such studies provide information on the incidence of PD-D. Furthermore, if a healthy control group is included, such studies can also deduce the relative increase in the risk of developing dementia related to PD. In addition, period prevalence, i.e. the total proportion of people with dementia in a PD cohort during a specified time, by combining prevalence, incidence and mortality rates, provides important information concerning the total proportion of PD patients who will eventually develop dementia.

Point prevalence

In an early review of 27 studies representing 4336 patients with PD, Cummings [2] found a mean prevalence of dementia of 40%. Although the studies were critically considered, most studies were based on patients referred to neurology clinics and may therefore not be representative of unselected PD populations. In addition, at that time, studies did not include the identification and exclusion of patients with DLB.

In a systematic review employing strict methodological inclusion and exclusion criteria, 13 studies with a total of 1767 patients were included. Of these, 554 were diagnosed with dementia, yielding a prevalence of 31.3% (95% confidence interval 29.2–33.6). This review also included 24 studies which explored the prevalence of dementia in the general population and included patients with PD. In this analysis 3–4% of patients with dementia in the general population were due to PD-D. The estimated prevalence of PD-D in the general population aged ≥65 years was found to be 0.3–0.5% [3]. The results of studies published after this review are in line with these findings, reporting PD-D rates of 48% [4], 23% [5] and 22% [6].

Incidence

Most studies on the incidence of dementia in PD have been based on longitudinal studies of community-based cohorts. In such studies, incidence rates of 95.3 [7] and 112.5 [8] in 1000 patient-years were reported, indicating that about 10% of a PD population will develop dementia per year. The relative risk for developing dementia in PD compared with non-PD subjects ranges from 1.7 [8], to 4.7 [6], 5.1 [4], and 5.9 [7]. There are several reasons for this variation, including case selection procedures, definitions of dementia, and the use of different estimates of risk.

Whereas most incidence studies have explored the probability of developing dementia in defined PD populations, frequency of dementia in patients with PD as part of a large, prospective, population-based cohort study of the general population was recently reported in two studies. In the MRC Cognitive Function and Ageing Study [9], all subjects aged ≥65 years in defined geographical regions of the UK were invited to participate, and more than 13 000 participants had a screening interview. Participants were assessed at baseline and two follow-up waves 2 and 6 years later. The proportion of PD was 2% and 3%, respectively, in those with dementia, compared to 1% in those without dementia, and the total adjusted odds ratio was 3.5 (1.3–9.3). The Rotterdam study was based on a door-to-door survey of nearly 8000 subjects aged ≥55 years at baseline in 1990–1993 [6]. Two follow-up visits were performed, and patients were diagnosed with prevalent PD at baseline ($n = 99$) and incident PD during follow-up ($n = 67$). The mean follow-up time was 6.9 years, and 4.3 years in the incident PD group. During follow-up, 15% of the prevalent PD group developed dementia compared with 4.9% of the control group, with a hazard ratio of 2.80 (1.79–4.38). In the incident cohort, the hazard ratio was 4.74 (2.49–9.02). The association of PD with dementia was more pronounced in those with at least one APOE *e4* allele, and especially with those with at least one *e2* allele, compared with *e3/e3* carriers.

The majority of 'incidence' studies of dementia in PD have been longitudinal studies of prevalence cohorts, meaning that patients with a variery of disease durations have been followed. Since the risk for developing dementia depends on the duration of disease, variations among cohorts in duration of PD will affect the incidence of dementia. Thus, following patients from onset of disease provides a more accurate and representative estimate of the incidence of dementia in PD. In the first study of dementia in PD based on an incident PD cohort, 180 PD patients were re-examined 3 and 5 years after baseline. The annual dementia incidence was 30 (16–53) per 1000 person-years [10]. In addition to the shorter duration of disease, the lower dementia incidence may also be related to the lower age at baseline in this cohort compared to most prevalence studies (Table 2.1).

Table 2.1 Studies of the incidence and relative risk for dementia in patients with PD

Study	Population	N-PD	Age at baseline	Duration of PD at baseline assessment	Rate/ 1000 pyr	Relative risk
Marder 1995	Community*	140	71	7	113	1.7(1.1-2.7)
Hughes 2000	Hospital	83	64	4	43	-
Aarsland 2001	Community	130	70	8.5	95	5.9(3.9-9.1)
Hobson 2005	Community*	86	74	7	107	5.1(2.1-12.5)
De Lau 2005	Incident[1]	67	-	-	-	4.7(2.5-9.0)
MRC CFAS[2]	Community[1]*	8	-	-	-	3.5(1.3-9.3)
Williams-Gray 2007	Incidence	126	70	Assessed at time of diagnosis	30	-

* 65+; 1) door-to-door survey of whole population

2) Age Ageing 2006

Period (cumulative) prevalence

Since the mortality is higher among demented than non-demented PD subjects [1], point prevalence is an underestimate of the true frequency of dementia in PD. Accordingly, reporting the cumulative proportion of PD patients who develop dementia with time provides a more accurate estimate of the frequency of dementia in PD. Some, but not all, longitudinal studies have controlled for the selected attrition due to death. Thus, merely adding up the number of patients who become demented before death will underestimate the true proportion with dementia. Another potential bias is the interval between assessments, since attrition due to death increases with the duration of the interval.

Only one study to date has prospectively followed newly diagnosed PD patients to assess the frequency of dementia over more than 10 years. In the Sydney study, 136 patients with carefully diagnosed PD were recruited from neurologists for inclusion in a clinical trial. Patients were assessed at baseline with a comprehensive neuropsychological assessment, and 17% were classified as having dementia, defined as impairment of memory and two additional cognitive domains [11]. As discussed above, several of these patients may have been classified as DLB today. After 3 and 5 years, 26% and 28% were demented [11]. After 15 years, 48% of the evaluated patients had dementia, a further 36% evidence of cognitive impairment and only 15% remained without evidence of cognitive impairment [12]. Recently, data from 20-year follow-up were presented [13], reporting that 83% of the 30 survivors had dementia after 20 years, and altogether 75% had developed dementia prior to death. No attempt to control for selective attrition due to death was made.

The Stavanger study was based on a prevalence cohort of people with PD in South-Western Norway, after a careful extensive search in the community. At baseline, the average duration of PD was 9 years, and 28% had dementia. After 8 years, after adjustment for mortality, the cumulative prevalence of dementia was found to be 78% [14]. Based on the 12-year follow-up period, Markov analysis was performed to enable a more precise estimate of the risk of developing dementia for an individual patient based on age, sex and duration of PD [15]. Without correcting for attrition due to death, the proportion that developed dementia has been stable at about 60%, but the cumulative prevalence steadily increased to 80–90% by age 90 years. More specifically, at age 70 years, a man with PD but no dementia has a life expectancy of 8 years, of which 3 years would be expected to be with dementia. At any age, the life expectancy after onset of dementia was substantially reduced. At 12-year follow-up, only 10% of the population were alive and without dementia, after having suffered from PD for an average of 19 years.

The majority of studies report that the mean duration from onset of PD to development of dementia is about 10 years [8,13,16]. There are, however, wide variations. In a study with two large community-based cohorts of patients with PD, we found a linear relationship between time from onset of PD to diagnosis of dementia (Figure 2.1). Whereas some patients develop cognitive impairment and subsequent dementia within a few years after onset of PD, others remain free from dementia for 20 or more years before developing dementia [8,17]. The time from onset of PD to dementia is related to clinical risk factors (see below) as well as to the type and extent of brain pathology [18]. Besides demonstrating a very high risk for developing dementia in people with PD, the Sydney and Stavanger studies on the other hand convincingly demonstrated that even after decades with PD, there are some people who remain free of dementia. Thus, in addition to identifying the risk factors for developing dementia in PD, a key research question is to identify factors which protect against dementia in long-standing PD. Similarly, since the

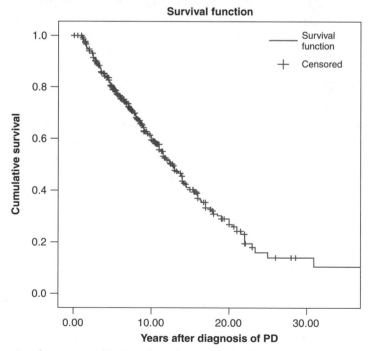

Fig. 2.1 The time from onset of Parkinson's disease to dementia diagnosis.

vast majority of PD patients will eventually develop dementia, another important question is to identify factors which are associated with the time to develop dementia in PD.

Risk factors for dementia in PD

Many demographic and clinical features have been assessed as potential risk factors for dementia in PD. The most consistent risk factors in longitudinal studies are more severe parkinsonism, higher age, and evidence of cognitive impairment at baseline.

Parkinsonism

Several longitudinal studies have confirmed that patients with more severe and advanced parkinsonism have a higher risk for dementia than those with less advanced PD. Particulary interesting is the report in several studies of association between specific motor symptoms and dementia. Symptoms such as rigidity, postural instability and gait disturbance predict more rapid cognitive decline and time to dementia. In one study, speech and axial impairment, indicative of predominantly non-dopaminergic deficiency, were found to predict incident dementia, whereas dopaminergic symptoms such as rigidity and akinesia were not [1]. Several studies have found that postural instability and gait disorder (PIGD) motor subtype are associated with dementia. The motor profile differs with time, the most common change being from tremor-dominant to PIGD type. We recently showed that in nearly all dementia cases, dementia was preceded by PIGD dominant, or by transition from tremor-dominant to PIGD type PD [19]. Similar findings were reported in another study [20]. In the CamPaign study of incident PD, severity of non-tremor type (i.e. mixed or PIGD type) motor symptom severity was associated with a higher risk for dementia independent of age [10].

Age

The majority of studies have found that age and age at onset are both associated with a higher risk of dementia. This is not surprising, given that age is the most prominent risk factor for dementia in the general population. Interestingly, age and severity of motor symptoms seem to have a combined rather than additive effect on the risk of dementia [1]. Age, duration of disease, and age at onset are highly correlated in PD cohorts, and thus it can be difficult to disentangle their relative importance, i.e. whether it is age, duration of disease or rather age of onset of PD that is driving the age-associated risk for dementia. There is evidence suggesting that age, but not age at onset or duration of disease, is the key risk factor for dementia in PD. Based on such evidence, a model of the relationship between age and disease-related processes in PD was proposed, suggesting that, on the background of the pathological process inherent to PD, ageing plays a substantial role in the pathogenesis through an interaction with the disease process in non-dopaminergic structures [1].

Mild cognitive impairment

A considerable proportion of non-demented PD patients have cognitive impairment, even early in the disease [21,22]. Impairment on neuropsychological tests, in particular tests of memory and executive functioning [1,23], were found to predict a shorter time to develop dementia. More recently, two groups have demonstrated that PD patients without dementia but with cognitive impairment, commonly labelled as mild cognitive impairment (MCI), have a higher risk for developing dementia over time than those with normal cognitive performance. First, in a cohort with advanced PD, Janvin *et al.* showed that after 4 years, more than 60% of PD patients with cognitive impairment had developed dementia compared with only 20% of those with normal cognition [23]. Similarly, in an incidence cohort, those with cognitive impairment at disease onset had a higher risk of dementia [10]. The validity of the concept of MCI is further supported by the imaging studies reporting some degree of cortical atrophy even in non-demented subjects with cognitive impairment [24].

The pattern of cognitive impairment in PD differs from that in Alzheimer's disease [25], but there is considerable cognitive heterogeneity even within PD. Some patients exhibit a typical executive-visuospatial impairment, whereas others show a more memory-dominant impairment. We found numerical evidence of some difference in the risk for dementia among patients with PD and different cognitive profiles [23], and this was confirmed recently in an incidence cohort. Patients with impairment in tests with a more posterior cortical basis, including semantic memory, had a higher risk for developing dementia than those with impairment of tests depending on frontal functions [10].

Visual hallucinations

Visual hallucinations (VH) are among the most characteristic neuropsychiatric features of PD, and may even aid in the differention of PD from other parkinsonian disorders [26]. VH are common in PD [27], particularly in patients with dementia [8]. In a longitudinal, community-based study, we found visual hallucinations to be associated both with a higher rate of cognitive decline [28] as well as a higher risk for development of dementia [14]. The association of VH with dementia is probably related to VH being associated both with Lewy body pathology in the temporal lobe, particularly in amygdala [29] as well as with cholinergic deficits [30]. Patients who develop hallucinations soon after initiation of dopaminergic treatment are also at higher risk to develop dementia [31].

Other factors

There is convincing evidence of an association between smoking and reduced risk for PD, possibly mediated by an effect upon nicotinic receptors. Nicotinic receptors are involved in learning and memory, and smoking may therefore theoretically protect against cognitive decline and dementia in PD. However, smoking also increases inflammation and oxidative stress and is associated with cardiovascular disease. Longitudinal studies have supported the hypothesis that smoking may reduce the risk for dementia and cognitive decline [32] in PD. However, another longitudinal study did not find an association between smoking and cognitive impairment [19].

A significant relationship between antiparkinson drug use and risk for dementia has not been convincingly demonstrated. However, an inverse relationship between use of amantadine and risk for dementia has been reported in a naturalistic longitudinal study [33]. Estrogen replacement therapy has been found to be associated with a decreased risk for dementia in PD, whereas risk factors for Alzheimer's disease and vascular dementia such as high cholesterol [34], head trauma, diabetes mellitus, and hypertension, were not associated with the risk for PD-D [1,35]. There is also conflicting evidence regarding whether hyperhomocysteinaemia, which is a well-known risk factor for cognitive decline in the general population, is associated with an increased risk for dementia in PD. Some studies have demonstrated this effect [36] whereas other studies have not found such an association [37]. However, cerebrovascular disease, although less common in PD than in the total population, seems to have a significant, but small, effect on the risk for dementia in PD [38].

Genetics

The study of genetics in PD has received much interest during the last decade, but few studies have systematically explored the potential relationship between genetics and dementia in PD. There is some evidence of an association between genes and risk of dementia in PD [39]. In a longitudinal community-based study, risk for dementia was not increased among the relatives of patients with PD compared with relatives of normal control subjects [40], although dementia in PD was associated with a family history of PD [40]. By contrast, in a recent large historical cohort study, a higher risk for cognitive impairment and dementia was found in relatives of PD patients compared with relatives of control subjects, particularly for PD patients with early age at onset [41].

The gene dosage of SNCA (the gene encoding alpha-synuclein) has been found to influence disease progression, including development of dementia [42,43].

The apolipoprotein (APOE) ε4 allele is associated with a higher risk and earlier disease onset of Alzheimer's disease, and several studies have explored the role of APOE in PD, with inconsistent results. An autopsy study suggested that the ε4 allele was associated with dementia in PD [44], and a similar conclusion was reached in a meta-analysis [45]. However, no association between PD-D and APOe ε4 could be seen when PD-D was more carefully defined [34].

A positive association of PD and PD-D with the *H1/H1* haplotype of tau (MAPT) gene has been reported in some [46], but not in all studies. In a recent prospective study based on an incidence cohort, an association between the *H1/H1* haplotype and increased risk for dementia was reported [47].

Conclusion

The point prevalence of dementia in PD is close to 30% and the incidence rate is increased 4–6 times compared with controls. The cumulative prevalence is very high – at least 75% of PD patients who survive for more than 10 years will develop dementia. The time from onset of PD to dementia varies considerably, however, and the most established risk factors are old age, severity of motor symptoms, in particular PIGD, MCI and presence of VH.

References

1 Levy G, Tang MX, Louis ED, *et al.* The association of incident dementia with mortality in PD. Neurology 2002; 59: 1708–13.

2 Cummings JL. Intellectual impairment in Parkinson's disease: clinical, pathologic, and biochemical correlates. J Geriatr Psychiatry Neurol 1988; 1: 24–36.

3 Aarsland D, Zaccai J, Brayne C. A systematic review of prevalence studies of dementia in Parkinson's disease. Mov Disord 2005; 20: 1255–63.

4 Hobson P, Meara J. Risk and incidence of dementia in a cohort of older subjects with Parkinson's disease in the United Kingdom. Mov Disord 2004; 19: 1043–9.

5 Athey RJ, Porter RW, Walker RW. Cognitive assessment of a representative community population with Parkinson's disease (PD) using the Cambridge Cognitive Assessment – Revised (CAMCOG-R). Age Ageing 2005; 34: 268–73.

6 de Lau LM, Schipper CM, Hofman A, Koudstaal PJ, Breteler MM. Prognosis of Parkinson disease: risk of dementia and mortality: the Rotterdam Study. Arch Neurol 2005; 62: 1265–9.

7 Aarsland D, Andersen K, Larsen JP, Lolk A, Nielsen H, Kragh-Sorensen P. Risk of dementia in Parkinson's disease: a community-based, prospective study. Neurology 2001; 56: 730–6.

8 Marder K, Tang MX, Alfaro B, *et al.* Risk of Alzheimer's disease in relatives of Parkinson's disease patients with and without dementia. Neurology 1999; 52: 719–24.

9 Yip AG, Brayne C, Matthews FE. Risk factors for incident dementia in England and Wales: The Medical Research Council Cognitive Function and Ageing Study. A population-based nested case–control study. Age Ageing 2006; 35: 154–60.

10 Williams-Gray CH, Foltynie T, Brayne CE, Robbins TW, Barker RA. Evolution of cognitive dysfunction in an incident Parkinson's disease cohort. Brain 2007; 130 (Pt 7): 1787–98.

11 Reid WG, Hely MA, Morris JG, *et al.* A longitudinal study of Parkinson's disease: clinical and neuropsychological correlates of dementia. J Clin Neurosci 1996; 3: 327–33.

12 Hely MA, Morris JG, Reid WG, Trafficante R. Sydney Multicenter Study of Parkinson's disease: non-L-dopa-responsive problems dominate at 15 years. Mov Disord 2005; 20: 190–9.

13 Hely MA, Reid WG, Adena MA, Halliday GM, Morris JG. The Sydney multicenter study of Parkinson's disease: the inevitability of dementia at 20 years. Mov Disord 2008; 23: 837–44.

14 Aarsland D, Andersen K, Larsen JP, Lolk A, Kragh-Sorensen P. Prevalence and characteristics of dementia in Parkinson disease: an 8-year prospective study. Arch Neurol 2003; 60: 387–92.

15 Buter TC, van den Hout A, Matthews FE, Larsen JP, Brayne C, Aarsland D. Dementia and survival in Parkinson disease: a 12-year population study. Neurology 2008; 70: 1017–22.

16 Hughes TA, Ross HF, Musa S, *et al.* A 10-year study of the incidence of and factors predicting dementia in Parkinson's disease. Neurology 2000; 54: 1596–602.

17 Aarsland D, Kvaløy JT, Andersen K, *et al.* The effect of age of onset of PD on risk of dementia. J Neurol 2007; 254: 38–45.

18 Halliday G, Hely M, Reid W, Morris J. The progression of pathology in longitudinally followed patients with Parkinson's disease. Acta Neuropathol 2008; 115: 409–15.

19 Alves G, Larsen JP, Emre M, Wentzel-Larsen T, Aarsland D. Changes in motor subtype and risk for incident dementia in Parkinson's disease. Mov Disorder 2006; 21: 1123–30.

20 Burn DJ, Rowan EN, Allan LM, Molloy S, O'Brien JT, McKeith IG. Motor subtype and cognitive decline in Parkinson's disease, Parkinson's disease with dementia, and dementia with Lewy bodies. J Neurol Neurosurg Psychiatry 2006; 77: 585–9.

21 Foltynie T, Brayne CE, Robbins TW, Barker RA. The cognitive ability of an incident cohort of Parkinson's patients in the UK. The CamPaIGN study. Brain. 2004; 127 (Pt 3): 550–60.

22 Muslimovic D, Post B, Speelman JD, Schmand B. Cognitive profile of patients with newly diagnosed Parkinson disease. Neurology 2005; 65: 1239–45.

23 Janvin CC, Larsen JP, Aarsland D, Hugdahl K. Subtypes of mild cognitive impairment in Parkinson's disease: progression to dementia. Mov Disord 2006; 21: 1343–9.

24 Beyer MK, Janvin CC, Larsen JP, Aarsland D. A magnetic resonance imaging study of patients with Parkinson's disease with mild cognitive impairment and dementia using voxel-based morphometry. J Neurol Neurosurg Psychiatry 2007; 78: 254–9.

25 Bronnick K, Emre M, Lane R, Tekin S, Aarsland D. Profile of cognitive impairment in dementia associated with Parkinson's disease compared with Alzheimer's disease. J Neurol Neurosurg Psychiatry 2007; 78: 1064–8.

26 Williams DR, Warren JD, Lees AJ. Using the presence of visual hallucinations to differentiate Parkinson's disease from atypical parkinsonism. J Neurol Neurosurg Psychiatry 2008; 79: 652–5.

27 Fenelon G, Mahieux F, Huon R, Ziegler M. Hallucinations in Parkinson's disease: prevalence, phenomenology and risk factors. Brain 2000; 123 (Pt 4): 733–45.

28 Aarsland D, Andersen K, Larsen JP, et al. The rate of cognitive decline in Parkinson disease. Arch Neurol 2004; 61: 1906–11.

29 Harding AJ, Broe GA, Halliday GM. Visual hallucinations in Lewy body disease relate to Lewy bodies in the temporal lobe. Brain 2002; 125 (Pt 2): 391–403.

30 Perry EK, Kerwin J, Perry RH, Blessed G, Fairbairn AF. Visual hallucinations and the cholinergic system in dementia. J Neurol Neurosurg Psychiatry 1990; 53: 88.

31 Factor SA, Feustal PJ, Friedman JH et al. Longitudinal outcome of Parkinson's disease patients with psychosis. Neurology 2003; 60: 1756–61.

32 Weisskopf MG, Grodstein F, Ascherio A. Smoking and cognitive function in Parkinson's disease. Mov Disord 2007 15; 22: 660–5.

33 Inzelberg R, Bonuccelli U, Schechtman E, et al. Association between amantadine and the onset of dementia in Parkinson's disease. Mov Disord 2006; 21: 1375–9.

34 Jasinska-Myga B, Opala G, Goetz CG, et al. Apolipoprotein E gene polymorphism, total plasma cholesterol level, and Parkinson disease dementia. Arch Neurol 2007; 64: 261–5.

35 Haugarvoll K, Aarsland D, Wentzel-Larsen T, Larsen JP. The influence of cerebrovascular risk factors on incident dementia in patients with Parkinson's disease. Acta Neurol Scand 2005; 112: 386–90.

36 Religa D, Czyzewski K, Styczynska M, et al. Hyperhomocysteinemia and methylenetetrahydrofolate reductase polymorphism in patients with Parkinson's disease. Neuroscience Lett 2006; 404 (1–2): 56–60.

37 O'Suilleabhain PE, Sung V, Hernandez C, et al. Elevated plasma homocysteine level in patients with Parkinson disease: motor, affective, and cognitive associations. Arch Neurol 2004; 61: 865–8.

38 Beyer MK, Aarsland D, Greve OJ, Larsen JP. Visual rating of white matter hyperintensities in Parkinson's disease. Mov Disord 2006; 21: 223–9.

39 Kurz MW, Schlitter AM, Larsen JP, Ballard C, Aarsland D. Familial occurrence of dementia and parkinsonism: a systematic review. Dementia Geriatr Cognitive Disorders 2006; 22: 288–95.

40 Kurz MW, Larsen JP, Kvaløy JT, Aarsland D. Associations between family history of Parkinson's disease and dementia and risk of dementia in Parkinson's disease: a community-based, longitudinal study. Mov Disord 2006; 21: 2170–4.

41 Rocca WA, Bower JH, Ahlskog JE, et al. Risk of cognitive impairment or dementia in relatives of patients with Parkinson disease. Arch Neurol 2007; 64: 1458–64.

42 Fuchs J, Nilsson C, Kachergus J, et al. Phenotypic variation in a large Swedish pedigree due to SNCA duplication and triplication. Neurology 2007 20; 68: 916–22.

43 Ross OA, Braithwaite AT, Skipper LM, et al. Genomic investigation of alpha-synuclein multiplication and parkinsonism. Ann Neurol 2008; 63: 743–50.

44 Papapetropoulos S, Farrer MJ, Stone JT, *et al.* Phenotypic associations of tau and ApoE in Parkinson's disease. Neurosci Lett 2007 6; 414: 141–4.

45 Huang X, Chen P, Kaufer DI, Troster AI, Poole C. Apolipoprotein E and dementia in Parkinson disease: a meta-analysis. Arch Neurol 2006; 63: 189–93.

46 Healy DG, Abou-Sleiman PM, Lees AJ, *et al.* Tau gene and Parkinson's disease: a case-control study and meta-analysis. J Neurol Neurosurg Psychiatry 2004; 75: 962–5.

47 Goris A, Williams-Gray CH, Clark GR, *et al.* Tau and alpha-synuclein in susceptibility to, and dementia in, Parkinson's disease. Ann Neurol 2007; 62: 145–53.

Chapter 3

General features, mode of onset and course of dementia in Parkinson's disease

Murat Emre

Introduction

Dementia associated with Parkinson's disease (PD-D) demonstrates characteristic features that make it a clinically recognizable entity, which is frequently associated with typical pathological changes. These features include its mode of onset, chronology and course of the symptoms, the profile of cognitive deficits and behavioural symptoms, the associated motor phenotype and other accompanying features. The characteristic symptoms and signs in each of these domains are described in detail in the subsequent chapters. The objective of this chapter is to describe the general features including the mode of onset, the course and prognosis of dementia associated with PD.

General features of PD-D

The prototypical form of dementia in PD can be described as a dysexecutive sydrome commonly associated with behavioural symptoms and a postural–imbalance–gait disability (PIGD) dominant motor phenotype [1]. The defining neuropscyhological deficits, described in detail in Chapter 4, include prominent and fluctuating impairment in attention, deficits in most aspects of the executive functions, early and prominent visuospatial deficits often disproportionate to the overall severity of dementia, usually retrival type and relatively milder memory impairment and largely preserved core language functions except for word-finding difficulties and impaired fluency. Behavioural symptoms include depression, hallucinations, apathy, delusions and anxiety [2]. Tremor is less frequent and a PIGD phenotype prevails; autonomic dysfunction, especially incontinence is common. Cognitive, bahavioural and motor features of PD-D are similar to dementia with Lewy bodies (DLB) and different from those seen in Alzheimer's disease (AD) [3].

As opposed to the majority of patients with AD, who deny that anything is wrong with their memory, insight as to their mental deficits is usually preserved in patients with PD-D; they would either complain themselves or admit when asked the presence of mental problems. Another defining feature is that patients who have initiation problems or frequent pauses during the performance of a task, would perform better when helped to initiate by providing guidance, or if external cues are given when they pause. In other words, internally driven performance is worse than that driven by external cues or help. This is similar to PD patients being able to walk better when visual guidance is provided. In this sense, cognitive deficits and dementia in PD (at least before the deficits become more advanced and severe) are more characterized with difficulties in the modulation of cognitive functions than with losses in their contents.

The sydrome described above is the prototypical form of dementia seen in patients with PD. There are, however, patients in which deviations from this pattern are observed. For example, the pattern of memory impairment is retrieval type in the majority of patients with relatively spared storage of new information, but some may develop a limbic type amnesia where the new information is not encoded, which is more typical for AD [4]. Likewise some patients may show a more AD-like 'cortical' pattern of deficits [5]. The extent and the topography of Lewy body (LB)-type degeneration as well as the magnitude of the coexistent AD-type pathology are likely to determine the profile, severity and the time course of cognitive and behavioural symptoms. In a clinico-pathological study, patients with a pure LB pathology had more a dysexecutive syndrome, those with pure AD pathology an amnestic syndrome, whereas those with both pathologies had a more mixed cognitive profile [6].

Mode and age of onset

Mode of onset

The mode of onset is inisidious; it is often diffucult for the patient and the family members to remember when the first signs of mental dysfunction became apparent. Not rarely, mental dysfunction may emerge or may be visible following a minor trauma, surgery, infection or dehydration; the symptoms may then not be fully reversible although the triggering insult has vanished. This represents an incipient dementia becoming overt, masquerading as prolonged 'acute confusion'. Such constellations may mislead the caregivers to the conclusion that the onset of mental dysfunction was acute. Conversely, acute confusion (delirium) due to systemic diseases or adverse effects of drugs may be mistaken for dementia. Therefore, an acute onset or acute worsening of mental dysfunction should always be suspicious for exogenous factors and necessitates a careful history, detailed clinical examination and appropriate laboratory investigations.

Age at onset of dementia and time from disease onset to dementia

Although marked cognitive dysfunction can be found in *de novo* populations or at the time of diagnosis [8% of newly diagnosed patients were found to have marked cognitive impairment defined as Mini-Mental State Examination (MMSE) score <24] [7], dementia at the onset of PD is a rare phenomenon. By current definitions, such cases would qualify for a diagnosis of DLB. A diagnosis of PD-D requires the preceding diagnosis of PD, followed by dementia developing on the background of established PD.

Hence, in the majority of patients cognitive dysfunctions are usually subtle at the onset of the disease and develop during the later stages. In a cohort of patients with newly diagnosed PD, 10% developed dementia at a mean 3.5 years from diagnosis; annual incidence of dementia was calculated to be 30 per 1000 person-years [8] (see Chapter 2). In the prospectively followed Sydney cohort the prevalence of dementia was 16% at baseline [9], whereas 84% of patients developed cognitive dysfunction, 48% severe enough to justify the diagnosis of dementia 15 years into the diagnosis [10]. In the same cohort, dementia was present in 83% of all surviving patients 20 years after the diagnosis [11]. In another prospective study, old age and longer duration of the disase were found to be strong determinants of dementia [12]. The reason for the delay to the onset of dementia may be the relatively late involvement of brain structures subserving mental functions in typical PD patients. This is suggested by staging of disease pathology as described by Braak *et al.* [13]. According to this hypothesis LB pathology in PD has its onset in certain susceptible nuclei of the brainstem, subsequently ascending to upper brainstem, limbic structures and finally to cerebral cortex, heteromodal association cortices succumbing first, followed by homomodal assocation and primary sensory-motor cortices. However, there seem also to be patients with greater burden of cortical pathology with a more malignant disease course and shorter time before dementia supervenes [14].

Average time to onset of dementia in PD was found to be about 9 years in one cohort [15]. An important determinant of time to occurrence of dementia is current age; the older the patient the more likely is a shorter time to the onset of dementia. Age-specific incidence estimates of cognitive impairment suggest that it is 2.7% per year at ages 55–64 years and increases to 13.7% at ages 70–79 years [16–18]. Similar effects of age were observed in the Sydney cohort: the prevalence of dementia at baseline was 5% aged <60 years, 14% aged 60–69 years and 35% in patients aged ≥70 years [9]. The effect of age at disease onset is, however, debated: whereas several studies reported that younger age of onset is associated with a lower risk of dementia, a recent analysis suggested that it is the age rather than age of onset which determines the risk [19].

Predictors and early signs

Several clinical and demographic features are associated with increased risk for dementia. These are described in detail in the Epidemiology section; the most important ones will be mentioned here. Among many reported associations three can be singled out: one demographic (age), one related to motor phenotype (PIGD-type), and the other cognitive performance at the time of assessment.

Predictors of dementia

Repeatedly confirmed in a number of studies, advanced age and severe motor symptoms are the most significant risk factors for dementia [18,20,21]. In a population-based cross-sectional study, dementia was not present in any of the patients aged <50 years, whereas 69% of all those aged >80 years were demented [22]. The combination of old age and severe motor symptoms seems to predict a particularly bleak prognosis, increasing the risk by almost tenfold compared with patients who are young and have mild disease [23]. There are certain constellations and clinical vignettes, which, when present render patients more susceptible to develop dementia. One such feature is the motor phenotype. Patients with more symmetrical signs, higher disability and bradykinesia scores, more impairment of gait and balance are more likely to develop dementia [9]. In contrast, patients with tremor-predominant subtype are less likely to develop dementia compared with those who suffer from a PIGD subtype [8]. In a group of patients who were prospectively followed up, those who suffered from a tremor-dominant subtype at baseline converted to a PIGD-predominat subtype by the time they developed dementia [24].

Neuropsychological test performance also provides clues as to the risk of developing dementia. Patients with low overall cognitive scores, mild deficits in executive functions, word-finding difficulties, mild impairment of memory, poor attentional function, reduced verbal fluency and impairments in picture completion tests are more likely to develop dementia than those patients with normal cognitive performance [18,21,25–27]. Letter and especially semantic fluency tests seem to be particularly sensitive measures as well as copying a figure of intersecting pentagons [8,25]. Appearance of visual hallucinations or confusion soon after initiation of dopaminergic medication may also be a harbinger of incipient dementia [28]. The reverse is also true: the main risk factor for appearence of hallucinations in treated PD patients is cognitive impairment [29]. Patients with a diagnosis of MCI at the time of examination have a higher risk of developing dementia compared to those without. In a prospective study, 62% of patients with mild cognitive impairment (MCI) at baseline converted to dementia as opposed to 20% of those who were cognitively intact. Single-domain non-memory MCI and multiple-domain slightly impaired MCI were associated with high risk of developing dementia, whereas amnestic MCI subtype was not; the numbers were, however, small in this latter group [30].

Early symptoms of incipient dementia

Before overt signs of dementia become visible to friends and family, many patients develop subtle symptoms (Box 3.1). One such symptom is disturbances of sleep–wake cycle. Caregivers notice that patients develop an increasing amount of daytime sleepiness, they often fall asleep when seated, reading a newspaper or watching television. Although excessive daytime sleepiness (EDS) can also be seen in PD patients without dementia, or sleep attacks may occur as a result of dopaminergic treatment, EDS is more frequent in patients with dementia [31] and is often an early sign. On awakening, patients may have a brief confusional episode, not realizing for a moment where they are, or have continuation of the dream they were just having by asking or searching for non-existing humans or animals.

Another sleep-related phenomenon is rapid eye movement sleep behaviour disorder (RBD), designating dream-enacting such as speaking, shouting or moving during sleep. Although it may occur also in non-demented patients and may precede the onset of the disease by many years, it is significantly more frequent in demented patients [32]. RBD has been found to predict cognitive decline in non-demented PD patients [33], especially

Box 3.1 Early signs and symptoms preceding dementia in Parkinson's disease

- ◆ Disturbances of sleep–wake cycle
- ◆ Excessive daytime sleepiness
- ◆ Brief confusion on awakening
- ◆ Feeling of presence, occasional hallucinations
- ◆ Disturbances of visual orientation
- ◆ Increasing forgetfulness
- ◆ Impaired attentiveness and concentration
- ◆ Apathy

if it is combined with hallucinations [34]. Thus, *de novo* emergence of RBD in a patient with PD may signal the onset of cognitive dysfunction.

Psychotic phenomena such as feeling of presence (the feeling that there is somebody in the room or in the house, although the patient does not actually see this person), the feeling that somebody is standing behind the patient, the sensation of passage of a shadow or of an animal, isolated brief episodes of visual hallucinations usually occurring at night time or on awakening can also precede the other signs of dementia. Hallucinations may develop on relatively low doses of dopamine agonists or levodopa, which the patient may have tolerated well previously.

Due to deterioration of attention, patients become more and more inattentive, they seem not to understand what is being told and their reactions become delayed. They become withdrawn and apathetic, they loose their spontaneity, doing less and less on their own. Visuospatial deficits are one of the earliest cognitive impairments in PD-D. Accordingly, having orientation problems in new environments can be an early symptom of mental dysfunction, to become worse as the disease progresses when the patients have also navigational problems in familiar places, mixing up rooms and not finding the direction to the toilet in their own home.

Course of dementia and rate of progression

The course of dementia in PD is relentlessly progressive over years – a reversible course has not been observed [35]. At times, patients may seem to have been stabilized for months; they may, however, also show episodes of rapid worsening without an obvious reason. Fluctuations during the day and from day to day, as they occur in DLB, are also frequent in patients with PD-D. When asked, family members would admit that the patient is clearly better on certain days or at certain times of the day, usually in the morning, and tending to perform worse particularly after a bad night's sleep. As dementia progresses patients become increasingly more confused, living almost in a continuous confusional state, with prolonged blank stares and signs of visual hallucinations, although these may not be verbalized. Speech and postural problems often worsen in parallel and patients become more and more dependent.

Rate of progression

There have been two studies in which rate of progression was evaluated prospectively in patients with PD-D, using MMSE as the cognitive measure. In one of these studies patients with PD-D were compared to those with AD and to healthy controls. Over a 4-year period the annualized decline was a mean score of 2.3 in the PD-D group compared with 2.6 in patients with AD; the change in the non-demented PD group was small and similar to that for non-demented control subjects [36]. The annualized decline in the PD-D group was variable across the patients and ranged from a score of 1 (18%) to >4 (16%). In the other study, cognitive decline was compared in patients with PD-D, DLB and controls. Over a 2-year period cognitive decline was a mean score of 4.5 in the PD-D, 3.9 in the DLB, 0.2 in the PD and 0.3 in the control group [37], thus yielding annual decline rates very similar to those in the previous study. Although these studies provide useful information, they may not reflect the true progression of the disease, as MMSE is rather insensitive for the assessment of executive dysfunction which is one of the core features of PD-D. Indirect evidence as to the rate of progression using other parameters, albeit over a shorter period, can also be deduced from placebo-controlled clinical trials. One such trial, performed in a large PD-D population with mild-to-moderate dementia, included a sizeable placebo arm. All cognitive and functional measures worsened in the placebo group; the decrease in the MMSE score over a period of 6 months was 0.2 (out of 20 at baseline), ADAS-cog decreased by 0.7 (out of 24 at baseline) and Alzheimer Disease Consortium Study ADL (activities of daily living) score decreased by 3.6 (out of 41 at baseline) [38]. These decreases were smaller compared with those observed in AD patients receiving placebo in clinical studies with comparable design and duration, suggesting a slower rate of progression in PD-D. Such comparisons, however, have limited value as they are indirect.

Determinants of progression rate

Patients with atypical neurological features such as early occurrence of autonomic failure, symmetrical disease presentation, and limited response to dopaminergic therapy tend to have more severe dementia [39]. In a prospective study spanning 2 years there was an association between PIGD subtype and increased rate of cognitive decline [37]. Likewise presence of major depression, visual hallucinations or of moderate-to-severe EDS predicts significantly greater or faster cognitive decline [31,36,40]. The amount of attentional deficits may also determine the severity of functional impairment. In a multiple regression analysis performed on the baseline data of a large patient population which participated in a clinical trial, the attention factor was the single strongest cognitive predictor of ADL status, matching the strength of the effects of motor functions on ADL status [41]. Disease prognosis is likely to be poorer and progression faster in patients who have mixed LB- and AD-type pathologies [6].

Survival

In a prospective study with follow-up of approximately 4 years, among those who died, 49% had become demented compared with 23% of those who remained alive. Incident dementia had an independent effect on mortality when controlling for extrapyramidal symptoms severity; the development of dementia was associated with a twofold increased mortality risk [42]. In another prospective 12-year study the cumulative incidence of dementia steadily increased with age and duration of PD, increasing to 80–90% by age 90 years conditional on survival. Women with PD lived longer than men and spent more years with dementia. At age 70 years, a man with PD without dementia was predicted to have a life expectancy of 8 years, of which 5 years would be expected to be dementia free followed by 3 years with dementia. In a 70-year-old patient with dementia the life expectancy is substantially reduced to 4.2 years for men and 5.7 years for women [12].

Pathological determinants of dementia in PD

An important question is why some patients with PD develop dementia relatively early whereas others do so late in the disease course, or not at all. It may be simply a matter of time, as the vast majority of surviving patients in the Sydney cohort did develop dementia 20 years into the diagnosis. This may be determined by how fast the disease pathology progresses to involve relevant brain structures. The predominance of the PIGD phenotype in demented patients, and conversion of initially tremor-dominant patients to PIGD phenotype by the time they developed dementia, indicate that involvement of certain brain structures subserving both postural–gait functions and cognition may be necessary for the development of dementia.

The amount and the topography of the alpha-synuclein pathology, the main component of LB, may be an important determinant. In families with a duplication of alpha-synuclein gene locus, dementia is not a common feature, whereas those carrying a triplication mutation frequently develop dementia (see Chapter 12). This indicates that total alpha-synuclein burden may be an important factor in determining which patients would develop dementia. It is, however, unlikely to be the only factor: in an autopsy study subjects with 'reasonable' burden of alpha-synuclein pathology in both brainstem and cortical areas had not developed motor or mental dysfunction during their lifetime. The distribution or load of alpha-synuclein pathology did not permit a dependable postmortem diagnosis of extrapyramidal symptoms or cognitive impairment [43]. The same group recently reported that around 55% of subjects with widespread alpha-synuclein pathology (Braak PD stages 5–6) lacked clinical signs of dementia or extrapyramidal signs antemortem [44]. Another clinico-pathological correlation study demonstrated that the presence of limbic or cortical LB may not always be associated with dementia in PD: nine out of 17 patients with a clinical diagnosis of PD and no history of cognitive impairment showed a neuropathological picture consistent with limbic and eight of them a pathology consistent with neocortical DLB [45]. It is unclear why some individuals appear to 'tolerate' high levels of synuclein deposition without developing symptoms. The specific pattern of LB distribution may be important for dementia to develop; in a multivariate analysis of various pathologies in the brains of patients with PD-D, only LB densities in the entorhinal and anterior cingulate cortex were significantly associated with cognitive scores [46]. Contribution of non-LB pathologies may be an additional factor, modifying or enhancing the impact of synuclein pathology. In an autopsy study, patients carrying both LB- and AD-type pathologies had a worse antemortem prognosis compared with patients with predominantly one type of pathology [6].

The severity and topography of cortical involvement seems to be another factor. Widespread areas of cortical atropy were found in patients with PD-D compared with normal controls, in both temporal and frontal lobes as well as in the left parietal lobe. Compared to PD patients with mild cogitive impairment but no dementia, grey matter reductions were found in frontal, parietal, limbic and temporal lobes of patients with PD-D [47]. In a comparative study of PD patients who developed dementia early versus late in the disease course, those with early dementia had more atrophy in certain brain areas, while the late dementia group had symmetrical reduction in grey matter in the insula bilaterally. The authors suggested that the early development of dementia in PD is associated with more severe degeneration of cortical and subcortical structures [48]. In another study, in which correlation between time to dementia and different type of cortical pathological findings was analysed, there was an association between longer duration of parkinsonism prior to dementia and less severe cortical alpha-synuclein pathology and lower plaque scores. There was an unexpected correlation between more pronounced cortical cholinergic deficits and longer duration of parkinsonism prior to dementia, implying greater loss of ascending cholinergic projections in this population before the onset of dementia [15]. By contrast, a more 'top-down' pathological process has also been described, with greater burden of cortical pathology in patients with a more malignant disease course and shorter time before dementia supervenes [14].

Conclusions

The typical profile of dementia in PD is characterized by a dysexecutive syndrome with prominent impairment of attention, visuospatial functions memory, and frequent behavioural symptoms. Dementia in PD has an insidious onset and slow progression, and overt symptoms are usually preceded by more subtle changes. The annual rate of decline is probably similar to that seen in AD. Old age, longer duration of disease and a PIGD subtype are associated with higher risk and faster progression. The severity and topography of LB-type degeneration, as well as the presence and amount of coexistent pathologies, may determine the risk of developing dementia, time to onset and the rate of progression.

References

1 Emre M, Aarsland D, Brown R, *et al*. Clinical diagnostic criteria for dementia associated with Parkinson's disease. Mov Disord 2007; 22: 1689–1707.
2 Aarsland D, Brønnick K, Ehrt U, *et al*. Neuropsychiatric symptoms in patients with Parkinson's disease and dementia: frequency, profile and associated care giver stress. J Neurol Neurosurg Psychiatry 2007; 78: 36–42.

3 Metzler-Baddeley C. A review of cognitive impairments in dementia with Lewy bodies relative to Alzheimer's disease and Parkinson's disease with dementia. Cortex 2007; 43: 583–600.

4 Weintraub D, Moberg PJ, Culbertson WC, Duda J, Stern MB. Evidence for impaired encoding and retrieval memory profiles in Parkinson disease. Cogn Behav Neurol 2004; 17: 195–200.

5 Aarsland D, Litvan I, Salmon D, et al. Performance on the dementia rating scale in Parkinson's disease with dementia and dementia with Lewy bodies: comparison with progressive supranuclear palsy and Alzheimer's disease. J Neurol Neurosurg Psychiatry 2003; 74: 1215–20.

6 Kraybill ML, Larson EB, Tsuang DW, et al. Cognitive differences in dementia patients with autopsy-verified AD, Lewy body pathology, or both. Neurlogy 2005; 64: 2069–73.

7 Foltynie T, Brayne CEG, Robbins TW, Barker RA. The cognitive ability of an incident cohort of Parkinson's patients in the UK. The CamPaIGN study. Brain 2004; 127: 1–11.

8 Williams-Gray CH, Foltynie T, Brayne CE, Robbins TW, Barker RA. Evolution of cognitive dysfunction in an incident Parkinson's disease cohort. Brain 2007; 130: 1787–98.

9 Reid WG, Hely MA, Morris JG, et al. A longitudinal study of Parkinson's disease: clinical and neuropsychological correlates of dementia. J Clin Neurosci 1996; 3: 327–333.

10 Hely MA, Morris JG, Reid WG, Trafficante R. Sydney Multicenter Study of Parkinson's disease: non-dopa responsive problems dominate at 15 years. Mov Disord 2005; 20: 190–9.

11 Hely MA, Reid WG, Adena MA, Halliday GM, Morris JG. The Sydney multicenter study of Parkinson's disease: the inevitability of dementia at 20 years. Mov Disord 2008; 23: 837–44.

12 Buter TC, van den Hout A, Matthews FE, Larsen JP, Brayne C, Aarsland D. Dementia and survival in Parkinson disease. Neurology 2008; 70: 1017–1022.

13 Braak H, Del Tredici K, Rub U, de Vos RA, Jansen Steur EN, Braak E. Staging of brain pathology related to sporadic Parkinson's disease. Neurobiol Aging 2003; 24: 197–211.

14 Halliday G, Hely M, Reid W, Morris J. The progression of pathology in longitudinally followed patients with Parkinson's disease. Acta Neuropathol 2008; 115: 409–415.

15 Ballard C, Ziabreva I, Perry R, et al. Differences in neuropathologic characteristics across the Lewy body dementia spectrum. Neurology 2006; 67: 1931–4.

16 Mayeaux R, Chen J, Mirabello E, et al. An estimate of the incidence of dementia in idiopathic Parkinson's disease. Neurology 1990; 40: 1513–1517.

17 Biggins CA, Boyd JL, Harrop FM et al. A controlled, longitudinal-study of dementia in Parkinson's disease. J Neurol Neurosurg Psych 1992; 55: 566–71.

18 Aarsland D, Andersen K, Larsen JP, Lolk A, Nielsen H, Kragh-Sorensen P. Risk of dementia in Parkinson's disease: a community-based, prospective study. Neurology 2001; 56: 730–6.

19 Aarsland D, Kvaloy JT, Andersen K, et al. The effect of age of onset of PD on risk of dementia. J Neurol 2007; 254: 38–45.

20 Hughes TA, Ross HF, Musa S, et al. A 10-year study of the incidence of and factors predicting dementia in Parkinson's disease. Neurology 2000; 54: 1596–602.

21 Hobson P, Meara J. Risk and incidence of dementia in a cohort of older subjects with Parkinson's disease in the United Kingdom. Mov Disord 2004; 19: 1043–9.

22 Mayeux R, Denaro J, Hemenegildo N, et al. A population-based investigation of Parkinson's disease with and without dementia. Relationship to age and gender. Arch Neurol 1992; 49: 492–7.

23 Levy G, Schupf N, Tang MX, et al. Combined effect of age and severity on the risk of dementia in Parkinson's disease. Ann Neurol 2002; 51: 722–9.

24 Alves G, Larsen JP, Emre M, et al. Changes in motor subtype and risk for incident dementia in Parkinson's disease. Mov Disord 2006; 21: 1123–30.

25 Jacobs DM, Marder K, Cote LJ, Sano M, Stern Y, Mayeux R. Neuropsychological characteristics of preclinical dementia in Parkinson's disease. Neurology 1995; 45: 1691–6.

26 Mahieux F, Fenelon G, Flahault A, Manifacier MJ, Michelet D, Boller F. Neuropsychologcial prediction of dementia in Parkinson's disease. J Neurol Neurosurg Psych 1998; 65: 804–5.

27 Taylor JP, Rowan EN, Lett D, O'Brien JT, McKeith IG, Burn DJ. Poor attentional function predicts cognitive decline in patients with non-demented Parkinson's disease independent of motor phenotype. J Neurol Neurosurg Psychiatry 2008; 79: 1318–23.

28 Stern Y, Marder K, Tang MX, Mayeux R. Antecedent clinical features associated with dementia in Parkinson's disease. Neurology 1993; 43: 1690–2.

29 Fenelon G, Mahieux F, Huon R, Ziegler M. Hallucinations in Parkinson's disease: prevalence, phenomenology and risk factors. Brain 2000; 123: 733–45.

30 Janvin CC, Larsen JP, Aarsland D, Hugdahl K. Subtypes of mild cognitive impairment in Parkinson's disease: progression to dementia. Mov Disord 2006; 21: 1343–49.

31 Gjerstad MD, Aarsland D, Larsen JP. Development of daytime somnolence over time in Parkinson's disease. Neurology 2002; 85: 1544–6.

32 Marion MH, Qurashi M, Marshall G, Foster O. Is REM sleeep behaviour disorder (RBD) a risk factor of dementia in idiopathic Parkinson's disease. J Neurol 2008; 255: 192–6.

33 Vendette M, Gagnon JF, Decary A, *et al.* REM sleep behavior disorder predicts cognitive impairment in Parkinson disease without dementia. Neurology 2007; 69: 1843–9.

34 Sinforiani E, Pacchetti C, Zangaglia R, Pasotti C, Mani R, Nappi G. REM behaviour disorder, hallucinations and cognitive impairment in Parkinson's disease: a two-year follow up. Mov Disord 2008; 23: 1441–5.

35 Aarsland D, Andersen K, Larsen JP, Lolk A, Kragh-Sorensen P. Prevalence and characteristics of dementia in Parkinson disease: an 8-year prospective study. Arch Neurol 2003; 60: 387–92.

36 Aarsland D, Andersen K, Larsen JP. The rate of cognitive decline in Parkinson disease. Arch Neurol 2004; 61: 1906–1911.

37 Burn DJ, Rowan EN, Allan LM, Molloy S, O'Brien JT, McKeith IG. Motor subtype and cognitive decline in Parkinson's disease, Parkinson's disease with dementia, and dementia with Lewy body disease. J Neurol Neurosurg Psychiatry 2006; 77: 585–589.

38 Emre M, Aarsland D, Albanese A, *et al.* Rivastigmine for dementia associated with Parkinson's disease. N Engl J Med 2004; 351: 2509–18.

39 Aarsland D, Tandberg E, Larsen JP, Cummings J. Frequency of dementia in Parkinson disease. Arch Neurol 1996; 53: 538–542.

40 Starkstein SE, Mayberg HS, Leiguarda R, Preziosi TJ, Robinson RG. A prospective longitudinal study of depression, cognitive decline, and physical impairments in patients with Parkinson's disease. J Neurol Neurosurg Psychiatry 1992; 55: 377–82.

41 Bronnick K, Ehrt U, Emre M, *et al.* Attentional deficits affect activities of daily living in dementia-associated with Parkinson's disease. J Neurol Neurosurg Psychiatry 2006; 77: 1136–42.

42 Levy G, Tang MX, Louis ED, *et al.* The association of incident dementia with mortality in PD. Neurology 2002; 59: 1708–13.

43 Parkkinen L, Kauppinen T, Pirttila T, Autere JM, Alafuzoff I. Alpha-synuclein pathology does not predict extrapyramidal symptoms or dementia. Ann Neurol 2005; 57: 82–91.

44 Parkkinen L, Pirttilä T, Alafuzoff I. Applicability of current staging/categorization of alpha-synuclein pathology and their clinical relevance. Acta Neuropathol 2008; 115: 399–407.

45 Colosimo C, Hughes AJ, Kilford L, Lees AJ. Lewy body cortical involvement may not always predict dementia in Parkinson's disease. J Neurol Neurosurg Psychiatry 2003; 74: 852–6.

46 Kovari E, Gold G, Herrmann FR, *et al.* Lewy body densities in the entorhinal and anterior cingulate cortex predict cognitive deficits in Parkinson's disease. Acta Neuropathol (Berl) 2003; 106: 83–8.

47 Beyer MK, Janvin CC, Larsen JP, Aarsland D. A magnetic resonance imaging study of patients with Parkinson's disease with mild cognitive impairment and dementia using voxel-based morphometry. J Neurol Neurosurg Psychiatry 2007; 78: 254–9.

48 Beyer MK, Aarsland D. Grey matter atrophy in early versus late dementia in Parkinson's disease. Parkinsonism Relat Disord 2008; 14: 620–5.

Chapter 4

Cognitive profile in Parkinson's disease dementia

Kolbjørn Brønnick

Introduction

Knowledge about the cognitive profile of patients with Parkinson's disease and dementia (PD-D) may serve several purposes. If PD-D is characterized with a specific cognitive impairment profile, cognitive assessment may be a useful tool in the diagnostic work-up of individual patients. Further, the pattern of cognitive deficits can contribute to knowledge about relationships between brain function, brain structure and cognitive processes in PD-D as related to other neurodegenerative dementias. Finally, the cognitive profile in PD-D is in itself a valuable insight regarding the phenomenology of PD-D.

Although there is a large literature on the cognitive features of PD in general [1], the research on cognition in PD-D is relatively scarce. Especially in several older studies, the diagnostic status of the PD patients regarding dementia was not reported according to explicit criteria. Further, studies preceding the first consensus criteria for dementia with Lewy bodies (DLB) proposed in 1996 [2] did not employ the 1-year rule concerning the interval between onset of parkinsonism and onset of cognitive dysfunction. In the literature review presented in the recently proposed criteria for PD-D [3], this problem was solved by restricting the reviewed papers to those investigating patients with PD and dementia according to clearly operationalized criteria. The same approach will be adopted in this chapter.

Cognitive domains and their assessment

When describing the 'cognitive profile' in PD-D, there are at least two implicit assumptions that should be elaborated on: (a) the existence of distinct cognitive 'functions' or 'domains', (b) that cognitive functions may be quantified and compared between groups of individuals. Assumption (a) has been extensively discussed in the cognitive neuropsychology literature. Although most researchers would probably agree that cognitive domains are separable, there is still some disagreement about the interrelationship between them. For instance, if there exist 'executive functions' that regulate all goal-directed behaviour, this would imply that these 'executive functions' should exert a global effect on tests that were designed to assess other cognitive domains, if those tests require executive control for optimal performance. This is problematic, however, considering that the 'double dissociation' method has often been used in order to analytically identify independent cognitive functions [4]. According to this method, it should be demonstrated that the hypothetical 'cognitive function A' could be impaired in some patients while 'cognitive function B' could be intact, and there should be patients where 'function B' is impaired while 'function A' is intact. However, as executive and attentional deficits by definition should have modulatory effects on a wide range of cognitive functions, the 'double dissociation' method does not always apply. Rather, it has been demonstrated that brain pathology in fronto-subcortical areas leads to a global deficit in all types of tests that require controlled attention. This is of particular relevance to PD-D, as it has been proposed that cognitive deficit in PD in general is caused by disruption of fronto-subcortical loops [1]. Another important issue concerns phenomena such as alertness and arousal. In DLB and PD-D, attentional 'fluctuation' is a feature of the cognitive profile. Possibly, such fluctuation could be related to changes of arousal or alertness, and this could exert a global effect on other cognitive and behavioural functions [5]. Thus, when interpreting patterns of cognitive dysfunctions in PD-D, one should be mindful of the possible influence of executive dysfunction and of reduced arousal/alertness. I will return to this issue later and discuss the term 'bradyphrenia' as related to arousal and alertness deficits.

Assumption (b), i.e. that it is possible to quantify and compare cognitive functions across groups, is more straightforward. Cognitive measures are constructed according to statistical psychometric principles and can be subjected to relative comparisons between groups. The fundamental 'gold standard' for describing a cognitive profile in a patient group is to compare with a healthy control group that matches the patients on background variables that are known to affect cognition, such as age, sex and education. Further, cognitive comparisons can be carried between patient groups.

The simplest way of comparing cognitive functions between different groups is to simply arrange them ordinally (e.g. group A worse than group B), as in qualitative reviews. This strategy was employed in two recent reviews on cognitive functions in PD-D and DLB [6,7]. Another method is to compare standardized effect-sizes to identify differences in group mean values (Cohen's d), a strategy used in quantitative meta-analysis. In this strategy, the differences of the means is divided by the weighted, pooled standard deviations of the groups, enabling a comparison of magnitude of differences in various cognitive domains, in this case between PD-D and the comparison groups. In the present review, this will be done for studies on cognition in PD-D that reported means, standard deviations and group sizes. Other studies will be described in a qualitative manner. The cognitive profile of patients with PD-D as compared to healthy control subjects (HC) will be described, representing the cognitive deficits in PD-D relative to healthy ageing. Further, the cognitive profile of PD-D as compared to other neurodegenerative dementias, i.e. PD-D vs Alzheimer's disease (AD) and PD-D vs DLB, will be presented.

Deficits in individual cognitive domains in PD-D

Attention and executive functions

The term 'executive functions' refers to a set of cognitive functions responsible for the planning, initiation, sequencing, and monitoring of complex goal-directed behaviour [8].

Historically, the term has been used in at least two different ways. The older use referred to 'higher', 'frontal' functions such as insight, will, abstraction and judgement. In the recent literature, the term usually means cybernetic 'control' functions [8] and is used more or less synonymously with concepts such as 'top-down' cognitive control, or attentional control functions [9].

Thus, attentional control refers to the same phenomena as the cybernetic executive control functions. However, the term 'attention' may also refer to 'bottom-up' phenomena such as orienting to stimulus novelty and startle, as well as to basic alertness or vigilance. Alertness and vigilance may be defined as readiness to detect and respond to stimuli, related to cortical arousal. Further, the term 'selective attention' refers to the ability to filter out task-irrelevant stimuli and to facilitate the processing of task-relevant stimuli [9]. Alertness and vigilance are basic requisites for behaviour involving processing of external events and have a global impact on behaviour and cognition [5]. Focus on the importance of alertness and vigilance has increased as the concept of 'fluctuating attention' has become a core feature in the diagnostic criteria for DLB [10], as such fluctuations could be viewed as a form of alertness deficit.

A problem in measuring executive functions and attention is that there are no pure tests of such functions. These functions are cognitive component-processes of both goal-directed behaviour and in bottom-up driven processing of external stimuli. This may pose a problem if only visual test-paradigms are used for measuring attention in a patient group with severe visuospatial impairment, for example. However, different tasks have different requirements for attention and executive functions, and executive and attentional deficits may be inferred if patients in general tend to perform worse on such tasks than on less demanding tasks.

An overview of studies in which PD-D was diagnosed according to explicit criteria is shown in Table 4.1. In the table columns, effect-sizes, measured with Cohen's d [11], defined as the difference of the means divided by the pooled standard deviations, are given for the comparisons of PD-D with different patient groups (DLB, AD and non-demented PD patients) and normal controls. The pooled standard deviation of the compared groups was calculated as recommended by Hedges and Olkin [12]. An effect size of 0.2 to 0.3 is considered small, 0.5 medium, and ≥0.8 a large effect [11]. A positive number indicates that the group represented by the column performed better than the PD-D group; a negative number indicates worse performance compared with the PD-D group. Data are given as means and standard deviations (or standard errors, which are convertible to standard deviations).

Attention and executive functions are clearly more severely affected in PD-D than in AD, with a medium average effect size of 0.4. It appears that attention and executive functions are more severely affected in DLB than in PD-D, but only with a small average effect size of −0.17. Caution should be exercised when interpreting these results, as there are few studies included and the effect-sizes are not weighted according to sample size. Also, studies that used several tests for executive functions are reported as separate findings, increasing the weight of these samples in the total results. Nevertheless, these results are more reliable than those in a qualitative review.

Table 4.1 Executive functions and attention

Test	NC	DLB	AD	PD
CAMCOG				
Attention [13]	1.71	−0.04	0.49	1.46
Verbal fluency				
Letter [14]		−0.13	0.52	
Letter [15]		0		
Letter [16]	1.91		0.43	
Letter [17]			0.23	
Category [14]		0.26	0.38	
Category [15]		−0.33		
Category [16]	1.65		−0.19	
Trail Making Test				
Part A [15]		−1.36[a]		
Part B [15]		−0.13[a]		
Dementia Rating Scale				
Initiation and perseveration [16]	2.04		0	
Attention [18]			0.03	
Initiation and perseveration [18]			0.30	
Wisconsin Card Sorting Test criteria [15]		−0.29		
Categories [16]	1.66		0.54	
Categories [17]			−0.04	
Cancellation				
Shape time [14]		−0.04[a]	1.06[a]	
TMX time [14]		−0.41	0.83	
Stroop				
Interference [15]		−0.41		
Frontal assessment battery [15]		0		
Digit span				
WAIS total [15]		0		
Forward [17]			−0.09	
Backward [17]			−0.10	
RBANS				
Attention [19]			0.72	1.46
Choice reaction time [20][b]	1.60[a]	0.04[a]	0.86[a]	1.20[a]
Cognitive reaction time [20][b]	0.74	−0.15[a]	0.47	0.46
Simple reaction time [20][b]	1.39	0.34[a]	0.74	1.21
Serial 7s [21]			0.72	
Average effect-size	1.59	−0.17	0.40	1.16

NC, normal controls; DLB, dementia with Lewy bodies; AD, Alzheimer's disease; PD, Parkinson's disease (non-demented); CAMCOG: Cambridge cognitive examination [22]; TMX: consonant trigram cancellation; WAIS, Wechsler Adult Intelligent Scale; RBANS: Repeatable Battery for the Assessment of Neuropsychological Status [23].

Numbers represent Cohen's d, relative to normal controls.

[a] Reaction time data reversed.

[b] This study had large MMSE and age differences.

There were a few studies that could not be included in Table 4.1 as the required statistics were not reported. In a study by Aarsland *et al.* [24], 60 patients with DLB, 35 with PD-D, 49 with progressive supranuclear palsy (PSP), and 29 with AD were compared using subscores from the Mattis dementia rating scale (DRS) [25]. The groups were not matched for age, education and severity of dementia, but statistical correction was used. Further, results were presented separately for mild-to-moderate vs severe dementia. The main findings were that patients with DLB and PD-D suffering from severe dementia had a similar cognitive profile. For mild-to-moderate dementia, the PD-D group had a higher conceptualization score than the DLB group. This subscale measures semantic language abilities and abstraction. No other differences were found. PD-D patients with mild-to-moderate dementia performed worse than AD patients on 'initiation and perseveration', a measure of executive functions. However, this subscale contains several complex motor tasks, possibly confounding the results.

There are two studies analysing components of attentional processes in PD-D using event-related potentials (ERPs). Perriol *et al.* investigated a sensory filtering mechanism, prepulse inhibition (PPI) in PD-D, DLB, AD and healthy controls (10 subjects in each group). PPI is calculated as the amplitude of N1/P2 event-related potentials (ERPs) to a startle stimulus after a preceding (about 120 ms in this case) non-startling stimulus. The authors found reduced PPI in DLB and PD-D as compared to the healthy controls, and the DLB group also showed reduced PPI when compared to the AD group. Thus, the authors concluded that sensory filtering was most severely affected in DLB, followed by PD-D, whereas the AD patients did not differ significantly from the healthy controls.

Brønnick *et al.* [26] investigated an auditory automatic stimulus change-detection mechanism by measuring the mismatch negativity (MMN) ERP [27] in PD-D, DLB, AD, PD and healthy control subjects. The amplitude of the MMN for the PD-D group was significantly attenuated compared with DLB, PD and healthy controls. Further, as compared with PD, DLB, AD and healthy controls, the PD-D group significantly more often missed target stimuli in an auditory 'oddball-distractor' task which significantly correlated with MMN amplitude. Thus, the authors concluded that the PD-D patients had a more severe auditory attention deficit than DLB and AD, related to automatic (bottom-up driven) detection of stimulus deviance. A notable finding was that the MMN of the PD group was equal to the healthy controls, there was not even a tendency towards amplitude-attenuation. Hence, there appears to be a qualitative difference in automatic stimulus detection in PD-D vs PD that may be associated with the development of dementia in PD. The more severe deficit in PD-D as compared to DLB was also surprising. A possible explanation could be that the attentional deficit in DLB is more pronounced in the visual modality, as most of the research on attentional deficits in DLB and PD-D has used visual tests. Clearly, it should not not be concluded that attention in general is impaired based on tests in a single sensory modality.

The finding that executive impairment is marked in PD-D is not surprising given that cognitive impairment in non-demented PD frequently is also characterized by a dysexecutive syndrome [1,28,29]. However, it is not clear how the cognitive deficits in PD progress to PD-D, i.e. if this process is one of a gradual change or of qualitative differences. Whereas in earlier studies progression of dopaminergic deficits was held responsible for cognitive impairment in PD-D, the role of other neural systems and neurotransmitters, including noradrenergic, serotonergic, and cholinergic systems, was subsequently emphasized [30].

The deficits of attention and executive functions in PD-D have a special significance, as it has been shown that attentional deficits in PD-D are the most important cognitive predictors of ability to perform activities of daily living (ADL) in a very large sample of PD-D patients [31]. Further, it has been shown that attention [32] and executive functions [33] appear to be the cognitive functions that are most closely associated with visual hallucinations in PD. There is a possibility that such attentional-executive deficits may partly underlie impairments in other cognitive domains, especially visuospatial dysfunction [34].

Attention and bradyphrenia

In 1922, the neurologist Neville introduced the concept of 'bradyphrenia', a condition characterized by slow cognition, apathy and impaired concentration [35]. The term originated in the context of an epidemic of encephalitis letargica in the 1920s which resulted in parkinsonism and the psychiatric syndrome that became to be known as bradyphrenia. In the older literature on cognitive deficits in PD, the term 'bradyphrenia' is frequently used. However, even initially there were conflicting results regarding the relationship between parkinsonism and bradyphrenia, as Worster-Drought and Hardcastle in 1924 found that reduced psychomotor speed, but not the increase in 'cerebration time' ('thinking time'), was associated with parkinsonism [35]. Authors such as Mayeux have suggested that slowed cognition is a cause of, or at least closely related to, deficits of alertness in PD [36].

In PD-D, there is consistent ERP-based evidence of slowed cognition. In a study investigating both auditory and visual ERPs in healthy controls, PD-D, AD and PD, auditory P300 and flash visual evoked potential latency measures were significantly increased in the PD-D group compared with controls [37]. Increased ERP latencies in PD-D have also been found in other studies [38]. Two studies have directly compared P300 latency in both PD-D and PD relative to normal controls. In both studies P300 latencies were normal in the PD groups, but increased in the PD-D groups [39,40].

Pate and Margolin [41], who used two reaction-time tasks, concluded that both motor as well cognitive slowing was present in both PD and PD-D, and that such slowing was disproportionate to the level of general cognitive impairment compared with a group of AD patients. However, Goldman *et al.* compared 22 patients with mild PD-D to 58 non-impaired PD patients and 48 healthy controls. They found slow movement time, but no increase in cognitive reaction time, in either PD or mild PD-D [42]. Nevertheless, the study of Ballard *et al.* [20] showed that cognitive reaction time was slower in PD-D than in PD and AD, being comparable to that in DLB. The non-demented PD patients had slower choice reaction time than the healthy controls, but similar variability of reaction time. Thus, this study indicates that slow cognition is associated with cognitive decline in PD, and its severity is disproportionately large in PD-D and DLB compared with that in AD.

The concept of bradyphrenia and 'slow cognition' may be problematic in relation both to the attention construct and to other cognitive functions. The study by Mayeux *et al.* [36]illustrates the problem. Poor performance on a vigilance task was deemed to be due to 'bradyphrenia'. What then is the relationship between 'bradyphrenia' and 'vigilance' or 'alertness'? A solution is offered in Salthouse's processing speed theory of adult age-differences in cognition [43]. Salthouse proposes that slowed cognition (bradyphrenia) is a general mechanism underlying age-related decline in cognitive performance. The assumption is that any complex mental task is executed by multiple cognitive component processes with associated neural underpinnings. If one or more of these processes runs more slowly because of pathology affecting the associated neural substrate(s), the mental task will either be solved more slowly, or not successfully solved at all if it depends on a timing restraint. This is the case in perceptual detection tasks, where the presentation of external stimuli cannot be slowed down by the perceiver. In this case, slowed cognition may for instance lead to missed target stimuli. Salthouse calls this phenomenon a 'limited time' mechanism. Slow component cognitive processes can also lead to deficits when the product of early processing stages is no longer available for use in a later processing stage. Salthouse calls this the 'simultaneity mechanism' [43]. The latter may for instance be the case in working memory tasks, where cognitive manipulation of working memory content is dependent upon active maintenance of this content. Thus, slow cognition and vigilance/alertness deficits are phenomena on different analytical levels. Slow cognition is a neural and mental mechanism, whereas vigilance/alertness deficits are behavioural manifestations of this mechanism. The evidence overall indicates that not all PD patients experience cognitive slowing, but that it is associated with cognitive decline and dementia and that it may be closely related to the aetiology of the cognitive decline in PD, to a larger degree than in AD.

In summary, the evidence convergently shows that executive and attentional dysfunction are cognitive hallmarks of PD-D when compared with AD. When compared with DLB, the deficits overall appear to be somewhat less severe. However, the studies that have compared 'fluctuations', defined as variability of reaction time [20,26], both showed that fluctuating attention was at least as severe in PD-D as in DLB.

Visuospatial functions

The term 'visuospatial functions' is used to describe a wide range of cognitive functions measured with several different tests. The unifying theme of the term is that these tests rely on visual perception, visual representation or a visual representational response, such as by drawing. The term can be misleading, as it lumps together very different cognitive processes, perhaps too broadly. After Ungerleider and Mishkin proposed two distinct cortical processing pathways of visual information, the occipito-temporal pathway (the 'what is it?' pathway) and the occipito-parietal pathway (the 'where is it?' pathway) [44], it has become clear that visual processing is performed in several widely distributed cortical areas [45,46] and that spatial cognition is very different from visual form perception and object categorization [45]. In the clinical neuropsychology literature, many 'visuospatial tests' are tests of the ability to draw complex figures (visual construction). Unfortunately, such tasks demand attentional/executive control as well as fine-motor control. In addition, such tests usually do not assess spatial cognition well. These issues are problematic in the research on PD-D, as it has been difficult to interpret findings. An overview of studies on PD-D where visuospatial functions were reported is given in Table 4.2.

PD-D patients have more pronounced visuospatial dysfunctions than patients with AD, with a medium effect-size (Cohen's d = 0.54). It is also evident that visuospatial functions are less severely affected in PD-D than in DLB, approaching a medium effect-size (Cohen's d = −0.39), a larger difference than for attention and executive functions. In some of the studies, perception tasks were used, requiring no eye–hand coordination and motor control, and less executive control; for instance, there was a larger deficit in PD-D compared with DLB on the CAMCOG construction task relative to the CAMCOG perception task [13]. Patients with PD-D also performed better than patients with DLB on other perception tasks [14,15].

The study by Mosimann *et al.* [13] is probably the most comprehensive so far published regarding visuospatial functions in PD-D compared with other patient groups.

Table 4.2 Visuospatial functions

Test	NC	DLB	AD	PD
Pentagon drawing [47]		−0.13	0.42	1.33
Dementia Rating Scale				
Construction [18]			0.53	
Rey–Osterrieth Complex Figure Test				
Copy [15]		−0.22		
Poppelreuter Test [15]		−0.64		
CAMCOG				
Construction [13]	3.16	−0.12	0.84	2.32
Perception [13]	1.60	−0.55	0.59	1.32
BVRT				
Matching [14]		−0.14	0.88	
Rosen drawing test [14]		−0.94	0.08	
ADAScog				
Construction [21]			0.49	
RBANS				
Visuospatial [19]			0.51	1.23
Average effect-size (SD)	2.38	−0.39	0.54	1.55

NC, normal controls; DLB, dementia with Lewy bodies; AD, Alzheimer's disease; PD, Parkinson's disease; CAMCOG: Cambridge cognitive examination [22]; BVRT, Benton Visual Retention Test [48]; ADAScog, cognitive part of Alzheimer's Disease Assessment Scale [49]; RBANS: Repeatable Battery for the Assessment of Neuropsychological Status [23].

Numbers represent Cohen's d, relative to normal controls.

In addition to the CAMCOG results listed in Table 4.2, the study included tests of visual object–form perception, space–motion perception and visual discrimination of various lengths and sizes. DLB, AD, PD and healthy controls were compared with PD-D, and separate analyses were conducted for patients with and without hallucinations. No statistically significant differences between DLB and PD-D patients were found on any tasks, and both these groups performed worse than patients with AD. Visual hallucinators performed worse than non-hallucinators in both the DLB and PD-D groups. While the authors concluded that the performance of the PD-D and DLB groups was worse in the object–form perception tasks than in the space–motion perception task, the very low error scores in the AD, PD and healthy control groups indicate a probable floor-effect that probably leads to underestimation of the real differences. Thus, it is difficult to draw conclusions regarding relative impairment in subdomains of visuospatial functioning in PD-D based on this study.

The previously mentioned study on PD-D, AD, DLB and PSP by Aarsland *et al.* [24] also showed that in the mild-to-moderate dementia groups, the DLB patients performed worse than the PD-D group on the Mattis DRS construction (drawing) tasks. No difference was found in the severe dementia groups.

In conclusion, PD-D is associated with visuospatial dysfunctions that are more severe than in AD, but possibly less severe than in DLB.

Memory

In several diagnostic manuals (DSM-IV, DSM-IIIR, ICD-10), memory impairment is required for the diagnosis of dementia. This requirement is arbitrary and a historical relic related to the importance of AD in earlier dementia research and in the clinic. In AD, the earliest sign of impairment is usually observed in episodic memory, related to pathology affecting the medial temporal lobes, most notably hippocampus and entorhinal cortex [50]. As AD is the most common cause of dementia, memory impairment has become a defining feature of dementia. However, in the most recent consensus criteria for diagnosing DLB, memory impairment is not essential [10], Likewise in the proposed clinical criteria for PD-D, memory impairment is not a preprequisite [3], impairment in 'free recall' is listed as one of the four core cognitive features, of which two are required to make a 'probable' PD-D diagnosis.

Like executive functions and visuospatial functions, memory is a broad term that encompasses several different phenomena that have little in common with each other. However, the present discussion will be restricted to declarative, episodic memory, which is the form of memory that has been commonly investigated. The basic features of this kind of memory are that (1) the memory content is consciously available for access and can be expressed verbally or by other means, such as drawing, and (2) the memory trace pertains to an experienced past event [51]. As mentioned above, this type of memory depends on the integrity of the medial temporal lobes, and episodic memory impairment is usually the first cognitive symptom of AD [50]. In Table 4.3, effect sizes for verbal memory in PD-D are presented. As visuospatial impairment in PD-D may affect the

Table 4.3 Verbal memory

Test	NC	DLB	AD	PD
Buschke selective reminding test				
Total recall [17]			−0.17	
Total recall [15]		−0.70		
Total recall [14]		−0.08	−0.26	
Delayed recall [14]		0.10	−1.26	
Total recall [52]	1.96		−0.08	1.12
Delayed recall [52]	1.74		−0.42	1.41
Total recall [53]	2.96		−0.08	
Delayed recall [53]	3.02		−0.15	
Delayed recognition [53]	1.99		−1.15	
ADAScog memory				
Recall [21]			−0.37	
Recognition [21]			−0.23	
Grober–Buschke procedure				
Total free immediate recall [54]			−2.05	
Long delay free recall [54]			−2.53	
Recognition correct [54]			−7.83[a]	
Recognition false positives [54]			−4.81[a]	
RBANS memory				
Immediate recall [19]			−0.08	1.01
Delayed memory [19]			−1.17	0.75
Rey Auditory Verbal Learning				
Free recall list A [55]	1.86		−0.16	
Recognition discriminability [55]	0.83		−0.94	
Luria memory test				
Immediate recall [53]	1.51		−0.32	
Delayed recall [53]	1.69		−0.82	
Story recall				
Short delay [53]	1.46		−0.84	
California Verbal Learning Test				
Short delay free recall [56]				1.75
Long delay free recall [56]				1.50
Short delay cued recall [56]				1.86
Long delay cued recall [56]				1.57
Recognition [56]				1.84
Average effect-size (SD)	1.90	−0.23	−0.68	1.42

NC, normal controls; DLB, dementia with Lewy bodies; AD, Alzheimer's disease; PD, Parkinson's disease; ADAScog, cognitive part of Alzheimer's Disease Assessment Scale [49]; RBANS: Repeatable Battery for the Assessment of Neuropsychological Status [23].

Numbers represent Cohen's d, relative to normal controls.

[a] These values are not normally distributed and are not included in the averages.

Table 4.4 Visual memory

Test	NC	DLB	AD	PD
Benton visual retention test				
Visual recognition [17]			0.21	
Visual recognition [15]		−0.78		
Visual recognition [14]		−0.25	0.74	
Visual recognition [52]	1.64		0.56	2.07
Delayed matching to sample				
Instant visual recognition [15]		−1.70		
Delayed visual recognition [15]		−1.5		
Rey–Osterrieth complex figure test				
Short delay, visual construction [15]		−0.18		
Average effect-size (SD)		−0.88	0.50	

NC, normal controls; DLB, dementia with Lewy bodies; AD, Alzheimer's disease; PD, Parkinson's disease.

Numbers represent Cohen's d, relative to normal controls.

memory performance for visual material, findings in visual memory tests are presented separately in Table 4.4.

As seen from these results, verbal memory performance in PD-D is severely deficient when compared with normal controls. The pooled data from 10 different studies show that patients with PD-D clearly have better verbal memory functioning than patients with AD, with an average effect-size of 0.68. Only two studies compared PD-D and DLB; the poorer performance in the DLB group is caused by the large difference in a single study [15].

In interpreting the findings in Table 4.4, it should be kept in mind that the average effect-sizes are calculated based on data from only two studies for the DLB vs PD-D comparison and from three studies for the AD vs PD-D comparison. Thus, the results may not be generalizable. Nevertheless, it is interesting to note that visual memory in PD-D is more deficient than in AD (Cohen's d = 0.50). The large average effect-size for the DLB vs PD-D comparison is caused by a single study showing a very large visual memory deficit in DLB as compared to PD-D [15].

Four studies have compared AD with PD-D using composite memory scales including both verbal and visual tasks. The average effect-size is very large (Cohen's d = −1.30), indicating that memory performance in AD overall is worse than in PD-D.

An important discussion concerning memory dysfunction in non-demented PD concerns whether there exists a genuine episodic memory deficit affecting learning (encoding) and retention of learned material, or if memory deficits are secondary consequences of executive/attentional deficits [57]. For instance, it has been claimed that patients with PD may show dysfunction on free recall measures of memory, but be able to recognize the material when it is presented to them [28]. Thus, the deficit could be related to deficient retrieval of memory content, and this has been called 'the retrieval deficit hypothesis'. It is still not clear whether there exists a recognition memory deficit in non-demented PD. In a quantitative meta-analytic review [58], the authors divided PD memory studies in three groups: (a) patients with dementia, (b) patients without dementia and (c) patients

Table 4.5 Composite memory scales

Test	NC	DLB	AD	PD
Dementia Rating Scale				
Memory [18]			−0.86	
Memory [16]	2.54		−1.51	
Wechsler memory scale				
Composite scale [16]	2.90		−1.19	
Composite scale [54]			−1.48	
CAMCOG memory				
Composite scale [13]	2.11	−0.37	−1.44	1.71
Average effect-size (SD)	2.52	−0.37	−1.30	1.71

NC, normal controls; DLB, dementia with Lewy bodies; AD, Alzheimer's disease; PD, Parkinson's disease; CAMCOG: Cambridge cognitive examination [22].

Numbers represent Cohen's d, relative to normal controls.

unselected according to cognitive status. A small effect-size of d = 0.16 for the patients without dementia suggested that there is a recognition memory deficit in PD, but that the magnitude is small, requiring studies with large samples to be detected. In the unselected patients, the effect-size was moderate (d = 0.52). The patients with PD-D had clear recognition memory deficits, as shown by a large effect-size (d = 1.3) when compared to the controls.

When averaging effect-sizes from all studies on memory in PD-D, we find that PD-D patients perform better than DLB (d = 0.63) and AD (d = 0.65), but show a severe memory dysfunction compared with healthy controls (d = 2.05) and non-demented PD patients (d = 1.51). Thus, while memory deficits are less pronounced than in AD and DLB, they are severe compared to those of non-demented subjects. However, as the included studies employed diagnostic criteria for dementia that required memory impairment, this may be an artefact of these criteria. Future research using the proposed criteria for PD-D [3] should be useful for gaining more accurate knowledge about memory impairment in PD-D.

Language

As shown in Table 4.1, several studies have assessed executive functions through verbal fluency tests, which may also be viewed as tests of expressive language. Patients with PD-D are not able to produce as many words within a given time-span as patients with AD, and they show a severe deficit when compared with healthy controls. However, these deficits have been interpreted as being caused by a more general executive control deficit [59], and few studies have focused on core language functions in PD-D.

Cummings *et al.* have published the most comprehensive study of language in PD-D to date [60]. In their study, 16 patients with PD-D, 35 with PD and 10 patients with AD were compared using a comprehensive language assessment battery derived from Boston Diagnostic Aphasia Examination [61] and Western Aphasia Battery [62]. Speech, writing, comprehension of spoken language, naming, verbal fluency, reading comprehension, reading aloud and repetition were assessed. The PD-D and AD patients did not differ on age, MMSE or disease duration. Several differences were found between AD and PD-D. The PD-D patients had more severe dysarthric speech deficits (loudness, pitch, articulation, rate and intelligibility), shorter phrase length, poorer speech melody, reduced grammatical complexity and poorer writing mechanics. Thus, the PD-D group mostly had deficits that could be attributed to the motor impairment. The PD-D patients showed less naming deficits (anomia), better word list generation, and had higher information content in spontaneous speech than the patients with AD.

Thus, the sparse research on language functions in PD-D indicates that language impairment is likely to be primarily due to executive/attentional deficits.

Conclusion: the overall cognitive profile in PD-D

In Figure 4.1 the data from Tables 4.1–4.5 are summarized and the cognitive profile of PD-D is shown graphically. Language functions are not shown as the literature does not warrant a quantitative comparison.

Perhaps somewhat surprisingly, visuospatial functions are most severely affected compared with healthy controls, followed by memory and finally attention and executive functions. Further, PD-D patients perform better than DLB on visuospatial functions and on memory, while being very similar on attention and executive functions. Compared with

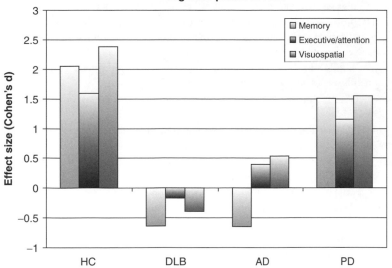

Fig. 4.1 Overall cognitive profile in Parkinson's disease with dementia (PD-D) compared with Alzheimer's disease (AD), dementia with Lewy bodies (DLB) and Parkinson's disease without dementia (PD). The bars represent average effect-size (Cohen's d) of comparisons between PD-D and healthy controls (HC), DLB, AD and PD (non-demented). A positive number indicates that the group performed better than PD-D patients, whereas negative numbers indicate poorer performance than in PD-D. See Plate 1.

AD, PD-D is characterized by clearly better memory functions, but poorer attention/ executive functions and worse visuospatial functions. Finally, we see that non-demented PD patients have a cognitive profile quite similar to that of healthy controls, but overall performing worse. When compared with PD-D, there is a more severe impairment of visuospatial and memory functions compared with attention and executive functions, possibly suggesting that the development of PD-D may be qualitatively different from the cognitive deficits seen in non-demented PD.

There is still considerable research required in order to clarify how PD-D develops from PD, and how the cognitive impairment seen in early PD [63] relates to PD-D, as there are very few studies that have dealt with these questions. The study by Janvin *et al.* suggests that mild cognitive impairment (MCI) in PD is associated with increased risk for developing dementia, but that amnestic-type MCI is not associated with increased risk for dementia [64]. Further, the same group have showed that there is heterogeneity in the cognitive profile of patients with PD-D, and it was suggested that some patients show a 'cortical' profile, whereas others demonsrate a 'subcortical' profile [65]. In the future, the impact of deficits in alertness and arousal should be systematically assessed, as such deficits could be important factors regarding the fluctuation of cognition in PD-D and the development of 'bradyphrenia'. The general impact of such deficits on other cognitive domains should also be more thoroughly assessed in future research.

References

1 Zgaljardic DJ, Borod JC, Foldi NS, Mattis P. A review of the cognitive and behavioral sequelae of Parkinson's disease: relationship to frontostriatal circuitry. Cogn Behav Neurol 2003; 16: 193–210.

2 McKeith IG, Galasko D, Kosaka K, *et al.* Consensus guidelines for the clinical and pathologic diagnosis of dementia with Lewy bodies (DLB): report of the consortium on DLB international workshop. Neurology 1996; 47: 1113–24.

3 Emre M, Aarsland D, Brown R, *et al.* Clinical diagnostic criteria for dementia associated with Parkinson's disease. Mov Disord 2007; 22:1689-707; quiz 837.

4 Van Orden GC, Pennington BF, Stone GO. What do double dissociations prove? Cognitive Science 2001; 25: 111–72.

5 Mesulam MM. A cortical network for directed attention and unilateral neglect. Ann Neurol 1981; 10: 309–25.

6 Troster AI. Neuropsychological characteristics of dementia with Lewy bodies and Parkinson's disease with dementia: differentiation, early detection, and implications for "mild cognitive impairment" and biomarkers. Neuropsychol Rev 2008; 18: 103–19.

7 Metzler-Baddeley C. A review of cognitive impairments in dementia with Lewy bodies relative to Alzheimer's disease and Parkinson's disease with dementia. Cortex 2007; 43: 583–600.

8 Royall DR, Lauterbach EC, Cummings JL, Reeve A, Rummans TA, Kaufer DI, *et al.* Executive control function: a review of its promise and challenges for clinical research. A report from the Committee on Research of the American Neuropsychiatric Association. J Neuropsychiatry Clin Neurosci 2002; 14: 377–405.

9 Parasuraman R. The attentive brain: Issue and prospects. In: Parasuraman R, editor. The attentive brain. Cambridge, MA: MIT Press, 1998; pp. 221–56.

10 McKeith IG, Dickson DW, Lowe J, *et al.* Diagnosis and management of dementia with Lewy bodies: third report of the DLB Consortium. Neurology 2005; 65: 1863–72.

11 Cohen J. Statistical power analysis for the behavioral sciences. Hillsdale, NJ: Laurence Erlbaum, 1988.

12 Hedges LV, Olkin I. Statistical methods for meta-analysis. Orlando: Academic Press, 1985.

13 Mosimann UP, Mather G, Wesnes KA, O'Brien JT, Burn DJ, McKeith IG. Visual perception in Parkinson disease dementia and dementia with Lewy bodies. Neurology 2004; 63: 2091–6.

14 Noe E, Marder K, Bell KL, Jacobs DM, Manly JJ, Stern Y. Comparison of dementia with Lewy bodies to Alzheimer's disease and Parkinson's disease with dementia. Mov Disord 2004; 19: 60–7.

15 Mondon K, Gochard A, Marque A, *et al.* Visual recognition memory differentiates dementia with Lewy bodies and Parkinson's disease dementia. J Neurol Neurosurg Psychiatry 2007; 78: 738–41.

16 Litvan I, Mohr E, Williams J, Gomez C, Chase TN. Differential memory and executive functions in demented patients with Parkinson's and Alzheimer's disease. J Neurol Neurosurg Psychiatry 1991; 54: 25–9.

17 Starkstein SE, Sabe L, Petracca G, *et al.* Neuropsychological and psychiatric differences between Alzheimer's disease and Parkinson's disease with dementia. J Neurol Neurosurg Psychiatry 1996; 61: 381–7.

18 Paolo AM, Troster AI, Glatt SL, Hubble JP, Koller WC. Differentiation of the dementias of Alzheimer's and Parkinson's disease with the dementia rating scale. J Geriatr Psychiatry Neurol 1995; 8: 184–8.

19 Beatty WW, Ryder KA, Gontkovsky ST, Scott JG, McSwan KL, Bharucha KJ. Analyzing the subcortical dementia syndrome of Parkinson's disease using the RBANS. Arch Clin Neuropsychol 2003; 18: 509–20.

20 Ballard CG, Aarsland D, McKeith I, O'Brien J, Gray A, Cormack F, *et al.* Fluctuations in attention: PD dementia vs DLB with parkinsonism. Neurology 2002; 59: 1714–20.

21 Bronnick K, Emre M, Lane R, Tekin S, Aarsland D. Profile of cognitive impairment in dementia associated with Parkinson's disease compared with Alzheimer's disease. J Neurol Neurosurg Psychiatry 2007; 78: 1064–8.

22 Roth M, Tym E, Mountjoy CQ, *et al.* CAMDEX. A standardized instrument for the diagnosis of mental disorder in the elderly with special reference to the early detection of dementia. Br J Psychiatry 1986; 149: 698–709.

23 Randolph C, Tierney MC, Mohr E, Chase TN. The repeatable battery for the assessment of neuropsycological status (RBANS): preliminary clinical validity. J Clin Exp Neuropsychol 1998; 20: 310–9.

24 Aarsland D, Litvan I, Salmon D, Galasko D, Wentzel-Larsen T, Larsen JP. Performance on the dementia rating scale in Parkinson's disease with dementia and dementia with Lewy bodies: comparison with progressive supranuclear palsy and Alzheimer's disease. J Neurol Neurosurg Psychiatry 2003; 74: 1215–20.

25 Mattis S. Dementia rating scale. In: Bellak L, Karasu TB (eds). Geriatric psychiatry. A handbook for psychiatrists and primary care physicians. New York: Grune & Stratton, 1976; p 108–21.

26 Bronnick KS, Nordby H, Larsen JP, Aarsland D. Disturbance of automatic auditory change detection in dementia associated with Parkinson's disease: a mismatch negativity study. Neurobiol Aging 2008, 4 April.

27 Naatanen R, Paavilainen P, Rinne T, Alho K. The mismatch negativity (MMN) in basic research of central auditory processing: a review. Clin Neurophysiol 2007; 118: 2544–90.

28 Dubois B, Pillon B. Cognitive deficits in Parkinson's disease. J Neurol 1997; 244: 2–8.

29 Zgaljardic DJ, Borod JC, Foldi NS, Mattis PJ, Gordon MF, Feigin A, *et al.* An examination of executive dysfunction associated with frontostriatal circuitry in Parkinson's disease. J Clin Exp Neuropsychol 2006; 28: 1127–44.

30 Braak H, Del Tredici K, Rub U, de Vos RA, Jansen Steur EN, Braak E. Staging of brain pathology related to sporadic Parkinson's disease. Neurobiol Aging 2003; 24: 197–211.

31 Bronnick K, Ehrt U, Emre M, De Deyn PP, Wesnes K, Tekin S, et al. Attentional deficits affect activities of daily living in dementia-associated with Parkinson's disease. J Neurol Neurosurg Psychiatry 2006; 77: 1136–42.

32 Meppelink AM, Koerts J, Borg M, Leenders KL, van Laar T. Visual object recognition and attention in Parkinson's disease patients with visual hallucinations. Mov Disord 2008; 23: 1906–12.

33 Barnes J, Boubert L. Executive functions are impaired in patients with Parkinson's disease with visual hallucinations. J Neurol Neurosurg Psychiatry 2008; 79: 190-2.

34 Miyake A, Friedman NP, Rettinger DA, Shah P, Hegarty M. How are visuospatial working memory, executive functioning, and spatial abilities related? A latent-variable analysis. J Exp Psychol Gen 2001; 130: 621–40.

35 Rogers D. Bradyphrenia in parkinsonism: a historical review. Psychol Med 1986; 16: 257-65.

36 Mayeux R, Stern Y, Sano M, Cote L, Williams JB. Clinical and biochemical correlates of bradyphrenia in Parkinson's disease. Neurology 1987; 37: 1130–4.

37 O'Mahony D, Rowan M, Feely J, O'Neill D, Walsh JB, Coakley D. Parkinson's dementia and Alzheimer's dementia: an evoked potential comparison. Gerontology 1993; 39: 228–40.

38 Matsui H, Nishinaka K, Oda M, Kubori T, Udaka F. Auditory event-related potentials in Parkinson's disease: Prominent correlation with attention. Parkinsonism Relat Disord 2007, 26 February.

39 Tanaka H, Koenig T, Pascual-Marqui RD, Hirata K, Kochi K, Lehmann D. Event-related potential and EEG measures in Parkinson's disease without and with dementia. Dement Geriatr Cogn Disord 2000; 11: 39–45.

40 Goodin DS, Aminoff MJ. Electrophysiological differences between demented and nondemented patients with Parkinson's disease. Ann Neurol 1987; 21: 90–4.

41 Pate DS, Margolin DI. Cognitive slowing in Parkinson's and Alzheimer's patients: distinguishing bradyphrenia from dementia. Neurology 1994; 44: 669–74.

42 Goldman WP, Baty JD, Buckles VD, Sahrmann S, Morris JC. Cognitive and motor functioning in Parkinson disease: subjects with and without questionable dementia. Arch Neurol 1998; 55: 674–80.

43 Salthouse TA. The processing-speed theory of adult age differences in cognition. Psychol Rev 1996; 103: 403–28.

44 Ungerleider LG, Mishkin M. Two cortical visual systems. In: Eagle DJ, Goodale MA, Mansfield RJ (eds). Analysis of visual behavior. Cambridge, MA: MIT Press, 1982; pp. 549–86.

45 Jeannerod M, Jacob P. Visual cognition: a new look at the two-visual systems model. Neuropsychologia 2005; 43: 301–12.

46 Gattass R, Nascimento-Silva S, Soares JG, Lima B, Jansen AK, Diogo AC, et al. Cortical visual areas in monkeys: location, topography, connections, columns, plasticity and cortical dynamics. Phil Trans R Soc Lond B Biol Sci 2005; 360 (1456): 709–31.

47 Cormack F, Aarsland D, Ballard C, Tovee MJ. Pentagon drawing and neuropsychological performance in dementia with Lewy Bodies, Alzheimer's disease, Parkinson's disease and Parkinson's disease with dementia. Int J Geriatr Psychiatry 2004; 19: 371–7.

48 Benton AL. A multiple choice type of the visual retention test. Arch Neurol Psychiatry 1950; 64: 699–707.

49 Rosen WG, Mohs RC, Davis KL. A new rating scale for Alzheimer's disease. Am J Psychiatry 1984; 141: 1356–64.

50 Dubois B, Feldman HH, Jacova C, et al. Research criteria for the diagnosis of Alzheimer's disease: revising the NINCDS-ADRDA criteria. Lancet Neurol 2007; 6: 734–46.

51 Baddeley AD. The psychology of memory. In: Baddeley AD, Kopelman MD, Wilson BA (eds). Memory disorders. Chichester: John Wiley & Sons, 2002.

52 Kuzis G, Sabe L, Tiberti C, Merello M, Leiguarda R, Starkstein SE. Explicit and implicit learning in patients with Alzheimer disease and Parkinson disease with dementia. Neuropsychiatry Neuropsychol Behav Neurol 1999; 12: 265–9.

53 Helkala EL, Laulumaa V, Soininen H, Riekkinen PJ. Different error pattern of episodic and semantic memory in Alzheimer's disease and Parkinson's disease with dementia. Neuropsychologia 1989; 27: 1241–8.

54 Pillon B, Deweer B, Agid Y, Dubois B. Explicit memory in Alzheimer's, Huntington's, and Parkinson's diseases. Arch Neurol 1993; 50: 374–9.

55 Tierney MC, Nores A, Snow WG, Fisher RH, Zorzitto ML, Reid DW. Use of the Rey Auditory Verbal Learning Test in differentiating normal aging from Alzheimer's and Parkinson's dementia. Psychol Assessm 1994; 6: 129–34.

56 Higginson CI, Wheelock VL, Carroll KE, Sigvardt KA. Recognition memory in Parkinson's disease with and without dementia: evidence inconsistent with the retrieval deficit hypothesis. J Clin Exp Neuropsychol 2005; 27: 516–28.

57 Higginson CI, King DS, Levine D, Wheelock VL, Khamphay NO, Sigvardt KA. The relationship between executive function and verbal memory in Parkinson's disease. Brain Cogn 2003; 52: 343–52.

58 Whittington CJ, Podd J, Kan MM. Recognition memory impairment in Parkinson's disease: power and meta-analyses. Neuropsychology 2000; 14: 233–46.

59 Bayles KA. Language and Parkinson disease. Alzheimer Dis Assoc Disord 1990; 4: 171–80.

60 Cummings JL, Darkins A, Mendez M, Hill MA, Benson DF. Alzheimer's disease and Parkinson's disease: comparison of speech and language alterations. Neurology 1988; 38: 680–4.

61 Goodglass H, Kaplan E. The assessment of aphasia and related disorders. Philadelphia: Lea & Febiger, 1976.

62 Kertesz A. Aphasia and associated disorders: taxonomy, localization and recovery. New York: Grune & Stratton, 1979.

63 Aarsland D, Bronnick K, Larsen JP, Tysnes OB, Alves G. Cognitive impairment in incident, untreated Parkinson disease: The Norwegian ParkWest Study. Neurology 2008, 19 Nov.

64 Janvin CC, Larsen JP, Aarsland D, Hugdahl K. Subtypes of mild cognitive impairment in Parkinson's disease: progression to dementia. Mov Disord 2006; 21: 1343–9.

65 Janvin CC, Larsen JP, Salmon DP, Galasko D, Hugdahl K, Aarsland D. Cognitive profiles of individual patients with Parkinson's disease and dementia: comparison with dementia with lewy bodies and Alzheimer's disease. Mov Disord 2006; 21: 337–42.

Chapter 5

Neuropsychiatric symptoms in Parkinson's disease dementia

Daniel Weintraub and Eugenia Mamikonyan

Introduction

Dementia affects about 30% of Parkinson's disease (PD) patients at any given time [1], with a long-term cumulative prevalence rate close to 80% [2]. In addition to clinically significant cognitive impairment that defines the disorder, dementia in PD (PD-D) is often accompanied by a range of psychiatric symptoms including psychosis, affective symptoms (e.g. depression and anxiety), apathy, and behavioural disturbances (e.g. aggression and agitation). This chapter provides an overview of the epidemiology and presentation, clinical impact, correlates and risk factors, neuropathophysiology, assessment, and clinical management of neuropsychiatric symptoms in PD-D (Table 5.1).

Epidemiology and clinical presentation

Prevalence of neuropsychiatric symptoms

The Neuropsychiatric Inventory (NPI) [3] is the most commonly used instrument to assess the range of neuropsychiatric symptoms that can occur in neurodegenerative diseases. In a placebo-controlled clinical trial of rivastigmine for the treatment of PD-D, 537 patients were assessed with the NPI at baseline and serially during the course of the study [4]. Almost all (≈90%) experienced at least one neuropsychiatric symptom, and 77% had two or more symptoms. In this study, five distinct NPI clusters were identified: one group with few and mild symptoms (52%); a mood cluster (11%; high depression, anxiety, and apathy scores); an apathy cluster (24%; high apathy score but low scores on other items); an agitation cluster (5%; high score on agitation and high total NPI score); and a psychosis cluster (8%; high scores on delusions and hallucinations).

In a community-based study that used the NPI to identify neuropsychiatric symptoms in 100 PD patients with (43%) and without (57%) dementia, five NPI clusters were identified [5]. The clusters with the highest representation of PD-D patients were a group characterized primarily by hallucinations (79% PD-D) and a group with high scores on several NPI items (57% PD-D).

In a study that used factor analysis to determine patterns of NPI symptoms in PD patients with (36%) and without (64%) dementia, the most common neuropsychiatric symptoms in the sample overall (demented and non-demented patients were not

Table 5.1 Summary of neuropsychiatric symptoms in Parkinson's disease dementia

Symptoms or disorder	Clinical description	Prevalence estimates	Symptom management
Aggression/agitation	Generally occurs in the context of psychosis; may be characterized by one or more of the following: irritability, emotional lability, aberrant motor behaviours, and disinhibited behaviours. Patients tend to have lower MMSE scores, and higher UPDRS and overall NPI scores. Predictive of caregiver distress.	30–40%	Rule out acute medical or neurological disorder. Consider decrease in PD medications. Off-label use of antipsychotics, and benzodiazepines (should be used with caution in PD-D patients). Off-label use of cholinesterase inhibitors and antidepressants.
Anxiety	More likely to occur in females and in patients with non-motor fluctuations (e.g. slowness of thinking, fatigue, and dysphoria).	Common, but specific prevalence rates for anxiety not provided; typically highly comorbid with other affective disorders, especially depression.	Adjustments made to PD medications to minimize off periods. Antidepressants (such as SSRIs). Low dose benzodiazepines (should be used with caution in PD-D patients).
Apathy	More likely to occur in males. Marked by diminished activity, motivation, and affect. Associated with severity of cognitive impairment (executive and verbal memory deficits, bradyphrenia).	15–50%	Off-label use of medications that increase dopamine or norepinephrine activity (e.g. bupropion, SNRIs). The efficacy of psychostimulants and stimulant-related compounds in PD-D is unknown.
Depression	More likely to occur in females. Occurs with increasing age and more severe disease. Risk factor for cognitive decline and development of PD-D. Comorbid with anxiety.	30–60%	Use of second generation antidepressants (SSRIs and SNRIs). Tricyclic antidepressants should be used with caution due to potentially significant adverse event profile. Beware of potential serotonin syndrome from combination of second generation antidepressants and MAO-B inhibitors.

Pseudobulbar affect (involuntary emotional expression disorder)	Repeated brief episodes of involuntary expression of either crying or laughing, with expressed emotion typically incongruent with patient's mood. May occur with or without a stimulus. May be mistakenly attributed to underlying depression.	5–10% (of PD patients, PD-D prevalence unknown)	No antidepressant studies with PD patients. Anecdotally SSRIs and mood stabilizers effective in treating PBA. Educate regarding the difference between pseudobulbar affect and depression.
Psychosis	Correlates include older age, more advanced disease, and exposure to PD medications. Associated with cognitive decline and development of dementia, and worsening of motor symptoms. Often comorbid with depression, anxiety, sleep disturbances, and apathy. Defined by either hallucinations or delusions Predictive of caregiver stress and nursing home placement.	Hallucinations: 45–65% Delusions: 25–30%	Consider adjustment to PD medications. Antipsychotic medications: quetiapine (first-line treatment in spite of lack of demonstrated efficacy), clozapine (efficacious but more adverse effects and impractical to use). Indirect evidence supports introduction of cholinesterase inhibitor.
Disorders of sleep and wakefulness	May be marked by one or more of the following: insomnia, hypersomnia, sleep fragmentation, sleep terrors, nightmares, nocturnal movements, REM behaviour disorder, restless legs syndrome, PLMS, sleep apnoea, and/or EDS, and sudden onset REM sleep.	90% of PD patients overall report some type of sleep disturbance. 15–50% of PD-D patients experience EDS/fatigue. Sudden-onset REM sleep not common in PD-D patients as it is reported in conjunction with DA treatment.	Insomnia: consider adjustment to PD medications, depending on specific disorder; consider sedative–hypnotic agent (must be used cautiously in PD-D patients). PLS and PLMS: dopaminergic medications. RBD: clonazepam (must be used cautiously in PD-D patients). EDS: consider modafinil or psychostimulants.

MMSE, Mini-Mental State Examination; UPDRS, Unified Parkinson's Disease Rating Scale; NPI, Neuropsychiatric Inventory; PD, Parkinson's disease; PD-D, PD with dementia; SSRI, selective serotonin reuptake inhibitor; SNRI, serotonin–norepinephrine reuptake inhibitor; MAO-B, monoamine oxidase-B inhibitor; PLMS, periodic leg movements in sleep; REM, rapid eye movement; RBD, REM behaviour disorder; EDS, excessive daytime sleepiness.

described separately) were depression (38%) and hallucinations (27%), and the least common were euphoria and disinhibition [6]. Factor analysis showed that hallucinations, delusions, and irritability clustered into one factor, and apathy and anxiety constituted another factor.

Comparison with other disease states

Several studies have also used the NPI to compare the frequency and patterns of neuropsychiatric symptoms in PD-D with other neurodegenerative diseases. In one study, neuropsychiatric symptoms overall were very common in both PD-D and Alzheimer's disease (AD), with hallucinations being more severe in PD-D, and aberrant motor behaviour, agitation, disinhibition, irritability, euphoria and apathy more common in AD [7]. In a comparative study of unselected PD patients with regard to their cognitive status and patients with progressive supranuclear palsy (PSP), PD patients had a higher frequency of hallucinations, delusions and depression, but less apathy and disinhibition than PSP patients [8].

PD-D and dementia with Lewy bodies (DLB) overlap to a great extent in terms of neuropathophysiology and clinical presentation. Regarding neuropsychiatric symptoms, a comparative study of PD-D and DLB found that delusions and hallucinations were more common in DLB, with little difference between the groups otherwise [9]. Another study found that cognitive fluctuations, visual and auditory hallucinations, depression and sleep disturbances were equally common in both PD-D and DLB, and all these symptoms were more common in PD-D and DLB than in an AD comparison group [10].

Clinical presentation

Depression and anxiety

Depression is common in PD-D, occurring in 30–60% of patients [4,6,7]. In addition, depression in non-demented PD patients is a risk factor for cognitive decline and development of PD-D [11–13]. This may be due in part to shared risk factors for dementia and depression in PD, including increasing age and more severe disease [12,14]. Although not specifically examined in PD-D patients, in PD there is high comorbidity between depression and anxiety disorders [15].

Most PD-D patients are on chronic levodopa treatment, and many experience motor fluctuations (MF), which involve 'off' periods characterized by worsening parkinsonism along with 'on' periods with better motor function. In addition to MF, non-motor fluctuations (NMF) also occur. Increasing anxiety and discrete anxiety attacks have been associated with motor fluctuations, particularly with the onset of 'off' periods, although this relationship does not hold for all patients [16]. When it does occur, patients often describe a sensation of feeling 'trapped' as they become increasingly immobilized, with anxiety symptoms typically resolving only after improvement in motor symptoms. Other NMF include slowness of thinking, fatigue, and dysphoria. NMF can be more disabling than MF for a substantial percentage of PD patients [17]. Patients may rarely experience hypomanic symptoms during 'on' periods [18].

Apathy

Apathy is another common comorbid condition in PD-D [1], one that overlaps with some motor symptoms of PD, but is a distinct clinical syndrome characterized by diminished spontaneous activity, motivation, and affect. It is common in a range of neurodegenerative diseases, including frontotemporal dementia (FTD) [19], progressive supranuclear palsy (PSP) [8], DLB [19], and AD [20], its frequency and severity increase with disease progression [20].

Recent studies have examined the prevalence of apathy in PD-D and determined that it affects 15–50% of patients [4,6–8,21]. In a study comparing PD patients with a similarly disabled group (e.g. osteoarthritis patients) [22], apathy was significantly more common in the PD group, was associated with cognitive impairment, but not associated with either depression or anxiety. Another study reported similar findings using the Lille Apathy Rating Scale [23,24], with apathy being more common in PD-D patients than in non-demented PD patients. All PD patients showed a decrease in action initiation compared with healthy controls, but PD-D patients were significantly more impaired in this regard. Additionally, they exhibited lower emotional responses and decreased self-awareness compared with non-demented PD patients.

Psychosis

Whereas disorders of affect in PD-D are common and clinically significant, psychosis may be the most clinically significant neuropsychiatric symptom in PD, as it is associated with cognitive decline and development of dementia, motor worsening, caregiver burden, and institutionalization [4,25,26]. Psychosis is defined by the presence of either hallucinations (i.e. false sensory perception) or delusions (i.e. fixed false beliefs). While hallucinations are common in PD overall, affecting about 25–44% of patients, the prevalence in PD-D is markedly higher than in non-demented PD patients [27], ranging from 45 to 65% [4,7,9]. Hallucinations are generally visual, well-formed, recurrent, and complex [9,28–30]; however, auditory [28,31], tactile [32], gustatory [29], and olfactory [33,34] hallucinations may also occur, although they are much rarer. Delusions are not as common as hallucinations, and typically co-occur with hallucinations. Most frequent forms are 'phantom boarder' phenomenon (the belief that a stranger is living in the patient's home), feeling of presence, and delusions of infidelity. Imposter phenomenon is rare but can occur. Prevalence rates for delusions are reported to be 17% in PD patients overall [6,8] and 25–30% in PD-D patients [4,7,9].

Agitation

PD-D patients may display agitation and other behavioural disturbances, often in the context of psychosis. Although not as common as depression, anxiety, or apathy [1], a large treatment study of PD-D patients found baseline agitation/aggression of some severity in 33% of PD-D patients, with one-third of those experiencing clinically significant symptoms. Of patients who had some degree of agitation/aggression, one-half of caregivers reported clinically significant distress [4]. In addition, about 30% of PD-D patients were reported to have some irritability or emotional lability, more than 20% had aberrant motor behaviour, and more than 10% demonstrated disinhibited behaviours.

Disorders of sleep and wakefulness

Disorders of sleep and wakefulness may be the most common non-motor symptoms in PD. Up to 90% of patients report insomnia, hypersomnia, sleep fragmentation, sleep terrors, nightmares, nocturnal movements, or rapid eye movement (REM) behaviour disorder (RBD) [6,35–37]. The latter is characterized by loss of normal skeletal muscle atonia during REM sleep resulting in dream-enacting behaviour, with speaking, shouting, and prominent motor activity associated with vivid, frequently scary dreams. Other sleep–wake cycle-related disorders in PD include restless legs syndrome (RLS) and periodic leg movements in sleep (PLMS). Patients with more advanced PD may have an increased frequency of obstructive or central sleep apnoea [38].

Excessive daytime sleepiness (EDS) or fatigue occurs in 15–50% of PD patients [39–41], and is more common in PD-D. Sudden-onset REM sleep (also known as daytime 'sleep attacks') may occur as well. It has usually been reported in conjunction with dopamine agonist treatment [38,42] and is expected to occur less in patients with PD-D as these patients are generally not prescribed dopamine agonists.

Pseudobulbar affect

Pseudobulbar affect (PBA), also known as involuntary emotional expression disorder (IEED) [43], is a specific form of affective lability that can occur in a variety of neurodegenerative diseases and neurological conditions, including PD. It is found in up to 10% of PD patients [44], its prevalence in PD-D, however, is not known. Clinically, PBA is repeated, brief episodes of involuntary expression of either crying or laughing, with the expressed emotion typically incongruent with the patient's underlying mood. If a stimulus is present, the emotional response is in excess of what would ordinarily be expected. For some patients, the episodes are embarrassing and distressing, and family members may mistakenly attribute crying episodes for an underlying depression.

Impulse control disorders

Impulse control disorders (ICDs), including pathological gambling, compulsive buying, compulsive sexual behaviour, and binge or compulsive eating, are increasingly recognized as common and clinically significant disorders in PD [45,46]. Case reports and cross-sectional studies have suggested an association between dopamine agonist treatment and ICDs in PD [47–49]; younger age is an additional risk factor [46]. Given that PD-D patients are typically older and not commonly prescribed dopamine agonists, it is expected that ICDs would be uncommon in patients with PD-D.

Impact of deep brain stimulation

The impact of deep brain stimulation (DBS), primarily bilateral subthalamic (STN DBS), on neuropsychiatric symptoms appears to be variable and complex [50]. Patients can experience transient postoperative psychiatric abnormalities such as confusional states [51], new-onset or worsening dementia. Recommendations to determine who is at increased risk of a poor postoperative prognosis include a neuropsychological evaluation prior to surgery and exclusion of those with significant baseline cognitive impairment [50].

The longer-term impact of DBS surgery includes executive dysfunction [52] and both overall improvement [50] and occasionally a worsening of depression, anxiety, psychosis, mania, and emotional lability [51,53]. In general, postsurgical neuropsychological decline has shown no correlation with postsurgical motor status [52,54], but it does appear to occur more often among patients with pre-existing neuropsychiatric disorders [53], a finding that further emphasizes the need for presurgical neuropsychological and psychiatric evaluation.

Clinical impact

Comorbid psychiatric symptoms in PD are predictive of caregiver stress, nursing home placement, more rapid cognitive decline, and mortality. In one study, caregivers of PD patients with depression, cognitive impairment, agitation, aberrant motor behaviour, or delusions experienced increased emotional or social distress [6]. In a subsequent study, these same researchers confirmed that agitation and depression are indicative of caregiver distress, and suggested that anxiety and apathy may also contribute, with nearly 60% of caregivers reporting at least one NPI symptom causing at least moderate distress [4].

Regarding individual disorders, there is ample research demonstrating that depression in PD is associated with worse long-term outcomes, including cognitive decline, worse motor function, greater functional impairment, and increased mortality [55–57]. Hallucinations tend to be particularly predictive of greater cognitive decline and development of PD-D over time [2,10,58,59], caregiver stress and burden [4,60,61], nursing home placement [6,60,62,63], and mortality [26,63,64]. One study in a population-based sample of PD patients found that the presence of dementia and hallucinations were independent predictors of nursing home placement [60,61]. What remains unclear is whether psychosis is an independent risk factor for cognitive decline or simply a clinical correlate of cognitive impairment and more rapidly progressive disease.

Correlates and risk factors

In a study that used the NPI to assess neuropsychiatric symptoms in PD-D patients [4], those with a Mini-Mental State Examination (MMSE) score <20 and Hoehn and Yahr stage ≥3 had significantly higher overall NPI scores. Females were more likely to be in the mood cluster, and males in the apathy cluster. The highest MMSE scores were found in the mood cluster, and the lowest in the agitation and psychosis clusters. In addition, patients with more advanced disease were more likely to be in a cluster with significant neuropsychiatric symptoms than those with mild disease. Other studies using the NPI have also reported that neuropsychiatric symptoms in general are associated with increasing severity of both PD and cognitive impairment [5–7,11]. Although depression is common in all stages of PD, its prevalence has been reported to be higher in PD-D patients than in non-demented PD patients [1,12]. Depression may also be a risk factor for, or a prodromal symptom of, PD-D [11,56,57]. The relationship between severity of apathy and severity of PD is unclear [22,23]; apathy, however, has been associated with a range of cognitive deficits and dementia in PD [21,23]. Although there is symptom overlap between depression and apathy, and patients meeting criteria for one disorder often meet criteria for the other, these appear to be distinct clinical syndromes [21,22].

Risk factors for, or correlates of, psychosis are a range of cognitive deficits [25,61,65,66], older age, advanced disease [28,29,61,67–71], and exposure to PD medication [61,62,66,72,73]. Until recently, exposure to dopaminergic therapy was implicated as the major cause of psychosis in PD [74]. Anecdotal claims have been made that certain agents are less likely than others to induce psychosis [75]. Despite the strong empirical association between medication exposure and psychosis in PD, some recent studies have reported that the dosage and duration of anti-parkinsonian treatment are not directly correlated with psychosis [29,67,76,77]. The aetiology of psychosis is complex and multifactorial, often including visual impairment and sleep disturbances [78,79]. Hallucinations are often comorbid with other neuropsychiatric conditions, including depression, anxiety, sleep disturbances, and apathy [30,61].

Agitated patients on average have lower MMSE and higher Unified Parkinson's Disease Rating Scale (UPDRS) motor (primarily akinesia and rigidity) scores [67]. Agitation is often associated with other psychiatric symptoms including delusions, hallucinations, and irritability [67]. In a factor analysis, irritability, hallucinations, and delusions clustered into one neuropsychiatric factor [6], and in a cluster analysis a small group of PD-D patients, displayed high agitation and overall NPI scores [4].

Clinical factors that are associated with sleep disruption are immobility due to nocturnal bradykinesia and rigidity, tremor, dyskinesia, cramps, micturia, pain, and excessive sweating [37,38,80]. Sleep disturbances are also correlated with psychosis [81], depression [37], and cognitive impairment [80]. EDS, and perhaps fatigue as well, have been attributed variably to impairment in the striatal-thalamic-frontal cortical system, exposure to dopaminergic medication (especially dopamine agonists), and to nocturnal sleep disturbances [38,41,80,82]. Clinical correlates of EDS include advanced disease, depression, cognitive impairment, and psychosis [39,40,83].

Pathophysiology of neuropsychiatric symptoms

Although there is extensive literature on the pathophysiology of both neuropsychiatric symptoms and cognitive impairment in PD, there has been almost no research on the pathophysiology of these symptoms in PD-D specifically.

In general, the high frequency of depression in PD has been explained by dysfunction in: (1) subcortical nuclei and the frontal lobes; (2) striatal-thalamic-frontal cortex circuits and limbic circuits, and; (3) brainstem monoamine and indolamine systems (i.e. dopamine, serotonin, norepinephrine, and acetylcholine). Impairments in the pathways connecting subcortical structures and the frontal cortex also are thought to be important [84]. Functional brain imaging studies have reported simultaneous pan-frontal cortex and caudate hypometabolism in depressed PD patients, changes which are presumed to reflect neurodegeneration of the cortical-striatal-thalamic-cortical circuits [85,86]. Regarding neurotransmitters, disproportionate degeneration of dopamine neurons in the ventral tegmental area has been reported in PD patients with a history of depression [87]. Functional imaging studies in depressed PD patients have found both a decrease in signal intensity of neural pathways originating from monoaminergic brainstem nuclei [88] and a negative correlation between depression scores and dorsal midbrain serotonin transporter (5-HTT) densities [89].

Goal-directed behaviour is associated with dopaminergic and noradrenergic function and with activation of the prefrontal cortex and basal ganglia [90]. Supporting the role of the frontal cortical-striatal impairments in the development of diminished goal-directed behaviour (i.e. apathy), studies of apathy in PD have reported associations with executive deficits, verbal memory impairment, and bradyphrenia [21,91].

As previously mentioned, the aetiology of psychosis in PD is complex and likely includes a complex interaction between medication exposure, PD pathology, aberrant REM-related phenomena, and comorbid conditions, particularly cognitive impairment and visual disturbances. Dopaminergic medication may lead to excessive stimulation or hypersensitivity of mesocorticolimbic D_2/D_3 receptors and induce psychosis [92]. However, the association between psychosis, cognitive impairment, and mood disorders suggests more widespread involvement of other neurotransmitter systems or neural pathways. For instance, cholinergic deficits and serotonergic/dopaminergic imbalance have also been implicated in the development of psychosis in PD [74,75,92–95].

RBD and other sleep disturbances in PD have been attributed both to progressive degeneration of the cholinergic pedunculopontine nucleus [96] and reduced striatal dopaminergic activity [97]. With regard to the pathophysiology of PBA, a final common pathway seems to be disinhibition of brainstem bulbar nuclei that control the expression of crying and laughing. PBA in PD probably results from impairment in neural pathways connecting the cortex and brainstem [98].

Assessment and diagnosis

As insight and memory are impaired in patients with PD-D, it is important to include an informed second party in the assessment of neuropsychiatric symptoms; patient self-completed assessments are not appropriate to assess such symptoms in PD-D. Although not validated yet, the new version of the UPDRS [99] has individual questions that can be used to screen for symptoms that are common in PD-D, including depression, anxiety, psychosis, apathy, and disorders of sleep and wakefulness.

The most commonly used global instrument to assess presence and severity of neuropsychiatric symptoms in PD-D is the NPI. The NPI was developed to overcome difficulties associated with assessing behavioural symptoms in patients with dementia, such as inaccurate reporting of symptom severity or frequency. The original NPI is comprised of a series of questions concerning 10 behavioural domains affected by dementia: delusions, hallucinations, agitation/aggression, depression, anxiety, euphoria, apathy, disinhibition, irritability/lability, and aberrant motor behaviour. A 12-item version was subsequently developed, which includes additional questions on night-time behavioural disturbances and appetite/eating changes. Domain-specific interview questions are administered to an informant, who is asked to assess the patient's behaviour in the past month. If a particular behaviour is endorsed, the severity (e.g. mild, moderate, or severe) and frequency (e.g. occasionally, often, frequently, or very frequently) are rated, and domain-specific scores are determined by multiplying severity and frequency. Subsequently, a brief caregiver-completed version of the NPI, the Neuropsychiatric Personality Inventory-Questionnaire (NPI-Q) [100] was also developed.

Management of neuropsychiatric symptoms

Depression and anxiety

There have been no controlled studies on the use of psychiatric medications for depression and anxiety symptoms specifically in PD-D. About 20–25% of PD patients in specialty care are on an antidepressant at any given time, most commonly a selective serotonin reuptake inhibitor (SSRI) [101,102], which is the recommended first-line antidepressant treatment class for geriatric depression [103]. Results of numerous open-label trials using SSRIs and other newer antidepressants in PD suggest a positive effect and good tolerability [104]. However, the only placebo-controlled SSRI study reported negative findings [105–107]. In addition, although apparently rare, the combination of an SSRI and a monoamine oxidase inhibitor (MAOI) can result in serotonin syndrome (i.e. development of symptoms such as mental confusion, hallucinations, agitation, headache, coma, shivering, sweating, hyperthermia, hypertension, tachycardia, nausea, diarrhoea, myoclonus (muscle twitching), hyperreflexia and tremor).

Interestingly, two placebo-controlled tricyclic antidepressant (TCA) studies were positive [107,108]; however, TCAs can be difficult for PD patients to tolerate due to aggravation of PD-associated orthostatic hypotension, constipation, and cognitive problems [109], thus in PD-D patients they must either be avoided or be prescribed with caution with close monitoring for cognitive worsening and increased confusion.

Regarding treatment of anxiety, there have been no controlled treatment studies in PD to inform clinical decision-making [110]. For patients who experience anxiety as part of an 'off' state, PD medication adjustments can be made in an attempt to decrease the duration and severity of these episodes. Anecdotally, newer antidepressants are commonly used for anxiety disorders, whether or not comorbid depression is present. However, anxiety in PD responds variably to antidepressants, and many patients require treatment with benzodiazepines (most commonly low-dose lorazepam, alprazolam, and clonazepam). Given that PD-D patients are cognitively and frequently physically impaired, benzodiazepines must be used cautiously due to their propensity to worsen cognition, sedation, and gait/balance. It remains to be seen if treatments shown to reduce severity or time of MF, such as catechol-O-methyltransferase (COMT) inhibitors or DA, also lead to improvements in severity or duration of NMF, including anxiety and dysphoria.

Apathy

There have been no treatment studies for apathy in PD. Comorbid psychiatric conditions (e.g. depression) should be treated initially. Anecdotally, psychostimulants (e.g. methylphenidate) and stimulant-related compounds (e.g. modafinil) are used in clinical practice, but their effectiveness for PD-D patients is not known. Based on the proposed pathophysiology of apathy, antidepressants and other medications that increase dopamine or norepinephrine activity (e.g. dopamine agonists, TCAs, dual reuptake inhibitor antidepressants, bupropion, and atomoxetine) may be beneficial [111]. In addition to pharmacologic treatment, it is important to educate patients and families on the distinction between apathy and depression and to encourage steps that overcome patient inertia that may lead to improved functioning and quality of life [112].

Psychosis and agitation

Several studies have found a relationship between exposure to PD medication and the presence of some neuropsychiatric symptoms, particularly psychosis and cognitive impairment [67,72,113–116]. If tolerated, a decrease in overall PD medication exposure may lead to an improvement in mental status in PD-D patients. Based on expert opinion, medications are usually discontinued (if tolerated from a motor standpoint) in the following order: anticholinergics, selegiline, amantadine, dopamine agonists, COMT inhibitors, and finally, a reduction in levodopa dosage [75,117]. In a recent description of clinical outcomes in a small number of PD patients with psychosis, it was reported that a decrease in PD medications commonly led to improvement in psychosis, and the authors estimated that 30% of psychotic PD patients may not require ongoing antipsychotic medication [118].

Cholinesterase inhibitors (donepezil, rivastigmine, and galantamine) have been studied as cognitive-enhancing treatments for PD-D, and indirectly for their effects on neuropsychiatric symptoms [119]. In an open-label study examining the psychiatric benefits of donepezil in DLB and PD-D patients [120], 35 PD-D patients who completed at least 12 weeks of treatment had an average 12.0 point decrease in total NPI score (about 50% decrease from baseline NPI score) and reduced caregiver distress. In contrast, a small placebo-controlled cross-over study of donepezil in PD-D did not report psychiatric benefits [121].

There is evidence that rivastigmine, approved for the treatment of PD-D based on the results of a large international study [122], may also have psychiatric benefits in this population. In this study, mean NPI scores decreased by 2.0 points in the rivastigmine-treated group over the course of treatment, compared with no change in the placebo-treated group ($P = 0.02$). In addition, significantly more patients in the rivastigmine group had an improvement of at least 30% in NPI score (45.4% vs 34.6%, $P = 0.03$). In a *post hoc* analysis of the data, it was found that those patients with visual hallucinations at baseline derived greater benefit from rivastigmine treatment relative to placebo treatment [123].

There is preliminary evidence that cholinesterase inhibitors may improve hallucinations in PD-D. A small open-label study of rivastigmine was conducted with PD patients with a range of neuropsychiatric symptoms and significant cognitive impairment. Total NPI score, the hallucinations and sleep disturbance subscales specifically, improved significantly in study completers (80% of sample) over the course of 6 weeks of maximal treatment, and caregivers reported significantly less distress over time [124]. Similarly, a small open-label study of galantamine in PD-D found benefit for neuropsychiatric symptoms overall and psychosis specifically [125].

When psychosis does not improve with the aforementioned clinical interventions, it is sometimes necessary to introduce antipsychotic treatment. Recent research shows that about one-third of older PD patients newly treated with dopaminergic agents will be prescribed an antipsychotic within a 7-year period [126]. There are four well-studied atypical antipsychotics that are used in the PD population: clozapine, risperidone, olanzapine, and quetiapine [72,113,114,116]. Only clozapine has been shown to be efficacious for psychosis in PD, with little adverse motor effects [72,113,116]. Unfortunately, clozapine has a rare but serious adverse effect, agranulocytosis [72,113,116], which necessitates routine blood monitoring.

Risperidone and olanzapine are not recommended for use in PD, due to limited research and evidence that their use is associated with worsening parkinsonism [72,113]. In one meta-analysis, motor symptom worsening was reported in 33% of risperidone-treated PD patients [127], and a similar meta-analysis found worsening of motor symptoms in 40% of olanzapine-treated patients [72,128].

Quetiapine has become the first-line antipsychotic treatment for PD psychosis, based on the results of open-label reporting of symptomatic improvement and good tolerability from a motor standpoint [72,113,116]. However, the two randomized, placebo-controlled quetiapine studies for psychosis in PD have been negative [129,130]. In addition, a retrospective chart review of quetiapine for the treatment of hallucinations in PD patients with and without dementia found that PD-D patients were as likely as PD patients without dementia to experience a decrease in psychotic symptoms, but were more likely to report worsening in motor symptoms [131]. Another retrospective analysis found that while about 80% of the PD patients experienced at least partial remission of psychotic symptoms with quetiapine treatment, presence of dementia was independently associated with non-response [132]. Finally, in an open-label quetiapine study for psychosis in PD patients with and without dementia, non-demented PD patients demonstrated a trend toward improvement on the Brief Psychiatric Rating Scale, whereas PD-D patients showed no improvement. In addition, PD-D patients were more likely to experience motor worsening, required a longer titration period, and were eventually treated with a higher mean (SD) quetiapine dosage, 151 (90) vs. 76 (59) mg/day [133].

Antipsychotic use in PD-D is of particular concern. In 2005 the US Food and Drug Adminstration issued an advisory letter warning regarding increased morbidity and mortality in patients with dementia associated with atypical antipsychotic use [134]. Specific causes of death reported were cardiovascular or infectious in nature, though prior studies did find significant linkages with cerebrovascular events [135,136]. In 2008, the warning was extended to include conventional (i.e. typical) antipsychotics based on recent research [137,138]. Thus, given the frequent occurrence of dementia in PD, the associated morbidity and mortality with antipsychotic use in PD-D is likely higher than previously thought [139].

For the reasons mentioned above, there has been interest in exploring other treatment options for psychosis and agitation in patients with dementia. Cholinesterase inhibitors, antidepressants, benzodiazepines, and mood stabilizers have all been studied to varying degrees for these indications, but there are no clear pharmacological alternatives to antipsychotics at this time [140,141].

Disorders of sleep and wakefulness

Treatment depends on the specific disorder and its etiology. Sleep disturbances that are due to nocturnal worsening of parkinsonism may respond to adjustments in the PD medication regimen. RLS and PLMS are commonly treated with dopaminergic medications, and RBD is typically treated with clonazepam. Preliminary studies suggest that EDS can be treated successfully with modafinil [142,143], and psychostimulants are also used in clinical practice. The role of other hypnotic or psychiatric medications in the treatment of sleep disturbances in PD has not been evaluated.

Pseudobulbar affect

Numerous small-scale studies have found both TCAs and SSRIs to be efficacious in the treatment of PBA, although none included PD patients [144]. Anecdotally, SSRIs and mood stabilizers (e.g. valproic acid) appear to be effective for this syndrome in PD; no reports specifically in PD-D patients are available. In addition, it is important to educate patients and family members on the distinction between PBA and depression.

Conclusions

Common psychiatric symptoms in PD-D range from disorders of affect to psychosis and agitation. The symptoms are problematic for both patients and caregivers alike, and are associated with numerous adverse outcomes. Given recent evidence that dementia is a very common long-term outcome in PD, there needs to be greater attention devoted to the assessment, diagnosis, and clinical management of the range of neuropsychiatric symptoms that occur in PD-D, including assessment of the role that PD treatments play either in the aetiology or treatment of these disorders.

References

1 Emre M, Aarsland D, Brown R, *et al.* Clinical diagnostic criteria for dementia associated with Parkinson's disease. Mov Disord 2007; 22: 1689–1707.

2 Aarsland D, Andersen K, Larsen JP, Lolk A, Kragh-Sørensen P: Prevalence and characteristics of dementia in Parkinson disease: an 8-year prospective study. Arch Neurol 2003; 60: 387–92.

3 Cummings JL, Mega M, Gray K, *et al.* The Neuropsychiatric Inventory: comprehensive assessment of psychopathology in dementia. Neurology 1994; 44: 2308–14.

4 Aarsland D, Brønnick K, Ehrt U, *et al.* Neuropsychiatric symptoms in patients with Parkinson's disease and dementia: frequency, profile and associated caregiver stress. J Neurol Neurosurg Psychiatry 2007; 78: 36–42.

5 Bronnick K, Aarsland D, Larsen JP. Neuropsychiatric disturbances in Parkinson's disease clusters in five groups with different prevalence of dementia. Acta Psychiatr Scand 2005; 112: 201–7.

6 Aarsland D, Larsen JP, Lim NG, Janvin C, Karlsen K, Tandberg E, Cummings JL. Range of neuropsychiatric disturbances in patients with Parkinson's disease. J Neurol Neurosurg Psychiatry 1999; 67: 492–6.

7 Aarsland D, Cummings JL, Larsen JP. Neuropsychiatric differences between Parkinson's disease with dementia and Alzheimer's disease. Int J Geriatr Psychiatry 2001; 16: 184–91.

8 Aarsland D, Litvan I, Larsen JP: Neuropsychiatric symptoms of patients with progressive supranuclear palsy and Parkinson's disease. J Neuropsychiatry Clin Neurosci 2001; 13: 42–9.

9 Aarsland D, Ballard C, Larsen JP, McKeith I. A comparative study of psychiatric symptoms in dementia with Lewy bodies and Parkinson's disease with and without dementia. Int J Geriatr Psychiatry 2001; 16: 528–36.

10 Galvin JE, Pollack J, Morris J. Clinical phenotype of Parkinson disease dementia. Neurology 2006; 67: 1605–11.

11 Lieberman A. Are dementia and depression in Parkinson's disease related? Neurological Sciences 2006; 248: 138–42.

12 Giladi N, Treves TA, Paleacu D, et al. Risk factors for dementia, depression and psychosis in long-standing Parkinson's disease. J Neural Transm 2000; 107: 59–71.

13 Emre M. What causes mental dysfunction in Parkinson's disease? Mov Disord 2003; 18 (Suppl 6): S63–S71.

14 Hoehn MH, Yahr MD. Parkinsonism: onset, progression, and mortality. Neurology 1967; 17: 427–42.

15 Menza MA, Robertson-Hoffman DE, Bonapace AS. Parkinson's disease and anxiety: comorbidity with depression. Biol Psychiatry 1993; 34: 465–70.

16 Richard IH, Justus AW, Kurlan R. Relationship between mood and motor fluctuations in Parkinson's disease. J Neuropsychiatry Clin Neurosci 2001; 13: 35–41.

17 Witjas T, Kaphan E, Azulay JP, et al. Nonmotor fluctuations in Parkinson's disease: frequent and disabling. Neurology 2002; 59: 408–13.

18 Racette BA, Hartlein JM, Hershey T, et al. Clinical features and comorbidity of mood fluctuations in Parkinson's disease. J Neuropsychiatry Clin Neurosci 2002; 14: 438–42.

19 Hirono N, Mori E, Tanimukai S, Kazui H, Hashimoto M, Hanihara T, Imamura T. Distinctive neurobehavioral features among neurodegenerative dementias. J Neuropsychiatry Clin Neurosci 1999; 11: 498–503.

20 Benoit M, Robert P, Staccini P, et al. One-year longitudinal evaluation of neuropsychiatirc symptoms in Alzheimer's disease. The REAL.FR Study. J Nutr Health Aging 2005; 9: 134–9.

21 Starkstein SE, Mayberg HS, Preziosi TJ, Andrezejewski P, Leiguarda R, Robinson RG. Reliability, validity, and clinical correlates of apathy in Parkinson's disease. J Neuropsychiatry Clin Neurosci 1992; 4: 134–9.

22 Pluck GC, Brown RG. Apathy in Parkinson's disease. J Neurol Neurosurg Psychiatry 2002; 73: 636–42.

23 Dujardin K, Sockeel P, Devos D, et al. Characteristics of apathy in Parkinson's disease. Mov Disord 2007; 22: 778–84.

24 Sockeel P, Dujardin K, Devos D, Deneve C, Destee A, Defbvre L. The Lille apathy rating scale (LARS), a new instrument for detecting and quantifying apathy: validation in Parkinson's disease. J Neurol Neurosurg Psychiatry 2006; 77: 579–84.

25 Santangelo G, Trojano L, Vitale C, et al. A neuropsychological longitudinal study in Parkinson's patients with and without hallucinations. Mov Disord 2007; 22: 2418–25.

26 Goetz CG, Stebbins GT. Risk factors for nursing home placement in advanced Parkinson's disease. Neurology 1993; 43: 2227–9.

27 Kulisevsky J, Pagonabarraga J, Pascual-Sedano B, García-Sánchez C, Gironell A, for the Trapecio Group Study. Prevalence and correlates of neuropsychiatric symptoms in Parkinson's disease without dementia. Mov Disord 2008; 23: 1889–96.

28 Fenelon G, Mahieux F, Huon R, Ziegler M. Hallucinations in Parkison's disease: prevalence, phenomenology and risk factors. Brain 2000; 123 (Pt 4): 733–45.

29 Holroyd S, Currie L, Wooten GF. Prospective study of hallucinations and delusions in Parkinson's disease. J Neurol Neurosurg Psychiatry 2001; 70: 734–8.

30 Mosimann UP, Rowan EN, Partington C, Collerton D, Littlewood E, O'Brien JT. Characteristics of visual hallucinations in Parkinson's disease dementia and dementia with Lewy bodies. Am J Geriatr Psychiatry 2006; 14: 153–60.

31 Inzelberg R, Kipervasser S, Korczyn AD. Auditory hallucinations in Parkinson's disease. J Neurol Neurosurg Psychiatry 1998; 64: 533–5.

32 Fenelon G, Thobois S, Bonnet AM, Broussolle E, Tison F. Tactile hallucinations in Parkinson's disease. J Neurol 2002; 249: 1699–1703.

33 Tousi B, Frankel M. Olfactory and visual hallucinations in Parkinson's disease. Parkinsonism Relat Disord 2004; 10: 253–54.

34 Goetz CG, Wuu J, Curgian L, Leurgans S. Age-related influences on the clinical characteristics of new-onset hallucinations in Parkinson's disease patients. Mov Disord 2006; 21: 267–70.

35 Arnulf I, Bonnet AM, Damier P, et al. Hallucinations, REM sleep, and Parkinson's disease: a medical hypothesis. Neurology 2000; 55: 281–8.

36 Pappert E, Goetz C, Niederman F. Hallucinations, sleep fragmentation and altered dream phenomena in Parkinson's disease. Mov Disord 1999; 14: 117–21.

37 Smith MC, Ellgring H, Oertel WH. Sleep disturbances in Parkinson's disease patients and spouses. J Am Geriatr Soc 1997; 45: 194–9.

38 Stacy M. Sleep disorders in Parkinson's disease. Drugs Aging 2002; 19: 733–9.

39 Tandberg E, Larsen JP, Karlsen K. Excessive daytime sleepiness and sleep benefit in Parkinson's disease: a community-based study. Mov Disord 1999; 14: 922–7.

40 Friedman J, Friedman H. Fatigue in Parkinson's disease. Neurology 1993; 43: 2016–18.

41 Hitten JJ, van Hoogland G, van der Velde EA, et al. Diurnal effects of motor activity and fatigue in Parkinson's disease. J Neurol Neurosurg Psychiatry 1993; 56: 874–7.

42 Olanow CW, Schapira AH, Roth T. Waking up to sleep episodes in Parkinson's disease. Mov Disord 2000; 15: 212–5.

43 Cummings JL, Arciniegas DB, Brooks BR, et al. Defining and diagnosing involuntary emotional expression disorder. CNS Spectrums 2006; 111–7.

44 Phuong L, Garg S, Duda JE, Stern MB, Weintraub D. Involuntary emotional disorder in Parkinson's disease. Parkinsonism Relat Disord (in press).

45 Galpern W, Stacy M. Management of impulse control disorders in Parkinson's disease. Curr Opin Neurol 2007; 9: 189–97.

46 Voon V, Fox SH. Medication-related impulse control and repetitive behaviors in Parkinson disease. Arch Neurol 2007; 64: 1089–96.

47 Weintraub D, Siderowf AD, Potenza MN, et al. Association of dopamine agonist use with impulse control disorders in Parkinson disease. Arch Neurol 2006; 63: 969–73.

48 Voon V, Hassan K, Zurowski M, et al. Prospective prevalence of pathological gambling and medication association in Parkinson disease. Neurology 2006; 66; 1750–2.

49 Voon V, Hassan K, Zurowski M, et al. Prevalence of repetitive and reward-seeking behaviors in Parkinson disease. Neurology 2006; 67; 1254–7.

50 Voon V, Kubu C, Krack P, Houeto JL, Tröster AI. Deep brain stimulation: neuropsychological and neuropsychiatric issues. Mov Disord 2006; 21 (Suppl 14): S305–S326.

51 Herzog J, Volkmann J, Krack P, et al. Two-year follow-up of subthalamic deep brain stimulation in Parkinson's disease. Mov Disord 2003; 18: 1332–7.

52 Smeding HM, Speelman JD, Koning-Haanstra M, et al. Neuropsychological effects of bilateral STN stimulation in Parkinson disease: a controlled study. Neurology 2006; 66: 1830–6.

53 Houeto JL, Mesnage V, Mallet L, et al. Behavioral disorders, Parkinson's disease and subthalamic stimulation. J Neurol Neurosurg Psychiatry 2002; 72: 701–7.

54 Berney A, Vingerhoets F, Perrin A, et al. Effect on mood of subthalamic DBS for Parkinson's disease: a consecutive series of 24 patients. Neurology 2002; 59: 1427–9.

55 Hughes TA, Ross HF, Mindham RH, et al. Mortality in Parkinson's disease and its association with dementia and depression. Acta Neurol Scand 2004; 110: 118–23.

56 Starkstein SE, Bolduc PL, Mayberg HS, Preziosi TJ, Robinson RG. Cognitive impairments and depression in Parkinson's disease: a follow up study. J Neurol Neurosurg Psychiatry 1990; 53: 597–602.

57 Starkstein SE, Mayberg HS, Leiguarda R, et al. A prospective longitudinal study of depression, cognitive decline, and physical impairments in patients with Parkinson's disease. J Neurol Neurosurg Psychiatry 1992; 55: 377–82.

58 Aarsland D, Andersen K, Larsen JP, et al. The rate of cognitive decline in Parkinson disease. Arch Neurol 2004; 61: 1906–11.

59 Ramirez-Ruiz B, Junque C, Marti M, Valldeoriola F, Tolosa E. Cognitive changes in Parkinson's disease patients with visual hallucinations. Dement Geriatr Cogn Disord 2007; 23: 281–8.

60 Aarsland D, Larsen JP, Karlsen K, et al. Mental symptoms in Parkinson's disease are important contributors to caregiver distress. Int J Geriatr Psychiatry 1999; 14: 866–74.

61 Marsh L, Williams JR, Rocco M, Grill S, Munro C, Dawson TM. Psychiatric comorbidities in patients with Parkinson disease and psychosis. Neurology 2004; 63: 293–300.

62 Salter B, Andersen KE, Weiner WJ. Psychosis in Parkinson's disease: case studies. Neurol Clin 2006; 24: 363–9.

63 Aarsland D, Larsen JP, Tandberg E, et al. Predictors of nursing home placement in Parkinson's Disease: a population-based, prospective study. J Am Geriatr Soc 2000; 48: 938–42.

64 Goetz CG, Tanner CM, Stebbins GT, Buchman A. Risk factors for progression in Parkinson's disease. Neurology 1988; 38: 1841–4.

65 Aarsland D, Andersen K, Larsen JP, et al. Risk of dementia in Parkinson's disease: a community-based, prospective study. Neurology 2001; 56: 730–6.

66 Graham J, Grunewald R, Sager H. Hallucinosis in idiopathic Parkinson's disease. J Neurol Neurosurg Psychiatry 1997; 63: 434–40.

67 Aarsland D, Larsen JP, Cummings JL, Laake K. Prevalence and clinical correlates of psychotic symptoms in Parkinson disease: a community-based study. Arch Neurol 1999; 56: 595–601.

68 Weintraub D, Moberg PJ, Duda JE, Katz IR, Stern MB. Effect of psychiatric and other non-motor symptoms on disability in Parkinson's disease. J Am Geriatr Soc 2004; 52: 784–8.

69 Biglan KM, Holloway RG J, McDermott MP, Richard I. Risk factors for somnolence, edema, and hallucinations in early Parkinson disease. Neurology 2007; 69: 187–95.

70 Biggins C, Boyd J, Harrop F, et al. A controlled, longitudinal study of dementia in Parkinson's disease. J Neurol Neurosurg Psychiatry 1992; 55: 566–71.

71 Alves G, Larsen JP, Emre M, Wentzel-Larsen T, Aarsland D. Changes in motor subtype and risk for incident dementia in Parkinson's disease. Mov Disord 2006; 21: 1123–30.

72 Wint DP, Okun MS, Fernandez HH. Psychosis in Parkinson's disease. J Geriatr Psychiatry Neurol 2004; 17: 127–36.

73 Weintraub D, Morales KH, Duda JE, Moberg PJ, Stern MB. Frequency and correlates of co-morbid psychosis and depression in Parkinson's disease. Parkinsonism Related Disord 2006; 12: 427–31.

74 Wolters ECh. Intrinsic and extrinsic psychosis in Parkinson's disease. J Neurol 2001; 248 (Suppl 3): 22–7.

75 Henderson MJ, Mellers JDC. Psychosis in Parkinson's disease: 'between a rock and a hard place'. Int Rev Psychiatry 2000; 12: 319–34.

76 Sanchez-Ramos JR, Ortoll R, Paulson GW. Visual hallucinations associated with Parkinson disease. Arch Neurol 1996; 53: 1265–8.

77 Merims D, Shabtai H, Korczyn AD, Peretz C, Weizman N, Giladi N. Antiparkinsonian medication is not a risk factor for the development of hallucinations in Parkinson's disease. J Neural Transm 2004; 111: 1447–53.

78 Onofrj M, Thomas A, Bonanni L. New approaches to understanding hallucinations in Parkinson's disease: phenomenology and possible origins. Expert Review of Neurotherapeutics 2007; 7: 1731–50.

79 Pacchetti C, Manni R, Zangaglia R, et al. Relationship between hallucinatons, delusions, and rapid eye movement sleep behavior disorder in Parkinson's disease. Mov Disord 2005; 20: 1439–48.

80 Phillips B. Movement disorders: a sleep specialist's perspective. Neurology 2004; 62 (Suppl 2): S9–S16.

81 Comella CL, Tanner CM, Ristanovic RK. Polysomnographic sleep measures in Parkinson's disease patients with treatment-induced hallucinations. Ann Neurol 1993; 34: 710–14.

82 Chaudhuri A, Behan PO. Fatigue and basal ganglia. J Neurol Sci 2000; 179: 34–42.

83 Karlsen K, Larsen JP, Tandberg E, et al. Fatigue in patients with Parkinson's disease. Mov Disord 1999; 14: 237–41.

84 Mayberg HS. Modulating dysfunctional limbic–cortical circuits in depression: towards development of brain-based algorithms for diagnosis and optimised treatment. Br Med Bull 2003; 65: 193–207.

85 Mentis MJ, McIntosh AR, Perrine K, et al. Relationships among the metabolic patterns that correlate with mnemonic, visuospatial, and mood symptoms in Parkinson's disease. Am J Psychiatry 2002; 159: 746–54.

86 Mayberg HS, Starkstein SE, Sadzot B, et al. Selective hypometabolism in the inferior frontal lobe in depressed patients with Parkinson's disease. Ann Neurol 1990; 28: 57–64.

87 Brown AS, Gershon S. Dopamine and depression. J Neural Transm 1993; 91: 75–109.

88 Berg D, Supprian T, Hofmann E, et al. Depression in Parkinson's disease: brainstem midline alteration on transcranial sonography and magnetic imaging. J Neurol 1999; 246: 1186-1193.

89 Murai T, Muller U, Werheid K, et al. In vivo evidence for differential association of striatal dopamine and midbrain serotonin systems with neuropsychiatric symptoms in Parkinson's disease. J Neuropsychiatry Clin Neurosci 2001; 13: 222–8.

90 Duffy JD. The neural substrates of motivation. Psychiatric Annals 1997; 27: 39–43.

91 Isella V, Melzi P, Grimaldi M, et al. Clinical, neuropsychological, and morphometric correlates of apathy in Parkinson's disease. Mov Disord 2002; 17: 366–71.

92 Wolters ECh. Dopaminomimetic psychosis in Parkinson's disease patients: diagnosis and treatment. Neurology 1999; 52 (Suppl 3): S10–S13.

93 Cheng A, Ferrier I, Morris C, et al. Cortical serotonin S-2 receptor-binding in Lewy body dementia, Alzheimer's and Parkinson's diseases. J Neurol Sci 1991; 106: 50–5.

94 Perry E, Marshall E, Kerwin J. Evidence of monoaminergic-cholinergic imbalance related to visual hallucinations in Lewy body dementia. J Neurochem 1990; 55: 1454–6.

95 Birkmayer W, Danielczyk W, Neumayer E, et al. Nucleus ruber and L-dopa psychosis: biochemical and post-mortem findings. J Neural Transm 1974; 3: 593–116.

96 Jellinger K. The pedunculopontine nucleus in Parkinson's disease. J Neurol Neurosurg Psychiatry 1988; 51: 540–3.

97 Eisensehr I, Linke R, Noachtar S, *et al.* Reduced striatal dopamine transporters in idiopathic rapid eye movement sleep behavior disorder. comparison with Parkinson's disease and controls. Brain 2000; 123: 1155–60.

98 Green RL. Regulation of affect. Semin Clin Neuropsychiatry 1998; 3: 195–200.

99 Goetz CG, Tilley BC, Shaftman SR, *et al.* Movement Disorder Society-sponsored revision of the Unified Parkinson's Disease Rating Scale (MDS-UPDRS): scale presentation and climimetric testing results. Mov Disord 2008; 23: 2129–70.

100 Kaufer DI, Cummings JL, Ketchel P, et al. Validation of the NPI-Q, a brief clinical form of the Neuropsychiatric Inventory. J Neuropsychiatry Clin Neurosci 2000; 12: 233–9.

101 Weintraub D, Moberg PJ, Duda JE, Katz IR, Stern MB. Recognition and treatment of depression in Parkinson's disease. J Geriatr Psychiatry Neurol 2003; 16: 178–83.

102 Richard IH, Kurlan R, Parkinson Study Group. A survey of antidepressant use in Parkinson's disease. Neurology 1997; 49: 1168–70.

103 Alexopoulos GS, Katz IR, Reynolds CF III, *et al.* The expert consensus guideline series: pharmacotherapy of depressive disorders in older patients. Postgraduate Medicine Special Report 2001 (October); 1–86.

104 Weintraub D, Morales KH, Moberg PJ, *et al.* Antidepressant studies in Parkinson's disease: a review and meta-analysis. Mov Disord 2005; 20: 1161–9.

105 Wermuth L, Sørensen PS, Timm S, *et al.* Depression in idiopathic Parkinson's disease treated with citalopram: a placebo-controlled trial. Nordic J Psychiatry 1998; 52: 163–9.

106 Leentjens AF, Vreeling FW, Luijckx GJ, *et al.* SSRIs in the treatment of depression in Parkinson's disease. Int J Geriatr Psychiatry 2003; 18: 552–4.

107 Menza M, Dobkin RD, Marin H, *et al.* A controlled trial of antidepressants in patients with Parkinson's disease and depression. Neurology 2009; 72: 886–92.

108 Andersen J, Aabro E, Gulmann N, *et al.* Anti-depressive treatment in Parkinson's disease: a controlled trial of the effect of nortriptyline in patients with Parkinson's disease treated with l-dopa. Acta Neurol Scand 1980; 62: 210–9.

109 Emre M. Treatment of dementia associated with Parkinson's disease. Parkinsonism Relat Disord 2007; 13 Suppl 3: S457–S461.

110 Walsh K, Bennett G. Parkinson's disease and anxiety. Postgrad Med J 2001; 7789–93.

111 Marin RS, Fogel BS, Hawkins J, *et al.* Apathy: a treatable syndrome. J Neuropsychiatry Clin Neurosci 1995; 723–30.

112 Shulman LM. Apathy in patients with Parkinson's disease. Int Rev Psychiatry 2000; 12: 298–306.

113 Friedman JH, Factor SA. Atypical antipsychotics in the treatment of drug-induced psychosis in Parkinson's disease. Mov Disord 2000; 15: 201–11.

114 Dewey RB, O'Suilleabhain PE. Treatment of drug-induced psychosis with quetiapine and clozapine in Parkinson's disease. Neurology 2000; 55: 1753–4.

115 Weiner WJ, Minagar A, Shulman LM. Quetiapine for l-dopa-induced psychosis in PD. Neurology 2000; 54: 1538.

116 Poewe W, Seppi K. Treatment options for depression and psychosis in Parkinson's disease. J Neurol 2001; 248 (Suppl 3): III12–III21.

117 Olanow CW, Watts RL, Koller WC. An algorithm (decision tree) for the management of Parkinson's disease (2001): treatment guidelines. Neurology 2001; 56 (Suppl 5): S1–S88.

118 Thomsen TR, Panisset M, Suchowersky O, Goodridge A, Mendis T, Lang AE. Impact of standard of care for psychosis in Parkinson disease. J Neurol Neurosurg Psychiatry 2008; 79: 1413–15.

119 Maidment I, Fox C, Boustani M. Cholinesterase inhibitors for Parkinson's disease dementia. Cochrane Database Syst Rev 2006; CD004747.

120 Thomas AJ, Burn DJ, Rowan EN, et al. A comparison of the efficacy of donepezil in Parkinson's disease with dementia and dementia with Lewy bodies. Int J Geriatr Psychiatry 2005; 20: 938–44.

121 Ravina B, Putt M, Siderowf A, Farrar JT, et al. Donepezil for dementia in Parkinson's disease: a randomised, double blind, placebo controlled, crossover study. J Neurol Neurosurg Psychiatry 2005; 76: 934–9.

122 Emre M, Aarsland D, Albanese A, et al. Rivastigmine for dementia associated with Parkinson's disease. N Engl J Med 2004; 351: 2509–18.

123 Burn D, Emre M, McKeith I, et al. Effects of rivastigmine in patients with and without visual hallucinations in dementia associated with Parkinson's disease. Mov Disord 2006; 21: 1899–1907.

124 Reading PJ, Luce AK, McKeith IJ. Rivastigmine in the treatment of parkinsonian psychosis and cognitive impairment: preliminary findings from an open trial. Mov Disord 2001; 16: 1171–95.

125 Aarsland D, Hutchinson M, Larsen JP. Cognitive, psychiatric and motor responses to galantamine in Parkinson's disease with dementia. Int J Geriatr Psychiatry 2003; 18: 937–41.

126 Marras C, Kopp A, Qiu F, et al. Antipsychotic use in older adults with Parkinson's disease. Mov Disord 2007; 22: 319–23.

127 Factor SA, Molho E, Friedman JH. Risperidone and Parkinson's disease. Mov Disord 2002; 17: 221–2.

128 Fernandez HH, Trieschmann ME, Friedman JH. Treatment of psychosis in Parkinson's disease: safety considerations. Drug Saf 2003; 26: 643–59.

129 Ondo WG, Tintner R, Voung KD, et al. Double-blind, placebo-controlled, unforced titration parallel trial of quetiapine for dopaminergic-induced hallucinations in Parkinson's disease. Mov Disord 2005; 20: 958–63.

130 Rabey JM, Prokhorov T, Miniovitz A, Dobronevsky E, Klein C. Effect of quetiapine in psychotic Parkinson's disease patients: a double-blind labeled study of 3 months' duration. Mov Disord 2007; 22: 313–18.

131 Reddy S, Factor SA, Molho E, Feustel PJ. The effect of quetiapine on psychosis and motor function in parkinsonian patients with and without dementia. Mov Disord 2002; 17: 676–81.

132 Fernandez HH, Trieschmann ME, Burke MA, Jacques C, Friedman JH. Long-term outcome of quetiapine use for psychosis among Parkinsonian patients. Mov Disord 2003; 18: 510–14.

133 Prohorov T, Klein C, Miniovitz A, Dobronevsky E, Rabey JM. The effect of quetiapine in psychotic Parkinsonian patients with and without dementia. An open-labeled study utilizing a structured interview. J Neurol 2006; 253: 171–5.

134 FDA Center for Drug Evaluation and Research. Information for Healthcare Professionals: Antipsychotics. 2008. Available at: http://www.fda.gov/cder/drug/InfoSheets/HCP/antipsychotics_conventional.htm (accessed 9 February 2009).

135 Schneider LS, Dagerman KS, Insel P. Risk of death with atypical antipsychotic drug treatment for dementia: meta-analysis of randomized placebo-controlled trials. J Am Med Assoc 2009; 294: 1934–43.

136 Setoguchi S, Wang PS, Brookhart MA, Canning CF, Kaci L, Schneeweiss S. Potential causes of higher mortality in elderly users of conventional and atypical antipsychotic medications. J Am Geriatr Soc 2008; 56: 1644–50.

137 Schneeweiss S, Setoguchi S, Brookhart A, Dormuth C, Wang PS. Risk of death associated with the use of conventional versus atypical antipsychotic drugs among elderly patients. Can Med Assoc J 2007; 176: 627–32.

138 Gill SS, Bronskill SE, Normand S-LT, et al. Antipsychotic drug use and mortality in older adults with dementia. Ann Intern Med 2007; 146: 775–86.

139 Friedman JH. Atypical antipsychotics in the elderly with Parkinson's disease and the "black box" warning. Neurology 2006; 67: 564–6.

140 Anonymous. Practice Guideline for the Treatment of Patients with Alzheimer's Disease and Other Dementias. Am J Psychiatry 2007; 164 (Suppl): 1–56.

141 Howard RJ, Juszczak E, Ballard CG, et al. Donepezil for the treatment of agitation in Alzheimer's disease. N Engl J Med 2007; 357: 1382–92.

142 Nieves AV, Lang AE: Treatment of excessive daytime sleepiness in patients with Parkinson's disease with modafinil. Clin Neuropharmacol 2002; 25: 111–14.

143 Adler CH, Caviness JN, Hentz JG, et al. Randomized trial of modafinil for treating subjective daytime sleepiness in patients with Parkinson's disease. Mov Disord 2003; 18: 287–93.

144 Arciniegas DB, Topkoff J. The neuropsychiatry of pathologic affect: an approach to evaluation and treatment. Semin Clin Neuropsychiatry 2000; 5: 290–306.

Chapter 6

Interaction between affect and executive functions in Parkinson's disease

Paolo Barone and Gabriella Santangelo

Introduction

The relationship between affect and cognition is a topic continuing to generate intense debate [1]. Affect and cognition are processes interconnected, related and mediated by a circuitry that is widely distributed throughout the brain and includes subcortical areas typically considered to be 'affective' (e.g. the amygdala and nucleus accumbens), as well as portions of the cortex that are typically considered 'cognitive' (e.g. the ventromedial prefrontal cortex/anterior cingulate and orbitofrontal cortex) [2] (Fig. 6.1).

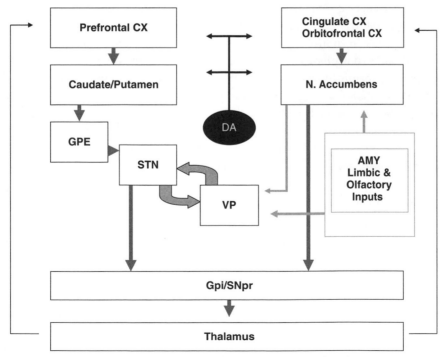

Fig. 6.1 Circuiting interconnections between affective and cognitive functions. GPE: external global pallidus; STN: subthlamic nucleus; VP: ventral pallidum; AMY: amygdala; GPi-SNpr: internal globus pallidus and substantia nigra pars reticulata; DA: dopamine.

Cognitive impairment in Parkinson's disease (PD) is common at all stages of the disease and may precede development of dementia. It includes impairments in attention, encoding memory, visuospatial and executive dysfunctions, the latter being mainly attributed to the disruption of the fronto-striatal circuitry (see Chapter 4) [3]. Affective disorders in PD include depression, apathy and anhedonia. Prevalence rates of depression in PD vary from 2.7% to more than 90%. This variability may be in part due to differences in study methods, presence of substantial overlap between symptoms of PD and symptoms of depression, and criteria used to diagnose depression [4]. When using the Diagnostic and Statistical Manual of Mental Disorders, Fourth Edition (DSM-IV), there is a particular problem because of the ambiguity between depression, apathy and dementia [5]. Furthermore, apathy and anhedonia, which are both included in DSM Criterion A.2, may be independent of depression and may reflect the decreased involvement of PD patients in their usual activities as a result of cognitive deficits rather than as a consequence of a depressive disorder.

Classically, dopamine denervation is associated with motor dysfunctions in PD. However, dopamine neurotransmission seems to have a relevant role in controlling both cognitive and emotional aspects of the disease. Depression in PD is associated with the loss of dopamine and noradrenaline innervation in the limbic system [6], and may fluctuate with motor functions, improving during the 'on' state and worsening during the 'off' state [7]. Similar fluctuations are reported for apathy in PD, suggesting that apathy is at least partly a dopamine-dependent syndrome [8]. Finally, neural substrate of anhedonia is suggested to be due to dysfunction of the dopaminergic–mesolimbic reward circuit involving ventral striatum and prefrontal cortex [9]. Along with the above observations supporting a role in controlling affect in PD, the dopamine system seems to be deeply involved also in controlling cognition related to frontal lobe functions. In particular, mesocortical dopamine inputs to prefrontal cortex regulate working memory function, planning and attention, suggesting that dopamine alterations may be responsible for executive dysfunctions in PD [10].

This review analyses the association between affective disorders and cognitive impairment in PD, with a special focus on the relationship between executive dysfunctions and depression, anhedonia and apathy (Table 6.1).

Depression and executive functions in PD

There is controversy about the relationship between depression and cognitive dysfunctions in PD patients. Three possible patterns emerge: (1) depression influences cognition in PD: in this case depression would mainly influence the severity (quantity) of cognitive impairment [11–22]; (2) depression and cognition are independent, though many symptoms of the two conditions might overlap in PD [23–27]; (3) cognitive dysfunctions, that are related to PD neuropathology, are the substrate of a depressive disorder in PD: in this case a distinct pattern of cognitive impairment (quality) would be associated with depression.

Evidence that depression affects cognition derives from both epidemiological studies indicating depression to be a risk factor for dementia [28] and from the observation that severely depressed PD (dPD) patients were cognitively more impaired than patients with mild depression. In particular, Starkstein *et al.* [7] found that PD patients with major depression (MD) reported a significantly worse performance in tasks assessing frontal lobe functions such as verbal fluency, set-shifting and attention compared with PD patients without MD. No significant difference on cognitive profile between PD patients with minor depression and non-depressed PD patients was found. Consistently, Troster *et al.* [22] found that depression exacerbates memory and language impairments in PD. However, difference in cognitive performance between depressed and non-depressed PD patients disappeared when patients were matched for total Mattis Dementia Rating Scale (MDRS), suggesting that depression influences the severity rather than the quality of cognitive impairment in PD. One limitation of the two studies mentioned above was the absence of a comparison group including patients with MD but without PD.

Kuzis *et al.* [14] compared cognitive profile of dPD and non-depressed PD patients and depressed patients without PD and found that all depressed patients (both with and without PD) reported poorer performance on tasks assessing verbal fluency and auditory attention than non-depressed PD patients. Moreover, dPD patients showed a significantly worse performance on frontal tasks evaluating concept formation and set-shifting as compared with non-depressed PD patients, patients with depression alone and normal subjects of a control group. This finding suggested that alteration of frontal lobe functions, such as concept formation and set-shifting, may result from an interaction between PD neuropathology and the mechanism of MD. Consistently, Costa *et al.* [20] found that PD patients with MD performed worse than non-depressed PD patients on long-term verbal episodic memory tasks, abstract reasoning tasks and tasks assessing executive functioning. They concluded that MD in PD is specifically associated with a qualitatively distinct neuropsychological profile that may be related to the alteration of prefrontal and limbic cortical areas.

Since duration of PD might be an important factor for both neuropathological and cognitive changes, Uekermann *et al.* [18] explored cognitive functions in early PD, finding poorer performance on short-term memory and lexical fluency task in dPD patients as compared to PD patients without depression, depressed patients without PD and control subjects. Similarly in early PD patients, Stefanova *et al.* [19] found that MD in PD patients was associated with cognitive impairment of specific domains (visuospatial memory, spatial working memory, language), and more profound executive and visuospatial deficits, whereas dysthymic disorder was associated only with the quantitative increase in executive dysfunctions observed in control PD. They concluded that cognitive impairment in early PD may be predicted by depression severity.

Evidence that depression and cognitive dysfunctions are independent derives from a variety of studies mainly focusing on general screening tools for dementia, such as the Mini-Mental State Examination [23–26]. In one study, executive dysfunctions, as explored by Stroop and Emotional Stroop Tests, were related neither to depression nor to PD severity [27].

The relationship between depression and executive dysfunctions is generally regarded as depression affecting severity of cognition. Conversely, executive dysfunction, which is

Table 6.1 Cognitive functions as assessed in Parkinson's disease (PD) patients with and without depression

Study	Cognitive tasks	Depressed PD patients	Non-depressed PD patients	Depressed patients without PD
Starkstein *et al.* (1989) [12]	Wisconsin Card Sorting Test	+	−	
	Controlled Word Association	+	−	
	Digit Span			
	Forwards	−	−	
	Backwards	−	−	
	Trail Making Test	+	−	
	Design Fluency Test	+	−	
	Symbol Digit Modalities	+	−	
	MMSE	+	−	
Troster *et al.* (1995) [22]	MDRS	+	−	
	Wisconsin Card Sorting Test	−	−	
	Boston Naming Test	+	−	
	Controlled Word Association	+	−	
	Animal Naming Test	+	−	
	WAIS-R		−	
	Digit span	−		
	Logical Memory I	+	−	
	Logical Memory II	−	−	
	When groups matched for mean MDRS:			
	Wisconsin Card Sorting Test	−	−	
	Boston Naming Test	−	−	
	Controlled Word Association	−	−	
	Animal Naming Test	−	−	
	WAIS-R			
	Digit span	−	−	
	Logical Memory I	−	−	
	Logical Memory II	−	−	
Kuzis *et al.* (1997) [14]	Raven Progressive Matrices	+	−	−
	Wisconsin Card Sorting Test		−	−
	Categories	+	−	−
	Perseverations	+	−	+
	Verbal fluency			
	Buschke – Total Recall Test	+	−	−
	Buschke – Delayed Recall Test	−	−	−
	Benton Visual Retention Test	−	−	−
	Digit Span Test			
	Forwards	−	−	−
	Backwards	+	−	+

Table 6.1 (continued) Cognitive functions as assessed in Parkinson's disease (PD) patients with and without depression

Study	Cognitive tasks	Depressed PD patients	Non-depressed PD patients	Depressed patients without PD
Costa *et al.* (2006) [20]	Digit Span Test			
	Forwards	–	–	
	Backwards	–	–	
	Corsi Test			
	Forwards	–	–	
	Backwards	–	–	
	Immediate visual memory	+	–	
	Word list recall			
	Immediate recall	–	–	
	Delayed recall	+	–	
	Word list recognition: correct items	+	–	
	Prose recall			
	Immediate recall	–	–	
	Delayed recall	–	–	
	Rey's figure	–	–	
	Immediate reproduction	–	–	
	Delayed reproduction	–	–	
	Freehand copying of drawings	–	–	
	Copying drawings with landmarks	–	–	
	Copying Rey's figure	–	–	
	Sentence construction	+	–	
	Raven's Progressive Matrices 47			
	Modified Card Sorting Test	+	–	
	Categories achieved	+	–	
	Perseverative errors	–	–	
	Non-perseverative errors	+	–	
	Lexical verbal fluency			
Uekermann *et al.* (2003) [18]	Digit Span Test			
	Forwards	–	–	–
	Backwards	+	–	–
	Benton Visual Retention Test	–	–	–
	Word List			–
	Immediate	–	–	–
	Delayed	–	–	–
	Semantic verbal fluency	–	–	–
	Lexical verbal fluency	+	–	–
	Hayling Test	–	–	

Table 6.1 (continued) Cognitive functions as assessed in Parkinson's disease (PD) patients with and without depression

Study	Cognitive tasks	Depressed PD patients	Non-depressed PD patients	Depressed patients without PD
Stefanova *et al.* (2006) [19]	WAIS-R			
	Verbal IQ	−	−	
	Performance of IQ	+	−	
	Rey Auditory Verbal Learning Test			
	Recall	−	−	
	Delayed recall	−	−	
	Letter (lexical) fluency	+	−	
	Category (semantic) fluency	+	−	
	Boston Naming Task	+	−	
	Hooper Test	−	−	
	Trail Making Test			
	Form A	−	−	
	Form B	−	−	
Silberman *et al.* (2006) [27]	Stroop Test	−	−	
	Emotional Stroop Test	−	−	

MMSE, Mini-Mental State Examination; MDRS, Mattis Dementia Rating Scale; WAIS-R, Wechsler Adult Intelligence Scale – Revised.

+, altered performance on cognitive tasks; −, normal performance on cognitive tasks.

related to neuropathology of PD, might be responsible for depressive symptoms, especially considering that DSM-IV criteria for MD diagnosis do not separate anhedonia from apathy (DSM-IVA, criterion 2). Santangelo *et al.* [29] subtyped PD patients with MD according to the occurrence of apathy/anhedonia (DSM-IVA, criterion 2). They found that dPD patients with high level of apathy and/or anhedonia scored significantly lower on frontal tasks than patients with depressed mood (DSM-IVA, criterion 1) and non-depressed patients. These findings suggest that the combination of apathy, anhedonia and frontal lobe dysfunctions might contribute to the overdiagnosis of depression in PD.

Apathy and executive functions in PD

Apathy is a primary loss of motivation, interest, and effortful behaviour. Studies in PD patients have shown that the presence of apathy is specifically associated with frontal lobe dysfunctions. Starkstein *et al.* [30] found that apathetic PD patients performed worse than non-apathetic PD patients on part B of the Trail Making Test and lexical fluency task. Consistently, Pluck and Brown [31] found that PD patients with apathy showed decreased performance compared with PD patients without apathy on tasks evaluating specific frontal lobe functions including verbal fluency, changing mental categories and inhibition. Isella *et al.* [32] confirmed the relationship between apathy and frontal lobe dysfunctions in PD patients; they found that apathetic patients showed a poorer performance than non-apathetic patients on tasks assessing verbal fluency set-shifting, sensitivity to interference, and ability to inhibit automatic behaviour. More recently, Zgaljardic *et al.* [33] demonstrated that patients with significant levels of apathy performed worse than patients with low apathy scores on measures of verbal fluency and verbal and non-verbal conceptualization. Low performance on cognitive tasks assessing verbal fluency, working memory, verbal abstraction and executive dysfunction significantly predict both the presence and the worsening of apathy.

Anhedonia and executive functions in PD

Anhedonia is an inability to experience pleasure from normally pleasurable life events such as eating, exercise, and social or sexual interaction. Findings about the relationship between anhedonia and frontal lobe dysfunctions are discordant. Isella *et al.* [34] carried out a study to formally assess prevalence and correlates of physical anhedonia in PD patients compared with normal controls. They found higher anhedonia levels in PD patients with respect to controls and no significant association of physical anhedonia with clinical, neuroradiological features or frontal lobe dysfunctions [34]. On the contrary, we found (personal observation) that in both PD and supranuclear palsy, anhedonia assessed by means of Snaith–Hamilton Pleasure Scale was associated with frontal lobe dysfunctions as evaluated by means of the Frontal Assessment Battery [35,36], a short neuropsychological tool aiming to assess executive functions at the bedside. Since there were controversial data about the relationship between anhedonia and frontal lobe dysfunctions, this topic should be investigated in further studies.

Conclusions

In PD, executive dysfunction is constantly associated with depression, apathy and anhedonia, though there is no definite agreement on the causative relationship between cognitive and affective disorders. Conceivably, they share a common neurochemical and neuroanatomical background consisting of degeneration of the mesocortical and mesolimbic dopaminergic projections. In the PD population, at least a subgroup of patients may be identified for the presence of specific characteristics: more severe executive dysfunction associated with apathy/anhedonia and depression, and increased risk for dementia. Thus, evaluations of both neuropsychological profile and the presence of depressed mood, apathy and anhedonia should be regarded as a routine procedure for an accurate prognosis and rational decision-making with regard to treatment.

References

1 Forgas JP. Affect in social thinking and behavior. New York: Psychology Press, 2006.
2 Duncun S, Barrett LF. Affect is a form of cognition: a neurobiological analysis. Cogn Emot 2007; 21: 1184–211.
3 Zgaljardic DJ, Borod JC, Foldi NS, Mattis P. A review of the cognitive and behavioral sequelae of Parkinson's disease: relationship to frontostriatal circuitry. Cogn Behav Neurol 2003; 16: 193–210.
4 Reijnders JS, Ehrt U, Weber WE, Aarsland D, Leentjens AF. A systematic review of prevalence studies of depression in Parkinson's disease. Mov Disord 2008; 23: 183–9.

5 Marsh L, McDonald WM, Cummings J, Ravina B, NINDS/NIMH Work Group on Depression and Parkinson's Disease. Provisional Diagnostic Criteria for Depression in Parkinson's disease: report of NINDS7NIMH Work Group. Mov Disord 2006; 21: 148–58.

6 Remy P, Doder M, Lees A, Turjanski N, Brooks D. Depression in Parkinson's disease: dopamine and noradrenaline innervation in the limbic system. Brain 2005; 128: 1314–22.

7 Kulisevsky J, Pascual-Sedano B, Barbanoj M, Gironell A, Pagonabarraga J, Garcìa-Sànchez C. Acute effects of immediate and controlled-release levodopa on mood in Parkinson's disease: A double-blind study. Mov Disord 2007; 22: 62–7.

8 Czernecki V, Pillon B, Houeto JL, Pochon JB, Levy R, Dubois B. Motivation, reward, and Parkinson's disease: influence of dopatherapy. Neuropsychologia 2002; 40: 2257–67.

9 Robbins T, Evritt B. Neurobehavioural mechanisms of reward and motivation. Curr Opin Neurobiol 1996; 6: 228–36.

10 Seamans JK, Yang CR. The principal features and mechanism of dopamine modulation in the prefrontal cortex. Prog Neurobiol 2004; 74: 1–58.

11 Mayeux R, Stern Y, Rosen J, Leventhal J. Depression, intellectual impairment, and Parkinson disease. Neurology 1981; 31: 645–50.

12 Starkstein SE, Preziosi TJ, Berthier ML, Bolduc PL, Mayberg HS, Robinson RG. Depression and cognitive impairment in Parkinson's disease. Brain 1989; 112: 1141–53.

13 Starkstein SE, Preziosi TJ, Bolduc PL, Robinson RG. Depression in Parkinson's disease. J Nerv Ment Dis 1990; 178: 27–31.

14 Kuzis G, Sabe L, Tiberti C, Leiguarda R, Starkstein SE. Cognitive functions in major depression and Parkinson disease. Arch Neurol 1997; 54: 982–6.

15 Cubo E, Bernard B, Leurgans S, Raman R. Cognitive and motor function in patients with Parkinson's disease with and without depression. Clin Neuropharmacol 2000; 23: 331–4.

16 Anguenot A, Loll PY, Neau JP, Ingrand P, Gil R. Depression and Parkinson's Disease: study of a series of 135 Parkinson's patients Can. J Neurol Sci 2002; 29: 139–46.

17 Norman S, Troster AI, Fields JA, Brooks R. Effects of depression and Parkinson's disease on cognitive functioning. J Neuropsychiatry Clin Neurosci 2002; 14: 31–6.

18 Uekermann J, Daum I, Peters S, Wiebel B, Przuntek H, Müller T. Depressed mood and executive dysfunction in early Parkinson's disease. Acta Neurol Scand 2003; 107: 341–8.

19 Stefanova E, Potrebic A, Ziropadja L, Maric J, Ribaric I, Kostic VS. Depression predicts the pattern of cognitive impairment in early Parkinson's disease. J Neurol Sci 2006; 248: 131–7.

20 Costa A, Peppe A, Carlesimo GA, Pasqualetti P, Caltagirone C. Major and minor depression in Parkinson's disease: a neuropsychological investigation. Eur J Neurol 2006; 13: 972–80.

21 Tröster AI, Paolo AM, Lyons KE, Glatt SL, Hubble JP, Koller WC. The influence of depression on cognition in Parkinson's disease: a pattern of impairment distinguishable from Alzheimer's disease. Neurology 1995; 45: 672–6.

22 Tröster AI, Stalp LD, Paolo AM, Fields JA, Koller WC. Neuropsychological impairment in Parkinson's disease with and without depression. Arch Neurol 1995; 52: 1164–9.

23 Beliauskas LA, Glantsz RH. Depression type in Parkinson's disease. J Clin Exp Neuropsychol 1989; 11: 597–604.

24 Santamaria J, Tolosa E, Valles A. Parkinson's disease with depression: a possible subgroup of idiopathic parkinsonism. Neurology 1986; 36: 1130–3.

25 Taylor AE, Saint-Cyr JA, Lang AE, Kenny FT. Parkinson's disease and depression: a critical reevaluation. Brain 1986; 109: 279–92.

26 Huber SJ, Paulson GW, Shuttleworth EC. Relationship of motor symptoms, intellectual impairment, and depression in Parkinson's disease. J Neurol Neurosurg Psychiatry 1988; 51: 855–8.

27 Silberman CD, Laks J, Capitão CF, *et al.* Frontal functions in depressed and nondepressed Parkinson's disease patients: impact of severity stages. Psychiatry Res 2007; 149: 285–9.

28 Stern Y, Marder K, Tang MX, Mayeux R. Antecedent clinical features associated with dementia in Parkinson's disease. Neurology 1993; 43: 1690–2.

29 Santangelo G, Vitale C, Trojano L, *et al.* Relationship between depression and cognitive dysfunctions in Parkinson's disease without dementia. J Neurol 2009; 256: 632–8.

30 Starkstein SE, Mayberg HS, Preziosi TJ, Andrezejewski P, Leiguarda R, Robinson RG. Reliability, validity, and clinical correlates of apathy in Parkinson's disease. J Neuropsychiatry Clin Neurosci 1992; 4: 134–9.

31 Pluck GC, Brown RG. Apathy in Parkinson's disease. J Neurol Neurosurg Psychiatry 2002; 73: 636–42.

32 Isella V, Melzi P, Grimaldi M, *et al.* Clinical, neuropsychological, and morphometric correlates of apathy in Parkinson's disease. Mov Disord 2002; 17: 366–71.

33 Zgaljardic DJ, Borod JC, Foldi NS, *et al.* Relationship between self-reported apathy and executive dysfunction in nondemented patients with Parkinson disease. Cogn Behav Neurol 2007; 20: 184–92.

34 Isella V, Iurlaro S, Piolti R, *et al.* Physical anhedonia in Parkinson's disease. J Neurol Neurosurg Psychiatry 2003; 74: 1308–11.

35 Dubois B, Slachevsky A, Litvan I, Pillon B. The FAB: a Frontal Assessment Battery at bedside. Neurology 2000; 12: 1621–6.

36 Santangelo G, Morgante L, Savica R, *et al.*, on behalf of the PRIAMO study group. Anhedonia and cognitive impairment in Parkinson's Disease: Italian validation of the Snaith–Hamilton Pleasure Scale and its application in the clinical routine practice during the PRIAMO study. Parkinsonism Relat Disord; 15: 576–81.

Chapter 7

Motor symptoms and phenotype in patients with Parkinson's disease dementia

David J. Burn

Introduction

Although considered primarily a disorder of movement, non-motor complications are now recognised to precede and to accompany the bradykinesia, rigidity and tremor of Parkinson's disease (PD). Given the frequency of these non-motor complications, they are assumed to be an intrinsic part of the pathophysiological process of PD, and presumably reflect multifocal cell dysfunction and loss in strategic subcortical and cortical structures. It therefore seems reasonable to assume that expression of the motor and non-motor phenotype in any individual with PD is unlikely to be an independent process, and that some inter-relationship may exist between the two.

This chapter specifically considers the association between motor phenotype and dementia associated with PD (PD-D). It will also briefly address related features, as part of this phenotype. The issue of motor phenotype as a predictive factor for incident dementia will be discussed, as well as the evidence for levodopa responsiveness and motor complications in PD-D. Finally, rate of progression of the extrapyramidal symptoms in PD-D will be described.

Motor phenotype in patients with PD-D

The notion of certain motor features being over-represented in people with PD and cognitive impairment is not new. The DATATOP study, which included 800 patients with early untreated PD, reported that bradykinesia, and postural instability and gait difficulty (PIGD), were more common at onset in patients with a rapid rate of disease progression as compared to those with a relatively slow rate of progression [1]. The authors described a means of classifying patients into tremor-dominant (TD), PIGD-dominant and indeterminate phenotypes on the basis of an equation derived from items in the Unified Parkinson's Disease Rating Scale (UPDRS) Parts II and III (this classification has been extensively revised subsequent to its initial publication). Comparisons of tremor-dominant PD ($n = 441$) with the PIGD-dominant type ($n = 233$) provided support for the existence of clinical subtypes, with the latter group reporting significantly greater subjective intellectual, motor, and occupational impairment than the tremor group. In the same year, Ebmeier *et al.* assessed a whole population cohort of 157 patients with Parkinsonism to determine prevalence figures for dementia and to examine the relationship between dementia, cognitive impairment and extrapyramidal signs [2]. Dementia, defined according to DSM-III-R criteria, was present in 23.3% of all patients. The authors reported that dementia and cognitive impairment were associated with overall measures of motor impairment and rigidity, but not tremor, even after controlling for age, sex and education. Gnanalingham *et al.* compared motor and cognitive function in patients with dementia with Lewy bodies (DLB), PD, or Alzheimer's disease [3]. PD-D cases were not specifically identified in this study. Compared with patients with PD, DLB patients had greater scores for rigidity and deficits in a finger-tapping test, but rest tremor and left/right asymmetry in extrapyramidal signs were more evident in PD. DLB patients were also less likely to present with left/right asymmetry in motor symptoms at the onset of their parkinsonism. In a later cross-sectional study, specifically aimed at comparing extrapyramidal features in PD, PD-D, and DLB patients, the PIGD phenotype was found to be more common in PD-D (88% of cases) and DLB (69% of cases) groups compared with the PD group (38% of cases), in which TD and PIGD phenotypes were more equally represented ($P < 0.001$) [4].

Poorer cognitive performance in PD is associated with greater impairment in motor and non-motor domains. Papapetropoulos *et al.* evaluated the impact of cognitive impairment on disease severity and motor function in 82 PD patients, 41 and 41 of whom did and did not have cognitive impairment, respectively, matched for age at onset and duration of the disease [5]. Those patients with cognitive impairment had overall poorer motor function, worse rigidity (both axial and limb) and bradykinesia, as well as worse performance in activities of daily living compared with PD patients without cognitive impairment. More recently, a cohort study of 400 PD patients reported that more severe cognitive impairment was associated with significantly more impairment in motor, autonomic, depressive and psychotic domains [6]. Furthermore, and in keeping with previous studies, patients with a PIGD-dominant phenotype showed more cognitive impairment compared with patients with a tremor-dominant phenotype.

In contrast to most previous studies which reported a greater risk for dementia in PD patients with predominant rigidity and akinesia, Vingerhoets *et al.* reported that older age and tremor at onset were significant predictors of poor cognitive performance in their retrospective cohort analysis [7]. Although the reasons for this disparity are unclear, it should be appreciated that tremor has uncommonly been related to PD-D and is not recognised *per se* as a risk factor for incident dementia (see below).

Studies attempting to relate cognitive impairment to asymmetry of motor symptoms in PD have found contradictory results. Thus, Tomer *et al.* examined 88 patients with unilateral onset of PD and found that patients whose motor signs began on the left side of the body consistently performed more poorly on a battery of cognitive measures than did patients with right-sided onset [8]. In a later study, PD patients with right-sided tremor onset performed significantly better than other PD subgroups in a neuropsychological battery and comparably to controls [9]. Williams *et al.* applied multiple regression analysis to examine UPDRS subscore contributions to cognitive function in 108 PD patients [10]. They found that right-sided symptoms (for laterality), axial symptoms (for region), and bradykinesia (for type of symptoms) were the best predictors of cognitive function in this patient group. In contrast, St Clair *et al.* found no difference in neuropsychological functioning between two groups of PD patients with either predominant left- or right-sided motor signs, matched for disease duration, severity of motor signs, and degree of lateralized motor deficits [11]. The results of these studies are therefore confusing and conclusions are limited in most cases by sample size, battery of tests chosen (hemispheric predilection) and natural hand dominance of patients tested versus the side of symptom dominance. The most parsimonious explanation would be that side of symptom dominance does not have a major influence upon cognitive function in PD or PD-D.

A data-driven approach to motor phenotype and cognition

The relationship between motor phenotype and dementia may also be examined by exploring heterogeneity within cohorts of PD using a data-driven approach. This approach is non-hypothesis driven and avoids arbitrary *a priori* subclassifications. Graham and Sagar explored heterogeneity in 176 patients with PD by using comprehensive demographic, motor, mood, and cognitive information [12]. Cluster analysis revealed three subgroups of patients, one subgroup with a disease duration of 5.6 years and two subgroups at 13.4 years. A 'motor only' subtype was characterized by motor symptom progression in the absence of intellectual impairment. Equivalent motor symptom progression was shown by a 'motor and cognitive' subtype which was accompanied by executive function deficits progressing to global cognitive impairment. A 'rapid progression' subtype was characterized by an older age at disease onset and rapidly progressive motor and cognitive disability. Lewis *et al.* subsequently investigated the heterogeneity of PD using a similar approach in a cohort of 120 patients in the early disease phase (Hoehn and Yahr stages I–III) [13]. The analysis revealed four main subgroups: (a) patients with a younger disease onset; (b) a tremor-dominant subgroup of patients; (c) a non-tremor-dominant subgroup with significant levels of cognitive impairment and mild depression; and (d) a subgroup with rapid disease progression but no cognitive impairment. Both studies suggest that, at least in cross-sectional analyses, distinct motor–cognitive phenotypes exist in PD, although these studies do not permit the assessment of change over time. In other words, motor phenotype is not necessarily stable, and patients who are initially tremor dominant may not remain so throughout their disease (see below). Most recently, Reijnders *et al.* performed an exploratory and confirmatory cluster analysis of motor and psychopathological symptoms in a randomized sample of 173 patients each, stemming from two research databases [14]. PD patients were robustly classified into four different subtypes: rapid disease progression subtype, young-onset subtype, non-tremor-dominant subtype with psychopathology and a tremor-dominant subtype. Cognitive deterioration, depressive and apathetic symptoms, and hallucinations all clustered within the non-tremor-dominant motor subtype, characterized by bradykinesia, rigidity, postural instability and gait disorder.

Expanding the motor phenotype

Dementia associated with PD is also an independent risk factor for falls. In a prospective study of 109 subjects with PD evaluated over 12 months, falls occurred in 68% of patients [15]. Previous falls, disease duration, loss of arm swing and notably dementia were independent predictors of falling. A subsequent meta-analysis of falling in PD was unable to include cognitive impairment and dementia as a predictive variable because this had not been quantified in all of the six studies included [16]. A more recent prospective study determined whether measures of attention were associated with falls in 164 PD patients [17]. A total of 103 (63%) subjects fell one or more times during the 12-month study period. Regression analysis revealed an association of fall frequency with poorer power of attention and increased reaction time variability (assessed using a computerized battery), which was retained after correcting for UPDRS scores. This finding therefore has implications for the identification of those PD patients most at risk of falling, and for the management and prevention of falls in this patient group.

PIGD phenotype has also been associated with more frequent excessive daytime sleepiness (EDS) in PD-D, although this association was lost over a 2-year follow-up period, suggesting that the pathophysiology of EDS and motor phenotype is anatomically and/or temporally distinct [18]. Intriguingly, in non-demented PD patients, rapid eye movement sleep behaviour disorder (RBD) is more common in patients with a PIGD phenotype and is associated with greater falls frequency and reduced levodopa responsiveness [19]. Moreover, the presence of RBD in PD has been strongly associated with more severe symptoms and signs of orthostatic hypotension [20,21]. A phenotypic pattern of PD associated with PD-D is thus emerging, characterized by a PIGD motor disturbance, RBD, EDS, greater autonomic disturbance and increased falls frequency.

Early cognitive impairment and motor function

In addition to motor phenotype in established PD-D, what evidence is there for differences in extrapyramidal signs in PD patients with mild cognitive impairment? Establishing differences at this point in the disease process could give greater insight into the underlying pathophysiological process. In a study of 60 consecutive patients with newly diagnosed, untreated PD and 37 matched, healthy control subjects, Cooper *et al.* reported that the PD group as a whole showed deficits in immediate recall of verbal material, language production and semantic fluency, set formation, cognitive sequencing, working memory and visuomotor construction. Motor disability correlated strongly with severity of depression but only weakly with cognitive impairment. Cognitive sequencing, set-formation and set-shifting deficits tended to associate with depression, but otherwise there was no association between cognition and depression. The authors suggested a dissociation of cognition and motor control in early PD [22]. More recently, Lyros *et al.* examined the relationship between motor phenotype and subtle cognitive dysfunction in PD [23]. A battery of neuropsychological tests was administered to two groups of non-demented patients with mild-to-moderate disease, classified either as PIGD or as non-PIGD. No significant differences were revealed between the two groups in the performance of any of the administered neuropsychological tests, leading the authors to suggest that diverse pathological processes may emerge later to account for the unequal incidence of dementia among different motor subtypes. Green *et al.* determined the nature and frequency of cognitive impairments in 61 non-demented patients with advanced PD and their relationship to other variables potentially predictive of neuropsychological performance [24]. Poorer performance on multiple neuropsychological measures was related to greater overall motor abnormality and increased bradykinesia on medication, as well as older age, longer disease duration and reduced education. Interestingly, non-demented PD patients with concomitant RBD also displayed significantly poorer performance on episodic verbal memory, executive functions, as well as visuospatial and visuoperceptual processing compared to PD patients without RBD [25].

Taken together, these observations suggest that the pathological processes determining motor phenotype may be dissociated from those determining cognition, either in temporal or spatial evolution, or both. By their cross-sectional nature, however, these studies were unable to address whether motor phenotype may be an independent risk factor for incident dementia in PD. This is addressed in the next section.

Motor phenotype as a risk factor for dementia

Although a number of risk factors for incident dementia in PD have been reported, three have been consistently found in almost all studies: advanced age, motor phenotype and baseline cognitive performance [26,27]. Advanced age is the single most significant risk factor, both in cross-sectional and prospective studies, although older age and more severe motor symptoms are synergistic in predicting dementia. When a cohort of patients was divided into four groups by dichotomizing around their median age and UPDRS motor scores, the group with older age and severe disease had a 12-fold increased risk for incident dementia as compared to the younger patients with mild disease [28]. As younger patients with greater disease severity and older patients with less severe motor symptoms did not show a significantly increased risk, a combined effect of age and disease severity was assumed. In addition to the overall severity of extrapyramidal features influencing the likelihood of developing PD-D, a non-tremor dominant motor phenotype also predicts a greater risk for incident dementia. In one prospective study of 40 PD patients, 25% of 16 PIGD phenotype patients developed dementia over 2 years, compared with none of 18 tremor-dominant or six indeterminate phenotype cases [29].

As mentioned above, predominant motor phenotype may not necessarily remain stable throughout the disease course. Thus a patient may evolve from a tremor dominant to a PIGD phenotype, presumably reflecting the underlying pathological progression. This, in turn, may influence risk of developing dementia. In a Norwegian community-based sample of 171 non-demented PD patients followed prospectively over 8 years, logistic regression was used to analyze the relationship between subtype of parkinsonism and dementia [30]. The transition from tremor dominant to PIGD subtype was associated with a more than threefold increase in the rate of Mini-Mental State Examination decline. Compared to patients with a persistent tremor dominant or indeterminate subtype, the odds ratio for dementia was 56.7 [95% confidence interval (CI): 4.0–808] for patients changing from TD or indeterminate subtype to PIGD subtype, and 80.0 (95% CI: 4.6–1400) for patients with persistent PIGD subtype. Furthermore, patients with a tremor-dominant subtype at baseline did not become demented until they developed a PIGD motor subtype, and dementia did not occur among patients with persistent tremor dominance. Although the CIs were wide for these estimates, reflecting relatively small numbers, this paper emphasizes the importance of current motor phenotype and associated dementia risk.

In a recent community-based study performed in Cambridgeshire, UK, incident cases of PD were recruited, thereby removing much of the bias associated with selective mortality in prevalence cohorts [31]. Bivariate comparisons of baseline demographic, clinical and neuropsychological variables versus rate of cognitive decline showed that, in addition to older age, a non-tremor-dominant motor phenotype, a higher UPDRS motor score, and below average performance on tests of semantic fluency, pentagon copying, spatial recognition memory and Tower of London were associated with a more rapid rate of cognitive decline. Multivariate analysis revealed that a non-tremor dominant motor phenotype together with poor semantic fluency and inaccurate pentagon copying were the most significant predictors of cognitive decline, independent of age. Patients with a non-tremor-dominant phenotype were 4.1 times more likely to develop dementia than tremor-dominant patients.

Axial symptoms and PD-D may have an overlapping pathogenesis, with distinct loci of dysfunction different from those underlying tremor-dominant PD. Specifically, the postural instability of PD tends to be refractory to dopaminergic therapy, and may relate to subcortical neuronal loss within the cholinergic system which also plays an important role in the cognitive and neuropsychiatric symptoms of PD-D [4]. This is further discussed below.

Response to levodopa and motor complications

The axial symptoms of PD are commonly viewed as being less levodopa responsive. They may be caused by 'non-dopaminergic' lesions, for example in the pedunculopontine nucleus. Levodopa responsiveness could therefore be expected to be reduced in PD-D where a PIGD phenotype predominates. One possibility, of course, is that previously levodopa-responsive symptoms become refractory as dementia develops [32]. To date, a majority of cross-sectional and longitudinal studies have failed to directly assess levodopa response in demented versus non-demented PD patients. Using a 200 mg single-dose levodopa challenge, one study failed to detect significant differences in mean improvement on UPDRS motor score, although more non-demented patients experienced >20% improvement compared to those with PD-D (90% vs 65%) [33]. A later study included patients with DLB, PD and PD-D and failed to detect differences in levodopa responsiveness between PD and PD-D [34]. Given the clinical (including motor phenotype) and pathological similarity between PD-D and DLB, it is also of potential relevance to consider the results of a study in 19 DLB subjects, where levodopa was increased and motor response assessed a mean of 3 months later [35] Motor improvement was found in only six of the 19 patients, despite a mean daily increase of 111 mg levodopa. A longitudinal study found greater cognitive decline over a 3-year period in those PD patients with less than 50% improvement of UPDRS score after a levodopa test performed at baseline [36]. More recently, a prospective study of 34 PD patients assessed annually over mean follow-up of 11.4 years from the point of commencement of levodopa found that the patients who developed dementia had a more rapid decline in motor function [37]. Moreover, although it was not formally commented upon by the authors, their data appeared to indicate that demented PD patients showed a reduced responsiveness to levodopa at the time of formal levodopa challenge compared with the non-demented patients.

Overall, it is not possible to draw firm conclusions on differences in the degree of levodopa responsiveness between PD subjects with and without dementia. The limited evidence available to date would suggest, however, an attenuated or dimininshed response.

Levodopa-induced motor complications

Whereas fewer dyskinesias were reported in demented PD patients in a cross-sectional study [38], a longitudinal study found greater mental deterioration in those patients exhibiting dystonic levodopa-induced dyskinesias at baseline [36]. Clissold *et al.* reported fluctuator versus non-fluctuator status in a longitudinal study of levodopa responsiveness in 22 surviving PD patients, in addition to latest Mini-Mental State Examination (MMSE) score [37]. When considering fluctuator status in those subjects with an MMSE score of ≤24, compared with those above this level (a threshold previously suggested to support a diagnosis of PD-D), only 15% of the fluctuators were classified as 'PD-D' versus 44% of the non-fluctuators. Although these data are insufficient to infer differences in the occurrence of levodopa-induced motor complications in PD-D, they lend some support to the notion that fluctuations may be less frequent.

Neuroleptic sensitivity

Although placebo-controlled studies have previously excluded patients with PD-D, open label studies with clozapine in PD-related psychosis have included PD-D subjects and found that the drug was similarly well-tolerated in demented and non-demented patients. Sedation and hypotension are the main side-effects described. One study evaluated severe neuroleptic sensitivity reactions (NSRs) according to an operationalized definition, blind to clinical and neuropathological diagnoses, in prospectively studied patients exposed to neuroleptics from two centres [39]. Severe NSR only occurred in patients with LBD—in 53% DLB, 39% PDD, and 27% PD patients—and did not occur in Alzheimer's disease. No other clinical or demo-graphic features predicted severe NSR. This high frequency of NSR in PD-D clearly has important implications for clinical practice, particularly as even so-called 'atypical neu-roleptics' are not exempt from causing this problem in the closely related DLB [40].

Rate of progression of motor symptoms in PD-D

Development of dementia may be associated with a more aggressive motor disease course [12,37,38]. Jankovic *et al.* determined overall rate of functional decline in 297 PD patients, followed up for an average of 6.4 (range: 3–17) years [41]. Patients were categorized as having tremor- or PIGD-dominant PD and the two categories were compared for progression of their total UPDRS scores. Patients with an older age at onset had more rapid progression of PD than those with a younger age at onset, while cognitive deterioration was greater in the older-onset group. Regression analysis of 108 patients whose symptoms were rated during their 'off' state showed a faster rate of cognitive decline as age at onset increased, and the annual rates of decline in the UPDRS scores, when adjusted for age at initial visit, were steeper for the PIGD-dominant group compared with the tremor-dominant group. Dementia at baseline was associated with more rapid motor decline in two studies [42,43], but this remained significant in only one study after adjusting for other baseline factors, where PD-D patients had a 7.9-point higher annual decline in UPDRS motor scores compared to those without dementia at baseline [43]. In a longitudinal study, a more rapid decline in UPDRS III scores was reported in PD-D compared with PD patients over 2 years (9.7 vs 5.1 points, respectively) [29]. Although not statistically significant, the absolute deterioration at 2 years was greater in the PIGD than the tremor-dominant PD subgroup. Rate of motor decline in the PD-D patients was independent of baseline disease duration. In a study of 232 PD patients followed for 8 years, population-averaged logistic regression models were used to describe annual disease progression and to analyse the influence of potential risk factors on functional decline [44]. Age, age at onset, disease duration, and excessive daytime somnolence at baseline were strong and independent predictors of greater impairment in motor function and disability, while cognitive impairment at baseline predicted higher disability and higher Hoehn and Yahr scores. Age at disease onset was, however, the main predictor of motor decline, indicating a slower and more restricted pathological process in patients with younger-onset PD.

Conclusions

A consistent motor phenotype associated with PD-D has emerged from observational studies. These patients are more likely to have symmetric disease and less tremor than their non-demented counterparts. The phenotype may be expanded to include a higher frequency of falls, sleep disorders (RBD and possibly EDS) and autonomic impairment. The demented PD patient may be less likely to experience levodopa-related dyskinesias and be more refractory to levodopa treatment overall, although more work is required to clarify these points and to control for potential confounders, including age, cumulative doses of levodopa received, and disease duration. Neuroleptics, including so-called 'atypical' agents, should be used with caution in PD-D, as the patients may be sensitized to potentially life-threatening extrapyramidal side-effects associated with these drugs. The PIGD phenotype is a robust predictor of incident dementia in PD, and conversion to this phenotype during the disease course appears to have sinister portent with regard to deterioration in cognition. Finally, the presence of dementia seems to herald a more rapid deterioration in motor function, which may contribute to the increased mortality observed in PD-D patients.

References

1 Jankovic J, McDermott M, Carter J, *et al.* Variable expression of Parkinson's disease: a baseline analysis of the DATATOP cohort. The Parkinson Study Group. Neurology 1990; 40: 1529–34.

2 Ebmeier KP, Calder SA, Crawford JR, Stewart L, Besson JA, Mutch WJ. Clinical features predicting dementia in idiopathic Parkinson's disease: a follow-up study. Neurology 1990; 40: 1222–4.

3 Gnanalingham KK, Byrne EJ, Thornton A, Sambrook MA, Bannister P. Motor and cognitive function in Lewy body dementia: comparison with Alzheimer's and Parkinson's disease. J Neurol Neurosurg Psychiatry 1997; 62: 243–52.

4 Burn DJ, Rowan EN, Minnett T, *et al.* Extrapyramidal features in Parkinson's disease with and without dementia and dementia with Lewy bodies: a cross-sectional comparative study. Mov Disord 2003; 18: 884–9.

5 Papapetropoulos S, Ellul J, Polychronopoulos P, Chroni E. A registry-based, case–control investigation of Parkinson's disease with and without cognitive impairment. Eur J Neurol 2004; 11: 347–51.

6 Verbaan D, Marinus J, Visser M, *et al.* Cognitive impairment in Parkinson's disease. J Neurol Neurosurg Psychiatry 2007; 78: 1182–7.

7 Vingerhoets G, Verleden S, Santens P, Miatton M, De Reuck J. Predictors of cognitive impairment in advanced Parkinson's disease. J Neurol Neurosurg Psychiatry 2003; 74: 793–6.

8 Tomer R, Levin BE, Weiner WJ. Side of onset of motor symptoms influences cognition in Parkinson's disease. Ann Neurol 1993; 34: 579–84.

9 Katzen HL, Levin BE, Weiner W. Side and type of motor symptom influence cognition in Parkinson's disease. Mov Disord 2006; 21: 1947–53.

10 Williams LN, Seignourel P, Crucian GP, *et al.* Laterality, region, and type of motor dysfunction correlate with cognitive impairment in Parkinson's disease. Mov Disord 2007; 22: 141–5.

11 St Clair J, Borod JC, Sliwinski M, Cote LJ, Stern Y. Cognitive and affective functioning in Parkinson's disease patients with lateralized motor signs. J Clin Exp Neuropsychol 1998; 20: 320–7.

12 Graham JM, Sagar HJ. A data-driven approach to the study of heterogeneity in idiopathic Parkinson's disease: identification of three distinct subtypes. Mov Disord 1999; 14: 10–20.

13 Lewis SJG, Foltynie T, Blackwell AD, Robbins TW, Owen AM, Barker RA. Heterogeneity of Parkinson's disease in the early clinical stages using a data driven approach. J Neurol Neurosurg Psychiatry 2005; 76: 343–8.

14 Reijnders JS, Ehrt U, Lousberg R, Aarsland D, Leentjens AF. The association between motor subtypes and psychopathology in Parkinson's disease. Parkinsonism Relat Disord 2008; 15: 379–82.

15 Wood BH, Bilclough JA, Bowron A, Walker RW. Incidence and prediction of falls in Parkinson's disease: a prospective multidisciplinary study. J Neurol Neurosurg Psychiatry 2002; 72: 721–5.

16 Pickering RM, Grimbergen YA, Rigney U, *et al.* A meta-analysis of six prospective studies of falling in Parkinson's disease. Mov Disord 2007; 22: 1892–1900.

17 Allcock LM, Rowan EN, Steen IN, Wesnes K, Kenny RA, Burn DJ. Impaired attention predicts falling in Parkinson's disease. Parkinsonism Relat Disord 2008; 15: 110–15.

18 Boddy F, Rowan EN, Lett D, O'Brien JT, McKeith IG, Burn DJ. Sleep quality and excessive daytime somnolence in Parkinson's disease with and without dementia, dementia with Lewy bodies and Alzheimer's disease: a comparative, cross-sectional study. Int J Geriatr Psychiatry 2007; 22: 529–35.

19 Postuma RB, Gagnon JF, Vendette M, Charland K, Montplaisir J. REM sleep behaviour disorder in Parkinson's disease is associated with specific motor features. J Neurol Neurosurg Psychiatry 2008; 79: 1117–21.

20 Allcock LM, Kenny RA, Burn DJ. Clinical phenotype of subjects with Parkinson's disease and orthostatic hypotension: autonomic symptom and demographic comparison. Mov Disord 2006; 21: 1851–5.

21 Postuma RB, Gagnon JF, Vendette M, Charland K, Montplaisir J. Manifestations of Parkinson disease differ in association with REM sleep behavior disorder. Mov Disord 2008; 23: 1665–72.

22 Cooper JA, Sagar HJ, Jordan N, Harvey NS, Sullivan EV. Cognitive impairment in early, untreated Parkinson's disease and its relationship to motor disability. Brain 1991; 114: 2095–2122.

23 Lyros E, Messinis L, Papathanasopoulos P. Does motor subtype influence neurocognitive performance in Parkinson's disease without dementia?. Eur J Neurol 2008; 15: 262–7.

24 Green J, McDonald WM, Vitek JL, et al. Cognitive impairments in advanced PD without dementia. Neurology 2002; 59: 1320–4.

25 Vendette M, Gagnon JF, Décary A, et al. REM sleep behavior disorder predicts cognitive impairment in Parkinson disease without dementia. Neurology 2007; 69: 1843–9.

26 Hughes TA, Ross HF, Musa S, et al. A 10-year study of the incidence of and factors predicting dementia in Parkinson's disease. Neurology 2000; 54: 1596–1602.

27 Levy G, Tang M-X, Cote LJ, et al. Motor impairment in PD: relationship to incident dementia and age. Neurology 2000; 55: 539–44.

28 Levy G, Schupf N, Tang MX, et al. Combined effect of age and severity on the risk of dementia in Parkinson's disease. Ann Neurol 2002; 51: 722–9.

29 Burn D, Rowan E, Allan L, Molloy S, O'Brien J, McKeith I. Motor subtype and cognitive decline in Parkinson's disease, Parkinson's disease with dementia, and dementia with Lewy bodies. J Neurol Neurosurg Psychiatry 2006; 77: 585–9.

30 Alves G, Larsen JP, Emre M, Wentzel-Larsen T, Aarsland D. Changes in motor subtype and risk for incident dementia in Parkinson's disease. Mov Disord 2006; 21: 1123–30.

31 Williams-Gray CH, Foltynie T, Brayne CEG, Robbins TW, Barker RA. Evolution of cognitive dysfunction in an incident Parkinson's disease cohort. Brain 2007; 130: 1787–98.

32 Joyce JN, Ryoo HL, Beach TB, et al. Loss of response to levodopa in Parkinson's disease and co-occurrence with dementia: role of D3 and not D2 receptors. Brain Res 2002; 955: 138–52.

33 Bonelli SB, Ransmayr G, Steffelbauer M, Lukas T, Lampl C, Deibl M. L-Dopa responsiveness in dementia with Lewy bodies, Parkinson's disease with and without dementia. Neurology 2004; 63: 376–8.

34 Molloy S, McKeith IG, O'Brien JT, Burn DJ. The role of levodopa in the management of dementia with Lewy bodies. J Neurol Neurosurg Psychiatry 2005; 76: 1200–3.

35 Goldman JG, Goetz CG, Brandabur M, Sanfilippo M, Stebbins GT. Effects of dopaminergic medications on psychosis and motor function in dementia with Lewy bodies. Mov Disord 2008; 23: 2248–50.

36 Caparros-Lefebvre D, Pecheux N, Petit V, Duhamel A, Petit H. Which factors predict cognitive decline in Parkinson's disease?. J Neurol Neurosurg Psychiatry 1995; 58: 51–5.

37 Clissold BG, McColl CD, Reardon KR, Shiff M, Kempster PA. Longitudinal study of the motor response to levodopa in Parkinson's disease. Mov Disord 2006; 21: 2116–21.

38 Elizan TS, Sroka H, Maker H, Smith H, Yahr MD. Dementia in idiopathic Parkinson's disease: variables associated with its occurrence in 203 patients. J Neural Transm 1986; 65: 285–302.

39 Aarsland D, Perry R, Larsen J, et al. Neuroleptic sensitivity in Parkinson's disease and parkinsonian dementias. J Clin Psychiatry 2005; 66: 633–7.

40 Burn DJ, McKeith IG. Current treatment of dementia with Lewy bodies and dementia associated with Parkinson's disease. Mov Disord 2003; 18(Suppl 6): S72–S79.

41 Jankovic J, Kapadia AS. Functional decline in Parkinson's disease. Arch Neurol 2001; 58: 1611–15.

42 Hely MA, Morris JGL, Reid WGJ, *et al*. Age at onset: the major determinant of outcome in Parkinson's disease. Acta Neurol Scand 1995; 92: 455–63.

43 Louis ED, Tang MX, Cote L, Alfaro B, Mejia H, Marder K. Progression of parkinsonian signs in Parkinson disease. Arch Neurol 1999; 56: 334–7.

44 Alves G, Wentzel-Larsen T, Aarsland D, Larsen JP. Progression of motor impairment and disability in Parkinson disease: a population-based study. Neurology 2005; 65: 1436–41.

Chapter 8

Interaction between cognition and gait in patients with Parkinson's disease

J. M. Hausdorff, G. Yogev-Seligman, M. Plotnik, A. Mirelman and N. Giladi

Introduction

Gait disturbances and falls are a frequent cause of morbidity and mortality among patients with Parkinson's disease (PD) [1–4]. This stems, in part, from the basal ganglia pathology and dopamine dysregulation [5] that causes impaired execution of automatic and repetitive movements such as those that are critical to walking. In addition to its effects on these so-called motor systems, PD also impacts cognition, most notably executive function and attention [6,7] (see also Chapter 4). In this chapter, we briefly describe the recent evidence which demonstrates that these cognitive deficits have a profound impact on the gait changes seen in PD.

Gait disturbances and fall risk

Gait disturbances in PD may be divided into two types: (1) continuous and (2) episodic or paroxysmal [8,9]. The continuous changes refer to alterations in the walking pattern that are more or less consistent from one step to the next, i.e. they persist and are apparent all the time. In contrast, the episodic gait disturbances occur occasionally, emerging in an apparently random, inexplicable manner. As further detailed below, both types of gait disturbances may be influenced by the cognitive changes associated with PD and both are associated with an increased fall risk.

   The continuous gait disturbances include slowed ambulation with decreased or absent arm swing, longer double limb support [1,10–12] and impaired postural control [13–16]. One of the keys to these gait problems is the inability of patients with PD to generate sufficient stride length [1,12,17]. Gait disturbances in PD also include features that are not always visible in routine clinical observation, but become apparent when gait is evaluated quantitatively with gait analysis systems, e.g. gait asymmetry, diminished left-right co-ordination [18], and a loss of consistency in one's ability to produce a steady gait rhythm, resulting in higher stride-to-stride variability [13,19–21]. These changes can be detected even in patients with very mild disease [19]. The continuous gait disturbances are strongly associated with instability, falls, and fear of future falls [22,23]. These symptoms, in turn, often lead to self-imposed restrictions of daily activities [22,24] which exacerbate reduced mobility, cause a further loss of independence, and deprive patients of social contacts, leading to isolation, depression [25], and overall reduced quality of life [26].

The episodic gait disturbances include festination, start hesitation, and freezing of gait (FOG) [2,24,27]. The latter is a debilitating phenomenon that is commonly experienced by patients with advanced PD [2,28–30]. FOG is typically a paroxysmal gait disturbance [28,31] with a 'sudden and transient'nature [32]. Patients who experience FOG frequently report that during the freezing episode, their feet are inexplicably 'glued' to the ground. Like some of the continuous gait disturbances, FOG episodes also increase the risk for falls [2,33] and have a considerable negative impact on the quality of life and wellbeing of affected PD patients [2,24,34–36]. FOG has been referred to as a 'motor' block and has been viewed as another PD motor symptom, but we shall see that its occurrence too is likely affected by the cognitive impairments common in PD.

Cognition, attention and executive function changes

Cognitive decline in PD patients occurs even in the early stages of the disease [37] and includes deficits in several cognitive domains. Executive function and attention are two of the most notable functions impaired by the disease [7,37,38]. Executive functions refers to a group of higher cognitive processes by which performance is optimized in situations requiring the operation of multiple cognitive functions [39–41]. Consequently, PD patients show diminished performance in tasks demanding planning, set-shifting and response inhibition, suggesting mental inflexibility or rigidity, slow generation of ideas, and reduced performance on tasks that involve attentional processes or divided attention [37,38,42,43]. As will be described, executive function and attention, two closely related cognitive domains, play an important role in gait and falls.

Cognitive function and continuous gait changes

A growing body of research has linked gait to cognitive function [44–48]. This association is commonly studied using dual-task paradigms, where a subject walks while simultaneously performing a secondary cognitive task (e.g. arithmetic calculations). In general, dual-tasking relies on frontal lobe function, in particular, executive function and the ability to divide attention [49,50]. The rationale behind using dual-tasking paradigms is, therefore, that if a gait feature is automated and does not require cognitive function, performance of a second task should not alter that aspect of gait. Alternatively, if that feature depends on cognitive function, then performance of one or both of the tasks will be affected [51]. Studies have demonstrated that dual-tasking affects certain aspects of gait in particular ways associated with specific populations. Healthy young adults reduce their gait speed during dual-tasking [52–55], while other aspects of gait are generally not affected [54,55]. Healthy older adults reduce both their gait speed and the duration of swing, increasing support time (stance); interestingly, gait variability, the stride-to-stride changes in the walking pattern that have been linked to fall risk, is not altered in healthy subjects, even when the dual-tasking becomes extremely challenging [55,56].

PD patients may use compensatory strategies to achieve a more normal gait, by recruiting attentional resources to correct for the reduced automaticity and to compensate for the continuous gait changes [12,57]. This ability to circumvent the impaired basal ganglia using cortical inputs is, however, limited because it may depend on higher-level cognitive function, i.e. executive function and attention. Executive function and attention are, however, also diminished in PD [58–60]. As a result, the overall effects observed in dual-tasking experiments with PD patients generally exceed those seen in healthy subjects. For example, in response to dual-tasking, PD patients walk more slowly and with a reduced swing time [56,61]. In addition gait dysrhthymicity [16] and asymmetry [62] increase, and bilateral co-ordination of gait decreases, much more than seen in age-matched controls [63] (Figs 8.1 and 8.2).

To better understand the role of attention on gait in PD, Hausdorff *et al.* tested the hypothesis that gait variability, a marker of fall risk, increases when subjects with PD walk while performing a cognitively challenging task [64]. Subjects with PD walked under normal

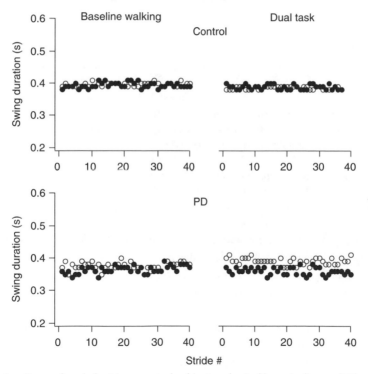

Fig. 8.1 Swing times of each foot in a control subject and a Parkinson's disease (PD) patient. The left and right columns show swing time and asymmetry during usual walking and during dual-tasking, respectively. The effect of dual-tasking is clearly apparent for the PD patient where right foot (○) values become further separated from the left foot (•) values. Such an effect was not present for the control subject, whose gait asymmetry values were 0.3 and 1.0 in the usual walking and the dual-task conditions, respectively. The corresponding values were 3.0 and 7.0 for the PD patient. From Yogev *et al.* [62].

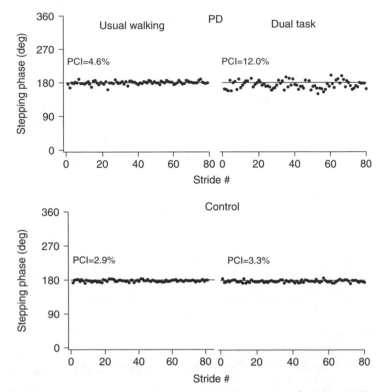

Fig. 8.2 Left–right stepping phase (φ) values are plotted for a series of strides. For the Parkinson's disease (PD) patient (top panels), the phase values became more scattered and more distanced from the 180° line during dual-tasking (right panel), as compared to the usual-walking (left panel). The data from the control subject showed only minor changes in the left–right stepping phase pattern in the presence of dual-tasking (lower panels). PCI, phase coordination index. Adapted from Plotnik *et al.* [63].

conditions and while performing another task simultaneously (i.e., serial 7 subtractions). When walking while cognitively challenged, gait variability increased significantly, more than two-folds ($P < 0.002$). These results highlighted the profound effects of attention and dual-tasking on walking, exacerbating gait variability and impairing the ability of patients with PD to maintain a stable walk.

In a follow-up study [16], Yogev *et al.* examined 30 patients with idiopathic PD (mean age: 70.9 years) with moderate disease severity (Hoehn and Yahr 2–3) and 28 age- and gender-matched healthy controls. Gait variability was measured under single and dual-tasking conditions (with different levels of cognitive loading). Compared to the controls, gait variability was significantly increased in the PD group under all conditions ($P < 0.01$; e.g. see Fig. 8.3). Further, as the degree of cognitive loading increased, so did gait variability, compared to usual walking, but only in the PD patients. Thus, the gap between the gait variability of the healthy controls and the patients grew as the cognitive loading level increased (see Fig. 8.4).

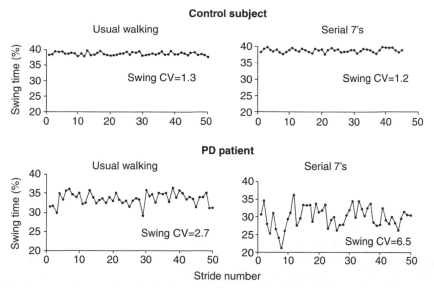

Fig. 8.3 Example of swing time series from a patient with Parkinson's disease (PD) and a control, under usual-walking conditions and when performing serial 7 subtractions. Under usual-walking conditions, variability is greater in the patient with PD [coefficient of variation (CV) = 2.7%] compared to the control (CV = 1.3%). Variability increases during dual-tasking in the subject with PD (CV = 6.5%), but not in the control (CV = 1.2%). Adapted from Yogev *et al*. [16].

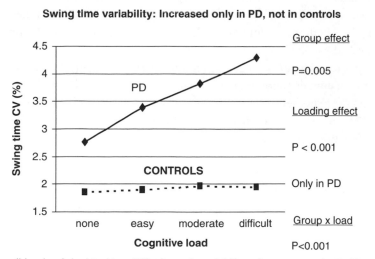

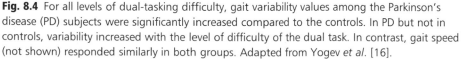

Fig. 8.4 For all levels of dual-tasking difficulty, gait variability values among the Parkinson's disease (PD) subjects were significantly increased compared to the controls. In PD but not in controls, variability increased with the level of difficulty of the dual task. In contrast, gait speed (not shown) responded similarly in both groups. Adapted from Yogev *et al*. [16].

Consistent with previous reports, executive function was significantly worse in the PD group ($P < 0.0002$) compared to aged-matched controls. However, memory, information processing, and scores on the Mini-Mental State Examination (MMSE), a general measure of cognitive function, were not different between the participants. Executive function and gait variability were moderately related during usual walking ($r = -0.39$; $P = 0.007$), and this association became stronger during cognitive loading ($r = 0.49$; $P = 0.002$). On the other hand, gait variability was not related to memory or to information processing abilities during any of the walking conditions. These findings demonstrate specific associations between executive function and gait variability and also suggest a cause-and-effect relationship. In the presence of the impaired executive function in patients with PD, greater attentional demands lead to greater reliance on executive function, and subsequently greater effects on gait variability.

Recent research further supports the association between cognitive changes in PD and the continuous gait changes. Several studies suggest that older adults who perform poorly under dual-task gait conditions are at increased risk for falls [65–67]. Similarly, a number of investigations have demonstrated a relationship between attentional abilities, gait, and fall risk in PD [56,61]. Indeed, Allock et al. recently demonstrated that attentional deficits are prospectively associated with future falls in patients with PD [68]. Deficits in attention and executive function apparently play an important role in the high fall risk observed in patients with PD.

The idea that disease-related alterations in executive function and attention influence the continuous gait changes and fall risk in PD is supported by intriguing preliminary work using pharmacological interventions. A number of pharmacological agents have been used to enhance cognitive function and attention in various populations [69]. Methylphenidate (MPH; Ritalin®) is a drug extensively used in therapy of attention deficits, mainly in children, but also in older adults [70–72]. Although the mechanism underlying MPH efficacy is not fully understood [73], its effects on attention has been well-established.

Assuming executive function and attention deficits alter gait, then enhancement of these cognitive domains should improve gait. An open label pilot study examined this idea, testing the hypothesis that MPH may improve gait and reduce fall risk in patients with PD [74]. Auriel et al. evaluated the effect of a single dose (20 mg) of MPH on cognitive function, gait performance and markers of fall risk in 21 patients with PD (mean age 70.2 ± 9.2 years). Patients took their anti-parkinsonian medications in the morning, performed baseline testing, received a single dose of MPH, and then were re-tested about 2 h later. Significant increases in a computerized battery index of attention ($P < 0.013$) and executive function ($P < 0.05$) were observed in response to MPH. In contrast, scores of memory, visuospatial orientation, and hand–eye co-ordination were unchanged. Significant improvements were also observed in the Timed Up and Go test, a classic measure of fall risk ($P < 0.001$), gait speed ($P < 0.005$) and stride time variability ($P < 0.013$) (see Table 8.1). The dual-tasking effect on stride-to-stride variability was also significantly reduced ($P < 0.05$), demonstrating that a single dose (20 mg) of MPH not

Table 8.1 Effects of methylphenidate (MPH) on gait and mobility in patients with Parkinson's disease

	Before MPH	After MPH	P-value
Timed up and go (s)	11.9 ± 3.8	10.6 ± 2.3	0.0001
Gait speed (m/s)	1.07 ± 0.19	1.13 ± 0.21	0.005
Average stride time (ms)	1114 ± 85	1100 ± 79	0.068
Stride time variability (%)	2.28 ± 0.63	2.00 ± 0.47	0.013

Adapted from Auriel *et al.* [74]

The positive response to MPH supports the idea that the gait disturbances in PD are related to executive function and attention.

only significantly improved attention and executive function in patients with PD, but also resulted in improvements in gait speed, gait variability and markers of fall risk. A similar study in healthy older adults where a placebo was also administered further supports this idea [75]. In addition, a 3-month open-label pilot study of MPH in patients with advanced PD found marked improvement in stride length and other measures of mobility [76], further supporting the association between executive function and gait in PD.

Freezing of gait and cognitive deficits

Only a limited number of studies have directly examined the relationship between the transient, episodic gait changes and the cognitive deficits in PD. Still, several lines of work suggest that there is indeed a connection and perhaps even a cause and effect relationship, with the cognitive alterations exacerbating or leading to the motor deficits. This work largely focuses on one of the episodic gait disturbances in PD, i.e. FOG.

As noted above, the mechanisms underlying FOG are largely unknown. Some have suggested that internal or external triggers (e.g. emotional reaction, change in walking environment) may operate on the background of an altered gait pattern to cause a further transient deterioration in locomotion control, which leads to FOG [30,77,78]. One possibility is that mental capacity and affect may play a role as triggers of FOG [30]. Indeed, 'panic attacks' have been associated with FOG [79] and Amboni *et al.* [80] observed that FOG was correlated with lower scores of cognitive tests related to frontal lobe and executive functions in patients with PD. In the study by Amboni *et al.*, PD patients who suffer from FOG (PD + FOG) scored lower on tests of executive functions including verbal fluency, the clock test, and the frontal assessment battery, whereas scores on the MMSE and the Unified Parkinson's Disease Rating Scale (UPDRS) motor scores were not different in the two groups. These findings support the possibility of exaggerated frontal impairment in PD + FOG patients.

How might these impairments affect FOG? It is helpful to examine the inter-ictal gait pattern of PD + FOG patients and compare it to that of patients who do not experience FOG (PD – FOG). Although the walking pattern of both groups appears to be similar between freezing episodes (i.e. inter-ical stride time and gait speed are not different in

PD – FOG and PD + FOG [81–83]), more subtle changes in the gait pattern of patients with FOG have been observed. These include an increased stride-to-stride variability [83], increased gait asymmetry [77], and altered bilateral co-ordination in walking periods isolated from freezing episodes [18] (see Fig. 8.5) in PD + FOG compared to PD – FOG. These latter findings might explain the relatively high incidence of FOG during turns [84], as turning is a task that demands a high level of bilateral co-ordination.

Support for the idea that turns are especially sensitive to cognitive loading comes from our recent analysis of data from 213 community-living, relatively healthy older adults (mean age: 76.6± 5.8 years). Subjects walked for 2 min at a self-selected pace, back and forth along a 25-m-long corridor, including 180° turns at each end with and without dual-tasking

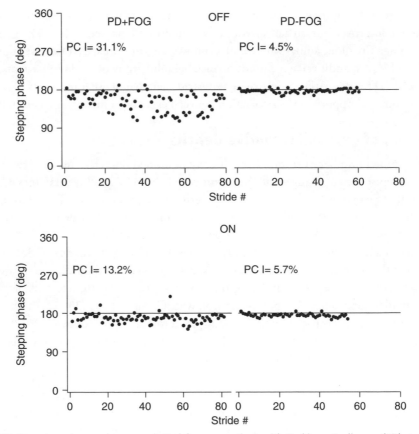

Fig. 8.5 Stepping phase values are plotted for one patient with Parkinson's disease (PD) + FOG and one patient from the PD – FOG group, both in the 'off' and 'on' states. A marked inability to consistently generate a 180° phase is observed in PD + FOG, but not in PD – FOG, during the 'off' state. The deviation in the phase, φ, from 180°, φ_ABS, was 29° for the PD + FOG and 3.8° for the PD – FOG patient. During the 'off' state, the PD + FOG was more inconsistent in phase generation (φ_CV = 15%) in comparison with the PD – FOG patient (φ_CV = 2.4%). In these examples, improvement is seen during the 'on' state for the PD + FOG patient, but not for the PD – FOG patient. Adapted from Plotnik *et al.* [18]. PCI, phase coordination index.

(i.e. serial 7 subtractions). During turns, but not during straight-line-walking, stride-to-stride time variability was significantly higher ($P < 0.008$) in the dual-tasking condition as compared to the baseline walking [85]. Apparently turns require more attention and cognitive resources than straight-line-walking. This may help to explain, in part, why turns are associated with FOG.

Three gait attributes (i.e. gait variability, gait asymmetry, and bilateral co-ordination of walking) are even more impaired in PD + FOG compared to PD − FOG patients [77,83,86]. Changes in gait variability, gait asymmetry, and the bilateral co-ordination of walking are associated with FOG. Taken together, these studies suggest that irregular central timing mechanisms of gait motor programs are associated with freezing. Since dual-tasking is known to have a large impact on these three aspects of gait in PD, one can speculate further that the dual-task effect will be even greater in PD patients with FOG whose executive function impairment is apparently even greater than that seen in PD patients who are not prone to FOG [80].

In one of the few studies on the effect of dual-tasking on gait in reference to susceptibility to FOG in PD, Camicioli *et al.* found that patients with FOG exhibited a greater increase in the number of steps to complete walking during dual-tasking [53]. The findings suggest that PD + FOG may be more dependent on attention and supports idea that the dual-task effects on gait are larger in PD + FOG compared with PD − FOG.

Recently, Dagan *et al.* investigated this issue in a study of 30 PD patients with motor response fluctuations during the 'on' state [87]. Twenty patients had a history of FOG and 10 were non-freezers. Patients walked 80 m at a comfortable pace and then repeated the walking task while performing serial 7 subtractions. Gait variability, gait asymmetry, and the phase co-ordination index tended to increase (i.e. become worse) in the PD + FOG during usual walking and became much worse during dual-tasking. The changes were accompanied by marked reduction in gait speed during dual-tasking. Multivariable regression showed that executive function and anxiety significantly contributed to this 'dual-task cost' in gait variability and gait speed. These findings further suggest that in advanced PD, poor emotional state and reduced executive function aggravate the effects of dual-tasking, especially in patients susceptible to FOG [87].

Some of the most intriguing evidence that links attention to FOG comes from the study by Devos *et al.* [76]. In addition to other changes in motor function and gait in response to the 3-month pilot study of the effects of methylphenidate (MPH) in patients with advanced PD, Devos *et al.* observed a reduction in the number of FOG episodes in response to MPH [76]. This reported reduction in FOG frequency could be explained in a number of different ways; one possibility is that MPH improved attentional abilities, and that this in turn led to a reduction in FOG, perhaps by enabling the patients to better allocate resources among competing tasks. Multiple pathways could account for this improvement; nevertheless, this finding further supports the association between executive function and this episodic gait disturbance in PD.

In patients with mild PD, recruitment of attentional resources may serve as a compensatory measure to improve gait [57,88]. This may be sufficient to help restore, to some degree, a functional gait pattern. In patients with advanced PD, however, both motor and cognitive function deteriorate further, potentially limiting the ability to utilize cognitive resources and attention to compensate for the impaired motor function. Gait may become even more 'fragile' and sensitive to external perturbations, increasing the demand for attentional resources. Perhaps this explains why cognitive challenges impact on gait (i.e. dual-tasking), especially during gait conditions known to be associated with FOG (i.e. turns) and how these conditions and the cognitive challenges combine to compound the likelihood that FOG will occur [78,86,89,90].

Conclusions

Patients with PD suffer from cognitive deficits, especially in executive function and attention. Gait disturbances, both continuous and episodic ones, are also common in PD. While many questions remain about the relationship between these symptoms, it appears that these are not distinct features. Rather, the characteristic cognitive changes apparently exacerbate the motor changes, in both the continuous and episodic gait disturbances. Recognition of this dependence may help to enhance the clinical treatment of gait disturbances that are common among patients with PD.

References

1 Morris ME, Iansek R, Matyas TA, Summers JJ. The pathogenesis of gait hypokinesia in Parkinson's disease. Brain 1994; 117(Pt 5): 1169–81.

2 Bloem BR, Hausdorff JM, Visser JE, Giladi N. Falls and freezing of gait in Parkinson's disease: a review of two interconnected, episodic phenomena. Mov Disord 2004; 19: 871–84.

3 Balash Y, Peretz C, Leibovich G, Herman T, Hausdorff JM, Giladi N. Falls in outpatients with Parkinson's disease: frequency, impact and identifying factors. J Neurol 2005; 252: 1310-5.

4 Pickering RM, Grimbergen YA, Rigney U, et al. A meta-analysis of six prospective studies of falling in Parkinson's disease. Mov Disord 2007; 22: 1892–900.

5 Ouchi Y, Kanno T, Okada H, et al. Changes in dopamine availability in the nigrostriatal and mesocortical dopaminergic systems by gait in Parkinson's disease. Brain 2001; 124(Pt 4): 784–92.

6 Yogev-Seligmann G, Hausdorff JM, Giladi N. The role of executive function and attention in gait. Mov Disord 2008; 23: 329–42.

7 Hausdorff JM, Doniger GM, Springer S, Yogev G, Giladi N, Simon ES. A common cognitive profile in elderly fallers and in patients with Parkinson's disease: the prominence of impaired executive function and attention. Exp Aging Res 2006; 32: 411–29.

8 Giladi N, Hausdorff JM, Balash Y. Episodic and continuous gait disturbances in Parkinson's disease. In: Galvez-Jimenez N editor. Scientific basis for the treatment of Parkinson's disease. 2 ed. London: Taylor & Francis, 2005; pp. 321–32.

9 Giladi N, Balash J. Paroxysmal locomotion gait disturbances in Parkinson's disease. Neurol Neurochir Pol 2001; 35(Suppl 3): 57–63.

10 Ebersbach G, Sojer M, Valldeoriola F, et al. Comparative analysis of gait in Parkinson's disease, cerebellar ataxia and subcortical arteriosclerotic encephalopathy. Brain 1999; 122(Pt 7): 1349–55.

11 Morris ME, Huxham FE, McGinley J, Iansek R. Gait disorders and gait rehabilitation in Parkinson's disease. Adv Neurol 2001; 87: 347–61.

12 Morris ME, Iansek R, Matyas TA, Summers JJ. Stride length regulation in Parkinson's disease. Normalization strategies and underlying mechanisms. Brain 1996; 119(Pt 2): 551–68.

13 Blin O, Ferrandez AM, Serratrice G. Quantitative analysis of gait in Parkinson patients: increased variability of stride length. J Neurol Sci 1990; 98: 91–7.

14 Hausdorff JM, Rios D, Edelberg HK. Gait variability and fall risk in community-living older adults: a 1-year prospective study. Arch Phys Med Rehabil 2001; 82: 1050–6.

15 Schaafsma JD, Giladi N, Balash Y, Bartels AL, Gurevich T, Hausdorff JM. Gait dynamics in Parkinson's disease: relationship to Parkinsonian features, falls and response to levodopa. J Neurol Sci 2003; 212: 47–53.

16 Yogev G, Giladi N, Peretz C, Springer S, Simon ES, Hausdorff JM. Dual tasking, gait rhythmicity, and Parkinson's disease: Which aspects of gait are attention demanding? Eur J Neurosci 2005; 22: 1248–56.

17 Morris ME, Iansek R, Matyas TA, Summers JJ. Ability to modulate walking cadence remains intact in Parkinson's disease. J Neurol Neurosurg Psychiatry 1994; 57: 1532–4.

18 Plotnik M, Giladi N, Hausdorff JM. A new measure for quantifying the bilateral coordination of human gait: effects of aging and Parkinson's disease. Exp Brain Res 2007; 181: 561–70.

19 Baltadjieva R, Giladi N, Gruendlinger L, Peretz C, Hausdorff JM. Marked alterations in the gait timing and rhythmicity of patients with de novo Parkinson's disease. Eur J Neurosci 2006; 24: 1815–20.

20 Frenkel-Toledo S, Giladi N, Peretz C, Herman T, Gruendlinger L, Hausdorff JM. Treadmill walking as an external pacemaker to improve gait rhythm and stability in Parkinson's disease. Mov Disord 2005; 20: 1109–14.

21 Hausdorff JM, Cudkowicz ME, Firtion R, Wei JY, Goldberger AL. Gait variability and basal ganglia disorders: stride-to-stride variations of gait cycle timing in Parkinson's disease and Huntington's disease. Mov Disord 1998; 13: 428–37.

22 Adkin AL, Frank JS, Jog MS. Fear of falling and postural control in Parkinson's disease. Mov Disord 2003; 18: 496–502.

23 Peretz C, Herman T, Hausdorff JM, Giladi N. Assessing fear of falling: can a short version of the Activities-specific Balance Confidence scale be useful? Mov Disord 2006; 21: 2101–5.

24 Bloem BR, Grimbergen YA, Cramer M, Willemsen M, Zwinderman AH. Prospective assessment of falls in Parkinson's disease. J Neurol 2001; 248: 950–8.

25 Schrag A, Jahanshahi M, Quinn NP. What contributes to depression in Parkinson's disease? Psychol Med 2001; 31: 65–73.

26 Chapuis S, Ouchchane L, Metz O, Gerbaud L, Durif F. Impact of the motor complications of Parkinson's disease on the quality of life. Mov Disord 2004; 20: 224–30.

27 Gray P, Hildebrand K. Fall risk factors in Parkinson's disease. J Neurosci Nurs 2000; 32: 222–8.

28 Fahn S. The freezing phenomenon in parkinsonism. Adv Neurol 1995; 67: 53–63.

29 Giladi N. Freezing of gait. Clinical overview. Adv Neurol 2001; 87: 191–7.

30 Giladi N, Hausdorff JM. The role of mental function in the pathogenesis of freezing of gait in Parkinson's disease. J Neurol Sci 2006; 248: 173–6.

31 Giladi N, McDermott MP, Fahn S, et al. Freezing of gait in PD: prospective assessment in the DATATOP cohort. Neurology 2001; 56: 1712–21.

32 Lamberti P, Armenise S, Castaldo V, et al. Freezing gait in Parkinson's disease. Eur Neurol 1997; 38: 297–301.

33 Lim I, van Wegen E, Jones D, et al. Identifying fallers with Parkinson's disease using home-based tests: who is at risk? Mov Disord 2008.

34 Ashburn A, Stack E, Pickering RM, Ward CD. A community-dwelling sample of people with Parkinson's disease: characteristics of fallers and non-fallers. Age Ageing 2001; 30: 47–52.

35 Koller WC, Glatt S, Vetere-Overfield B, Hassanein R. Falls and Parkinson's disease. Clin Neuropharmacol 1989; 12: 98–105.

36 Wood BH, Bilclough JA, Bowron A, Walker RW. Incidence and prediction of falls in Parkinson's disease: a prospective multidisciplinary study. J Neurol Neurosurg Psychiatry 2002; 72: 721–5.

37 Dubois B, Pillon B. Cognitive deficits in Parkinson's disease. J Neurol 1997; 244: 2–8.

38 Caballol N, Marti MJ, Tolosa E. Cognitive dysfunction and dementia in Parkinson disease. Mov Disord 2007; 22(Suppl 17): S358–S366.

39 Goethals I, Audenaert K, Van de WC, Dierckx R. The prefrontal cortex: insights from functional neuroimaging using cognitive activation tasks. Eur J Nucl Med Mol Imaging 2004; 31: 408–16.

40 Lezak MD. Executive function. New York: Oxford University Press, 1983.

41 Stuss DT, Bisschop SM, Alexander MP, Levine B, Katz D, Izukawa D. The Trail Making Test: a study in focal lesion patients. Psychol Assess 2001; 13: 230–9.

42 Nieoullon A. Dopamine and the regulation of cognition and attention. Prog Neurobiol 2002; 67: 53–83.

43 Stam CJ, Visser SL, Op de Coul AA, et al. Disturbed frontal regulation of attention in Parkinson's disease. Brain 1993; 116(Pt 5): 1139–58.

44 Hausdorff JM, Yogev G, Springer S, Simon ES, Giladi N. Walking is more like catching than tapping: gait in the elderly as a complex cognitive task. Exp Brain Res 2005; 164(4), 541–8.

45 Marquis S, Moore MM, Howieson DB, et al. Independent predictors of cognitive decline in healthy elderly persons. Arch Neurol 2002; 59: 601–6.

46 Verghese J, Lipton RB, Hall CB, Kuslansky G, Katz MJ, Buschke H. Abnormality of gait as a predictor of non-Alzheimer's dementia. N Engl J Med 2002; 347: 1761–8.

47 Alexander NB, Hausdorff JM. Linking thinking, walking, and falling. J Gerontol A Biol Sci Med Sci 2008; 63: 1325–8.

48 Hausdorff JM, Schweiger A, Herman T, Yogev-Seligmann G, Giladi N. Dual-task decrements in gait: contributing factors among healthy older adults. J Gerontol A Biol Sci Med Sci 2008; 63: 1335–43.

49 Della SS, Baddeley A, Papagno C, Spinnler H. Dual-task paradigm: a means to examine the central executive. Annal NY Acad Sci 2008; 769: 161–71.

50 Szameitat AJ, Schubert T, Muller K, Von Cramon DY. Localization of executive functions in dual-task performance with fMRI. J Cogn Neurosci 2002; 14: 1184–99.

51 Pashler H. Dual-task interference in simple tasks: data and theory. Psychol Bull 1994; 116: 220–44.

52 Brauer SG, Woollacott M, Shumway-Cook A. The influence of a concurrent cognitive task on the compensatory stepping response to a perturbation in balance-impaired and healthy elders. Gait Posture 2002; 15: 83–93.

53 Camicioli R, Howieson D, Lehman S, Kaye J. Talking while walking: the effect of a dual task in aging and Alzheimer's disease. Neurology 1997; 48: 955–8.

54 Woollacott M, Shumway-Cook A. Attention and the control of posture and gait: a review of an emerging area of research. Gait Posture 2002; 16: 1–14.

55 Springer S, Giladi N, Peretz C, Yogev G, Simon ES, Hausdorff JM. Dual-tasking effects on gait variability: the role of aging, falls, and executive function. Mov Disord 2006; 21: 950–7.

56 O'Shea S, Morris ME, Iansek R. Dual task interference during gait in people with Parkinson disease: effects of motor versus cognitive secondary tasks. Phys Ther 2002; 82: 888–97.

57 Rubenstein TC, Giladi N, Hausdorff JM. The power of cueing to circumvent dopamine deficits: a review of physical therapy treatment of gait disturbances in Parkinson's disease. Mov Disord 2002; 17: 1148–60.

58 Brown RG, Marsden CD. Dual task performance and processing resources in normal subjects and patients with Parkinson's disease. Brain 1991; 114(Pt 1A): 215–31.

59 Rowe J, Stephan KE, Friston K, Frackowiak R, Lees A, Passingham R. Attention to action in Parkinson's disease: impaired effective connectivity among frontal cortical regions. Brain 2002; 125(Pt 2): 276–89.

60 Uekermann J, Daum I, Bielawski M, *et al.* Differential executive control impairments in early Parkinson's disease. J Neural Transm Suppl 2004; 68: 39–51.

61 Bond JM, Morris M. Goal-directed secondary motor tasks: their effects on gait in subjects with Parkinson disease. Arch Phys Med Rehabil 2000; 81: 110–6.

62 Yogev G, Plotnik M, Peretz C, Giladi N, Hausdorff JM. Gait asymmetry in patients with Parkinson's disease and elderly fallers: when does the bilateral coordination of gait require attention? Exp Brain Res 2007; 177: 336–46.

63 Plotnik M, Giladi N, Hausdorff JM. Bilateral coordination of gait and Parkinson's disease: the effects of dual tasking. J Neurol Neurosurg Psychiatry 2009; 80: 347-50.

64 Hausdorff JM, Balash J, Giladi N. Effects of cognitive challenge on gait variability in patients with Parkinson's disease. J Geriatr Psychiatry Neurol 2003; 16: 53–8.

65 Verghese J, Buschke H, Viola L, *et al.* Validity of divided attention tasks in predicting falls in older individuals: a preliminary study. J Am Geriatr Soc 2002; 50: 1572–6.

66 Faulkner KA, Redfern MS, Cauley JA, *et al.* Multitasking: association between poorer performance and a history of recurrent falls. J Am Geriatr Soc 2007; 55: 570–6.

67 Zijlstra A, Ufkes T, Skelton DA, Lundin-Olsson L, Zijlstra W. Do dual tasks have an added value over single tasks for balance assessment in fall prevention programs? A mini-review. Gerontology 2008; 54: 40–9.

68 Allcock LM, Rowan EN, Steen IN, Wesnes K, Kenny RA, Burn DJ. Impaired attention predicts falling in Parkinson's disease. Parkinsonism Relat Disord 2008; 25: 110–5.

69 Vale S. Current management of the cognitive dysfunction in Parkinson's disease: how far have we come? Exp Biol Med (Maywood) 2008; 233: 941–51.

70 Galynker I, Ieronimo C, Miner C, Rosenblum J, Vilkas N, Rosenthal R. Methylphenidate treatment of negative symptoms in patients with dementia. J Neuropsychiatry Clin Neurosci 1997; 9: 231–9.

71 Homsi J, Walsh D, Nelson KA, LeGrand S, Davis M. Methylphenidate for depression in hospice practice: a case series. Am J Hosp Palliat Care 2000; 17: 393–8.

72 Whyte J, Hart T, Vaccaro M, *et al.* Effects of methylphenidate on attention deficits after traumatic brain injury: a multidimensional, randomized, controlled trial. Am J Phys Med Rehabil 2004; 83: 401–20.

73 Auriel E, Hausdorff JM, Giladi N. Methylphenidate for the treatment of Parkinson disease and other neurological disorders. Clin Neuropharmacol 2008; 32: 75–81.

74 Auriel E, Hausdorff JM, Herman T, Simon ES, Giladi N. Effects of methylphenidate on cognitive function and gait in patients with Parkinson's disease: a pilot study. Clin Neuropharmacol 2006; 29: 15–7.

75 Ben-Itzhak R, Giladi N, Gruendlinger L, Hausdorff JM. Can methylphenidate reduce fall risk in community-living older adults? A double-blind, single-dose cross-over study. J Am Geriatr Soc 2008; 56: 695–700.

76 Devos D, Krystkowiak P, Clement F, *et al.* Improvement of gait by chronic, high doses of methylphenidate in patients with advanced Parkinson's disease. J Neurol Neurosurg Psychiatry 2007; 78: 470–5.

77 Plotnik M, Giladi N, Balash Y, Peretz C, Hausdorff JM. Is freezing of gait in Parkinson's disease related to asymmetric motor function? Ann Neurol 2005; 57: 656–63.

78 Plotnik M, Hausdorff JM. The role of gait rhythmicity and bilateral coordination of stepping in the pathophysiology of freezing of gait in Parkinson's disease. Mov Disord 2008; 23(Suppl 2): S444–S450.

79 Lieberman A. Are freezing of gait (FOG) and panic related? J Neurol Sci 2006; 248: 219–22.

80 Amboni M, Cozzolino A, Longo K, Picillo M, Barone P. Freezing of gait and executive functions in patients with Parkinson's disease. Mov Disord 2008; 23: 395–400.

81 Willems AM, Nieuwboer A, Chavret F, *et al.* The use of rhythmic auditory cues to influence gait in patients with Parkinson's disease, the differential effect for freezers and non-freezers, an explorative study. Disabil Rehabil 2006; 28: 721–8.

82 Willems AM, Nieuwboer A, Chavret F, *et al.* Turning in Parkinson's disease patients and controls: the effect of auditory cues. Mov Disord 2007; 22: 1871–8.

83 Hausdorff JM, Schaafsma JD, Balash Y, Bartels AL, Gurevich T, Giladi N. Impaired regulation of stride variability in Parkinson's disease subjects with freezing of gait. Exp Brain Res 2003; 149: 187–94.

84 Schaafsma JD, Balash Y, Gurevich T, Bartels AL, Hausdorff JM, Giladi N. Characterization of freezing of gait subtypes and the response of each to levodopa in Parkinson's disease. Eur J Neurol 2003; 10: 391–8.

85 Weiss A, Gruendlinger L, Plotnik M, *et al.* Is turning during walking on automated motor task, or is it a complex cognitive action? Parkinsonism Relat Disord 2008; Suppl I: S41.

86 Plotnik M, Giladi N, Hausdorff JM. Bilateral coordination of walking and freezing of gait in Parkinson's disease. Eur J Neurosci 2008; 27: 1999–2006.

87 Dagan K, Plotnik M, Gruendlinger L, Giladi N, Hausdorff JM. Emotion, cognition, freezing of gait and dual tasking in patients with advanced Parkinson's disease: a volatile mixture. Parkinsonism Relat Disord 2008; 14: S6.

88 Rochester L, Hetherington V, Jones D, *et al.* The effect of external rhythmic cues (auditory and visual) on walking during a functional task in homes of people with Parkinson's disease. Arch Phys Med Rehabil 2005; 86: 999–1006.

89 Moreau C, Defebvre L, Bleuse S, *et al.* Externally provoked freezing of gait in open runways in advanced Parkinson's disease results from motor and mental collapse. J Neural Transm 2008; 115: 1431–6.

90 Plotnik M, Bartsch R, Yogev G, Hausdorff J, Havlin S, Giladi N. Synchronization of right–left stepping while walking is compromised in patients with Parkinson's disease during mental loading. Mov Disord 2006; 21: S592.

Chapter 9

Disorders of sleep and autonomic function in Parkinson's disease dementia

Eduardo Tolosa and Alex Iranzo

Introduction

Dementia is common in the advanced stages of Parkinson's disease (PD), when other non-motor symptoms (NMS) are also frequently present. Here, we review the available literature on the predictive value, prevalence and nature of sleep abnormalities, such as REM sleep behaviour disorder (RBD) and excessive daytime sleepiness (EDS), as well as symptoms of autonomic dysfunction in PD patients with cognitive impairment and dementia. The symptoms discussed here are frequently disabling and have a negative impact on the quality of life. Their treatment is beyond the scope of this chapter.

Sleep disturbances and cognition in PD

REM sleep behaviour disorder

REM sleep behaviour disorder (RBD) is characterized by dream-enacting behaviours (e.g. kicking, talking, swearing, shouting, jumping out of bed, etc.) linked to unpleasant dreams (e.g. being attacked, chased or robbed) and increased electromyographic activity during REM sleep. The pathophysiology of RBD is thought to be related to dysfunction of the brainstem REM sleep centres (e.g. locus subceruleus, nucleus gigantocellularis, etc.) and their indirect and direct anatomic connections (e.g. amygdala, pallidum, neocortex, etc.) [1]. These structures are frequently impaired in patients with PD and PD patients with dementia (PD-D) [2].

RBD may be idiopathic or linked to several neurodegenerative diseases, particularly PD, dementia with Lewy bodies (DLB) and multiple system atrophy. Patients with idiopathic RBD (IRBD) have no cognitive complaints and their neurological examination is unremarkable [1]. Long-term follow-up of patients with IRBD, however, frequently reveals the development of characteristic motor and cognitive features of PD, PD-D, mild cognitive impairment (MCI) and DLB [3–5]. This suggests that RBD may be an early manifestation of a neurodegenerative disease characterized by motor and cognitive impairment. In the text that follows we review the cognitive abnormalities that occur in patients with IRBD, RBD associated with MCI, and PD associated with RBD.

Cognitive performance in idiopathic RBD

Patients with IRBD report no cognitive problems. However, several studies using neuropsychological tests and quantitative cortical electroencephalogram (EEG) analysis found signs of asymptomatic cognitive dysfunction in IRBD. In a first study neuropsychological assessment of 17 consecutive IRBD patients disclosed visuospatial constructional dysfunction in 7 (44%) and altered visuospatial learning in 14 (82%) [6]. In another study involving 23 IRBD patients, neuropsychological assessment demonstrated poor visuoconstructional abilities (74%) and verbal memory (22%) [7]. Another report involving 14 IRBD patients showed executive dysfunction, as well as attentional and memory impairment on neuropsychological testing [8]. The cognitive profile found in patients with IRBD, namely impairment of visuospatial abilities, verbal memory, attention and executive function, is similar to what is seen in DLB, PD-D, and PD even in the early stages of the disease [2,9,10]. IRBD subjects had no abnormalities in semantic memory and language, two cognitive domains usually impaired in Alzheimer's disease [6–8].

Several studies using quantitative EEG analyses of waking and REM sleep found that IRBD patients had marked cortical EEG slowing (higher delta and theta power) in frontal, temporal and occipital regions [8,11,12]. This is in line with a study using brain SPECT that showed decreased blood flow in the frontal, temporal and parietal lobes in patients with IRBD [13]. Of note, a similar pattern of EEG slowing and reduced cortical perfusion has been described in subjects with PD and DLB [14–17].

Cognitive performance in RBD patients with MCI

MCI is a transitional stage between normal ageing and dementia, characterized by cognitive deficits that do not notably interfere with daily activities. Patients with MCI frequently convert to dementias such as Alzheimer's disease, DLB, and PD-D when parkinsonism preceded dementia [18].

There are no studies evaluating the prevalence and nature of RBD among patients diagnosed with MCI. In contrast, a few studies have reported the frequency and characteristics of MCI in patients initially diagnosed with IRBD. We first reported that MCI may develop in patients initially diagnosed with IRBD [4]. We showed that 20 of 44 (45%) IRBD patients diagnosed at our sleep centre developed a neurological disorder after a mean follow-up of 5 years. Emerging disorders were PD without dementia in seven patients, PD-D in two, DLB in six, multiple system atrophy in one and MCI in four. Neuropsychological assessment in three of these four MCI patients showed a pattern characterized by visuoperceptual dysfunction or memory impairment characterized by deficits in short-term free recall that benefited from external cues. The remaining MCI patient had impairment on both visuoperceptual abilities and memory. We hypothesized that these patients with MCI had an increased risk for developing DLB because: (1) the cognitive pattern was similar, albeit less severe, to that found in DLB and different from that seen in other dementias [9]; (2) MCI commonly converts to dementia [18]; and (3) RBD preceding dementia is suggestive of DLB [19]. In a second study from the same series we reported that after two additional years of follow-up, two of the four patients with MCI converted to DLB, seven with IRBD developed MCI, one with IRBD developed PD, and two IRBD patients previously diagnosed with PD developed MCI [20]. Overall, 28 of 44 (64%) of the IRBD patients from our centre developed a neurological disorder after a mean clinical follow-up of 7 years; PD without dementia in 10, PD-D in four, DLB in eight, multiple system atrophy in one, and MCI in nine [20].

In our sleep centre we further identified 15 patients with IRBD who later developed MCI at a mean age of 72 years. Eleven patients (73.3%) presented visuoperceptual dysfunction. In five of them this was the only cognitive domain affected. In the other six patients other domains were impaired: two patients failed in memory, one in executive functions, one in both memory and language, one in praxis, and one in both executive functions and praxis. In the remaining four patients, neuropsychological profile was the following: one had executive dysfunction, one had memory impairment, one had memory, executive and language deficits, and one had both executive and memory impairment. Memory deficit was again characterized by impaired short-term free recall that benefited from semantic clues. We concluded that in most IRBD patients who develop MCI, visuoperceptive function is altered but other cognitive domains may also be impaired, particularly memory and executive functions [21]. This cognitive profile of MCI in patients initially diagnosed with IRBD is similar to what is seen in PD with or without MCI [10,22], PD-D [2], MCI preceding DLB [23], DLB [9], and different from Alzheimer's disease.

A recent study evaluated the frequency and subtypes of MCI in 32 patients with IRBD, 22 PD patients with RBD, 18 PD patients without RBD and 40 healthy controls [24]. MCI was diagnosed in 50% of the IRBD patients, 73% of the PD patients with RBD, and only in 11% of the PD patients without RBD and in 8% of the controls. The main MCI subtype in IRBD was single domain non-amnestic MCI with impaired executive functions and attention and relatively preserved visuoconstructional and visuoperceptual functions. The two main MCI subtypes identified in PD patients with RBD were single domain non-amnestic MCI and multiple domain amnestic MCI, both characterized by predominant impairment of executive functions and attention. The authors concluded that, in both association with PD and its idiopathic form, RBD is an important risk factor for MCI and, subsequently, for the later conversion to dementia.

In addition, we have found that on quantitative EEG spectrum analysis, cortical EEG slowing is more marked in those IRBD patients who later develop MCI than in those in whom RBD remains idiopathic (unpublished data). Overall, studies assessing cognitive performance and cortical EEG activity in MCI patients with IRBD [4,21,24] showed similar results to that observed in IRBD [6–8,11,12], PD without cognitive complaints [10], PD with MCI [14, 22], PD-D [2] and DLB [9,17,23]. This indicates that patients with IRBD, and particularly those who develop MCI, are at high risk for developing dementia linked to PD and DLB. It has been hypothesized that cortical EEG slowing and cognitive deficits occurring in patients initially diagnosed with IRBD may be caused either by cortical pathology or damage of the brainstem structures that regulate REM sleep and activate the neocortex, thereby leading to cortical dysfunction [8,24]. The latter hypothesis, however, does not explain the fact that in MSA cognitive function is usually intact and RBD is universal [25,26].

Cognitive performance in PD patients with RBD

RBD occurs in 46–58% of the PD patients, antedating the onset of motor symptoms by several years in 20–40% of the subjects [26–29]. In PD, RBD may precede, coincide or follow the onset of parkinsonism [1,26]. In patients with PD-D and RBD, dementia may follow or antedate the onset of RBD [4,30]. It is thus unclear whether RBD is linked to PD-D. The majority of articles that evaluated RBD in PD excluded patients with dementia [26–29]. There have been no longitudinal studies assessing whether RBD is a risk factor for PD-D. Published studies have provided contradictory or not compelling data regarding a possible association between RBD and PD-D. It should be noted that in other neurodegenerative diseases characterized by dementia the presence of RBD is not uniform. RBD is rare in Alzheimer's disease [31] but very common in DLB [1]. One study showed that 34 of 37 patients with RBD and degenerative dementia met clinical criteria for DLB [19]. Three of these patients underwent autopsy where Lewy pathology was found in the cortex and limbic regions [19]. Conversely, RBD is almost universal in multiple system atrophy, a disease usually not associated with cognitive impairment [25,26]. Here we briefly review the small amount of available data regarding a possible pathophysiological link between RBD and dementia in the setting of PD.

1   RBD occurs in PD patients with associated MCI and dementia [4,24]. However, RBD also occurs in PD patients without cognitive deficits [4,26–29] and some PD-D patients do not have RBD (our personal observation). RBD occurs in PD secondary to Parkin mutations, a condition which has not been reported to be associated with dementia [32].

2   Some risk factors associated with dementia in PD such as the akinetic–rigid motor subtype [33], hallucinations [34], longer PD duration [27,28], EEG slowing [35], and male gender [1,26] have been associated with RBD in PD. In contrast, other risk factors for PD-D such as advanced age [27,28,36] and depression [37] have not been related to RBD in PD.

3   A study in 65 consecutive PD patients showed that the presence of RBD-like symptoms was significantly higher in PD-D (10/13, 77%) than in PD without dementia (14/52, 27%) [38]. In all 10 PD-D cases with symptoms suggestive of RBD, this parasomnia developed after onset of parkinsonism. In PD-D subjects, the interval between onset of motor symptoms and onset of cognitive symptoms was shortened in the presence of RBD, where 10 of the 24 RBD-like patients developed dementia with a median of 8.5 years and only 3 of the 41 non-RBD-like patients developed dementia with a median of 12 years. The authors of this study suggested that PD patients with RBD have a higher risk for developing dementia, which occurs earlier in the course of their disease [38]. However, another study found that the presence of dementia was numerically higher, but not statistically different in PD patients with symptoms suggestive of RBD (22/81, 27%) compared to those without symptoms suggestive of RBD (9/69, 13%) [39].

It has been suggested that RBD may be a marker for the development of dementia in PD because non-demented PD patients with RBD are more likely to exhibit EEG slowing

[35] and poorer performance in executive function, verbal memory and visuospatial abilities in neuropsychological tests [34,40]. However, it has been argued that these findings may simply reflect a more widespread neurodegenerative disease affecting the brainstem and the cortex rather than a pathophysiological explanation of a link between RBD and cognitive dysfunction [41].

In summary, available data are not conclusive and too small to assess whether RBD is linked to dementia in PD. Long-term follow-up of non-demented PD patients with and without RBD is necessary to elucidate whether this sleep disorder is associated with a high risk for dementia.

Excessive daytime sleepiness

Excessive daytime sleepiness (EDS) is common in PD with potentially serious consequences; it may lead to social problems, automobile accidents, and it exerts a negative impact on quality of life [42]. EDS in PD may be the initial manifestation of the disease [43] and its frequency increases as the disease progresses [44,45]. Since disease duration is associated with development of dementia in PD [46–50] it can be speculated that EDS is a common manifestation in PD-D. However, there are only a few reports that have specifically evaluated the frequency and nature of EDS in PD-D. One of these showed that the frequency of EDS in PD-D (57%) was greater than in PD without dementia (41%) and in DLB (50%) [51].

Clinical presentation and origin of excessive daytime sleepiness in PD

There are two possible clinical presentations of EDS in the setting of PD. One is a state of continuous and persistent EDS which is recognized by the patient, allowing him/her to fight against it, but eventually leading to unavoidable napping. The other is the occurrence of sudden onset of sleep (SOS) episodes ('sleep attacks') similar to those classically described in narcolepsy [1]. SOS episodes have been reported to occur at any age or stage of the disease. The most common variables associated with SOS are treatment with any dopaminergic agent, higher scores on the Epworth scale of sleepiness and three factors associated with dementia in PD; namely duration of parkinsonism, advanced age and male sex [47,48]. There is a subgroup of sleepy PD subjects with a narcolepsy-like phenotype where somnolence is due to REM sleep intrusions during daytime [49,50]. When compared with PD patients with non-narcoleptic features, those in the narcoleptic-like group have longer disease duration and more frequently experience daytime hallucinations [49,50], again two risk factors for dementia in PD.

The mechanism of EDS in PD involves multiple factors, the effects of dopaminergic medication and the disease pathology itself being the most relevant [1]. Predisposing factors for developing sleepiness in PD include dementia, disease severity, disease duration, hallucinations, circadian sleep–wake cycle disruption, nocturnal sleep quantity and quality, obstructive sleep apnoea, depression and genetic susceptibility [1]. The individual contribution of each of these factors, including dementia, has not yet been fully elucidated.

Excessive daytime sleepiness and dementia in PD

It is thought that development of EDS in PD is related to progressive cell loss in the dopaminergic and non-dopaminergic brain structures and networks that modulate the sleep–wake cycle. This is in line with the observed association between EDS and advanced stage of parkinsonism [52–54] and longer duration of the disease [52–54] suggesting that more severe and widespread brain damage leads to the development or worsening of EDS. Longitudinal studies showed that the prevalence of EDS in PD increases over time in parallel with cognitive decline and disease progression [44,45]. A longitudinal study showed that PD patients develop EDS at a rate of 6% per year and that this development is associated with dementia and more advanced parkinsonism [44]. A study using the Epworth sleepiness scale as a subjective measure of EDS showed that the frequency of PD-D patients reporting EDS increased from 57% to 81% after 2 years of follow-up [51]. The findings of two other studies showed that EDS in PD is linked to dementia, advanced stage of disease and hallucinations, suggesting an association between EDS with a more severe and diffuse brain pathology [45,53]. Of note, when compared with PD patients without EDS, those with EDS had cortical hypoperfusion and worse cognitive function, especially in the attentional domain [55].

Patients with idiopathic narcolepsy exhibit severe EDS and undetectable or reduced lumbar cerebrospinal fluid (CSF) levels of hypocretin secondary to almost complete loss of hypothalamic hypocretin-producing cells. Given that a narcolepsy-like phenotype is seen in some PD subjects with EDS [49,50,56] it is tempting to speculate that damage of the hypothalamic hypocretin-producing cells contributes to the occurrence of EDS in PD. Lumbar CSF levels of hypocretin, however, are normal in PD with and without dementia [57]. Two retrospective studies in postmortem PD brains have shown a moderate hypocretin cell loss (23–62%) in the hypothalamus [58,59]. In one of these studies loss of hypocretin neurons was correlated with the clinical stage of the disease, as measured by the Hoehn and Yahr scale, but not with disease duration [57]. Similarly, there was a loss of hypothalamic melanin-concentrating hormone cells (12–74%), which are also involved in the regulation of the sleep–wake cycle and are intact in idiopathic narcolepsy. Unfortunately, the occurrence before death of sleep symptoms such as EDS, dementia and cognitive complaints were not assessed in these two studies [57,58]. It is unclear to what extent the loss of hypocretin cells contributes to development of EDS in PD and if it is related or not to the occurrence of dementia or to other clinical variables. In an animal model of narcolepsy, loss of more than 70% of hypocretin cells results in a 50% decline in the CSF concentration and an increase in REM sleep [60]. It can be argued that in PD the hypocretin cell loss is simply a non-specific finding reflecting widespread neurodegeneration in advanced stages of the disease rather than the explanation for the occurrence of EDS.

Autonomic dysfunction in PD-D

Autonomic disturbances are common in PD, causing significant discomfort to patients and negatively affecting their quality of life [61]. Most common autonomic symptoms

(AS) are cardiovascular, gastrointestinal, genitourinary and thermoregulatory disturbances. It is well known that such disturbances can occur in the early stages of PD, presenting at the time of diagnosis or even antedating the onset of motor symptoms. Such is the case, for example, for constipation, bladder and erectile dysfunction, and for some cardiovascular abnormalities. Early and premotor autonomic dysfunction has been reviewed elsewere [62].

The prevalence of AS increases with disease progression [63–65]. James Parkinson already indicated the progressive worsening of constipation in advanced PD. Ano-rectal function was recently found to be more impaired in patients with longer disease duration and higher Hoehn and Yahr stages [66]; there is also a correlation between increasing severity of the disease and increasing bladder problems [67]. In another study, orthostatic hypotension was found to be related to the duration and severity of the disease and to the use of higher daily levodopa and bromocriptine doses [68]. In a recent study by Verbaan *et al.* [69], older, more severely affected, and more heavily medicated subjects had more autonomic involvement.

Autonomic symptoms

Dementia occurs generally in the advanced stages of PD. Although it has been considered to be an inevitable development, some patients die without severe cognitive deterioration despite longstanding disease and severe parkinsonism. Demented PD patients generally suffer from advanced parkinsonism with severe motor disability related to bradykinesia, freezing, poor balance and falls. Since autonomic symptoms are frequent in advanced PD and dementia develops also in these late stages, one can logically expect autonomic symptoms to be prominent in patients with PD-D. This conjecture, however, has not been systematically and comprehensively evaluated, and data on the relative frequency of autonomic symptoms in demented as compared to non-demented PD patients is scarce.

Assessing autonomic function in patients with severe parkinsonism and dementia has limitations. Because of severe motor impairment and the cognitive disturbance, collaboration of the patient cannot be obtained for some tests or in answering questionnaires, most of which have been validated in patients without dementia. In fact, in many studies on autonomic function in PD, patients with dementia have been specifically excluded.

A few studies have specifically assessed autonomic symptoms in PD patients with cognitive impairment. In the study by Idiaquez *et al.* [70], 40 PD patients and 30 age-matched controls were assessed for cognitive and behavioural manifestations using standardized neuropsychological tools. The subjects were also assessed for orthostatic hypotension (OH), postprandial hypotension, heart rate responses to deep breathing and autonomic symptoms using the Scale for Outcomes in Parkinson's disease for Autonomic symptoms (SCOPA-AUT). Eleven of the 40 PD patients fulfilled DSM-IV criteria for dementia. The authors found a higher incidence of cardiovascular symptoms in PD patients with dementia than those without. The presence of OH or postprandial hypotension did not correlate with the severity of cognitive impairment, and there was no correlation between gastrointestinal or urologicalsymptoms and cognitive impairment. According to the authors the lack of correlation between AS with cognitive impairment suggests that cognitive and autonomic involvement progress independently from each other and variably among PD patients.

A recent clinical study by Peralta *et al.* [71] provided some evidence that, when tested in an autonomic function laboratory, OH is more frequent in PD patients with dementia as compared to those without, but the difference failed to reach statistical significance. Drop in systolic blood pressure was significantly greater in the PD-D than in the PD group. In this study, attention, assessed with the 'Test of Everyday Attention', deteriorated significantly during tilt in the PD-D group, correlating with blood pressure response and suggesting that OH may exacerbate attentional dysfunction in PD-D. Allen *et al.* [72] assessed cardiovascular autonomic function in 39 patients with Alzheimer disease (AD), 30 with vascular dementia, 30 with dementia with Lewy bodies (DLB), 40 with PD-D and 38 elderly controls by Ewing's battery of autonomic function tests and power spectral analysis of heart rate variability. Autonomic dysfunction occurred in all common dementias, but was especially prominent in PD-D and DLB. PD-D patients showed consistent impairment of both parasympathetic and sympathetic function tests in comparison with controls and AD. Patients with advanced PD but without dementia were not studied. Graham and Sagar [73] also reported a higher frequency of symptomatic orthostasis, presumably a treatment complication, in association with cognitive impairment in PD.

The presence of autonomic dysfunction in advanced PD has been documented in the Sidney Multicenter Study of PD [74]. In this study a cohort of newly diagnosed patients have been followed longitudinally. At 15-year follow-up symptomatic postural hypotension occurred in 35%, and there were 22 people (41%) who had urinary incontinence. This condition became more frequent with increasing Hoehn and Yahr stage, from 14% at Stage 2 to 62% at Stage 5 patients. At 20-year follow-up [75] dementia was present 83% of the survivors. Autonomic symptoms were also common: symptomatic postural hypotension in 48% (6 required fludrocortisone), urinary incontinence in 71%. Fecal incontinence occurred in 5 (17%), and constipation requiring daily laxatives was present in 12 (40%). These findings illustrate how common and clinically important these NMS are in patients with advanced PD. However, it was not specified whether autonomic symptoms were more common or severe in patients with dementia.

Pathophysiology of autonomic symptoms

Clinicopathological studies have revealed that in PD typical synuclein pathology can be seen throughout the central and peripheral autonomic nervous system: hypothalamus, brainstem, pre- and post-ganglionic neurons and plexi, suggesting that autonomic dysfunction is integral to disease pathology and may underlie autonomic symptoms. Both pre- and post-ganglionic neurons and plexi as well as central autonomic structures are thought to become involved early in the disease process [76]. This explains why autonomic symptoms are common in PD with or without dementia, the later associated with synuclein pathology extending rostrally beyond the brainstem. The neuropathological substrate of dementia in PD can be heterogeneous [77–80]. Extension of synuclein pathology to the limbic and cerebral cortices is the characteristic finding in many instances of PD-D; these cortical lesions may contribute to the worsening of autonomic symptoms since several of these areas such as the amygdala, anterior cingulate, insular and ventromedial prefrontal cortices, among others, control the tonic, reflex and adaptive activities of the sympathetic and parasympathetic nervous systems. Degeneration of neurons in the frontal cortex, for example, may disinhibit the pontine bladder control centre and could play an important role in incontinence in PD-D [81].

In trying to define the neural substrate of autonomic dysfunction in PD, it becomes difficult to disentangle the role of central vs peripheral lesions. Constipation, for example, could be considered to be a consequence of lesions in the enteric neurons, but involvement of central structures such as the medullary raphe which projects to spinal nuclei such as Onuf's nucleus may be an important contributing factor [82]. Urinary dysfunction can be ascribed to the involvement of abdomino-pelvic plexuses by the neurodegenerative process. On the other hand degeneration in the nigro-striatal dopamine system that causes disinhibition of the micturition reflex may result in detrusor overactivity and may explain worsening of detrusor function with increasing Hoehn and Yahr stages [83,84]. Studies in PD have also revealed significant loss of neurons in the intermediolateral cell column which inhibits detrusor muscle function [85].

Comorbidities must also be considered in the pathophysiology. The presence of symptoms such as urinary incontinence or constipation may not always reflect direct involvement of the autonomic nervous system by PD related pathology, but may result, at least in part, from other conditions such as physical inactivity, or from defecatory dysfunction due to motor impairment; for example constipation may in part be due to severe immobility and to anal sphincter dystonia [86]. Other factors that can cause or contribute to dysautonomia in PD-D are advanced age, comorbid conditions (e.g. prostatic hypertrophy, cerebrovascular pathology), or use of numerous medications known to cause autonomic dysfunction. Dopaminergic drugs, for example, frequently cause OH, profuse sweating spells occur in association with levodopa-related on-off fluctuations, and anticholinergic drugs can cause constipation and bladder dysfunction. Cholinesterase inhibitors and atypical antipsychotics can also induce autonomic symptoms. Finally, symptoms such as urinary and fecal incontinence or sexual dysfunction may be due in part to behavioural symptoms such as hallucinations or excessive daytime sleepiness, which are frequently associated with PD-D.

Conclusions

RBD may be a feature of neurological conditions where cognitive impairment is common such as MCI, PD and DLB. Patients with the idiopathic form of RBD have no cognitive complaints, but neuropsychological tests and quantitative EEG analysis show subtle asymptomatic cognitive deficits and cortical EEG slowing. The cognitive profile in patients with IRBD and IRBD with MCI is characterized by impairment in visuol-perceptual and executive functions, two features seen in PD, PD-D and DLB. It is not clearly established if RBD represents a risk factor for dementia in PD, and if RBD is more common in

PD-D than in PD without cognitive impairment. Likewise there is little evidence regarding a possible link between EDS and dementia in PD. Longitudinal studies have shown that the prevalence of EDS in PD increases over time in parallel with cognitive decline and disease progression. The origin of EDS in PD is multifactorial. One of the main contributing factors is the disease pathology itself, damaging the nuclei and networks involved in the regulation of the sleep-wake cycle. It is unclear if the hypocretinergic cell loss found in PD contributes to the development of EDS or represents a non-specific finding reflecting widespread cell loss, particularly in advanced stages of the disease.

Studies on autonomic dysfunction in PD-D are scarce. The available information indicates that urinary incontinence, constipation, fecal incontinence and postural hypotension are common in patients with PD-D. This is to be expected since autonomic symptoms are more prevalent and severe in advanced disease and dementia usually occurs in the late stages of PD. Whether they are more common in demented vs non demented patients in advanced stages remains, however, unclear. Information on other autonomic symptoms such as thermal dysregulation or sexual dysfunction is hardly available for patients with PD-D. The cause of autonomic dysfunction is probably multifactorial and may be difficult to uncover in a given patient. The involvement of peripheral and central autonomic systems plays a central role, but behavioural and motor problems, severe immobility, advanced age and adverse effects of drugs can all contribute to the presence and severity of AS. In PD-D higher autonomic symptom scores are associated with poorer outcomes in all measures of physical activity, activities of daily living, affect and quality of life [87]. Symptoms of autonomic dsyfunction have important treatment implications and need to be addressed in all patients with advanced PD in order to minimize their consequences for the patient and the carer [88].

References

1 Iranzo A, Santamaria J, Tolosa E. The clinical and pathophysiological relevance of REM sleep behavior disorder in neurodegenerative diseases. Sleep Med Rev (in press).

2 Emre M. Dementia associated with Parkinson's disease. Lancet Neurology 2003; 2: 229–37.

3 Schenck CH, Bundlie SR, Mahowald MW. Delayed emergence of a parkinsonian disorder in 38% of 29 older men initially diagnosed with idiopathic rapid eye movement sleep behavior disorder. Neurology 1996; 46: 388–93.

4 Iranzo A, Molinuevo JL, Santamaria J, et al. Rapid-eye-movement sleep behaviour disorder as an early marker for a neurodegenerative disease: a descriptive study. Lancet Neurol 2006; 5: 572–7.

5 Postuma RB, Gagnon JF, Vendette M, Fantini ML, Massicotte-Marquez J, Montplaisir J. Quantifying the risk of neurodegenerative disease in REM sleep behavior disorder. Neurology 2009; 72: 1296–300.

6 Ferini-Strambi L, Di Gioia MR, Castronovo V, et al. Neuropsychological assessment in idiopathic REM sleep behavior disorder. Neurology 2004; 62: 41–5.

7 Terzaghi M, Sinforiani E, Zucchella C, et al. Cognitive performance in REM sleep behaviour disorder: a possible early marker of neurodegenerative disease?. Sleep Med 2008; 9: 343–51.

8 Massicotte-Marquez J, Décary A, Gagnon JF, et al. Executive dysfunction and memory impairment in idiopathic. REM sleep behavior disorder 2008; 70: 1250–7.

9 McKeith I, Mintzer J, Aarsland D, et al. Dementia with Lewy bodies. Lancet Neurol 2004; 3: 19–28.

10 Aarsland D, Bronnick K, Larsen JP, *et al.* Cognitive impairment in incident, untreated Parkinson disease. The Norwegian Park West Study. Neurology 2009; 72: 1121–6.

11 Fantini ML, Gagnon JF, Petit D, *et al.* Slowing of electroencephalogram in rapid eye movement sleep behavior disorder. Ann Neurol 2003; 53: 774–80.

12 Massicotte-Marquez J, Carrier J, Décary A, *et al.* Slow-wave sleep and delta power in rapid eye movement sleep behavior disorder. Ann Neurol 2005; 57: 277–82.

13 Mazza S, Soucy JP, Gravel P, *et al.* Assessing whole brain perfusion changes in patients with REM sleep behavior disorder. Neurology 2006; 67: 1618–22.

14 Caviness JN, Hentz JG, Evidente VG, *et al.* Both early and late cognitive dysfunction affects the electroencephalogram in Parkinson's disease. Parkinsonism Relat Disord 2007; 13: 348–54.

15 Kai T, Asai Y, Sakuma K, Koeda T, Nakashima K. Quantitative electroencephalogram analysis in dementia with Lewy bodies and Alzheimer's disease. J Neurol Sci 2005; 237: 89–95.

16 Huang C, Mattis P, Perrine K, *et al.* Metabolic abnormalities associated with mild cognitive impairment in Parkinson disease. Neurology 2008; 70: 1470–7.

17 Inui Y, Toyama H, Manabe Y, *et al.* Evaluation of probable or possible dementia with Lewy bodies using 123I-IMP brain perfusion SPECT, 123I-MIBG, and 99mTc-MIBI myocardial SPECT. J Nucl Med 2007; 48: 1641–50.

18 Gauthier S, Reisberg B, Zaudig M, *et al.* Mild cognitive impairment. Lancet 2006; 367: 1262–70.

19 Boeve BF, Silber MH, Ferman TJ, *et al.* REM sleep behavior disorder and degenerative dementia. An association likely reflecting Lewy body disease. Neurology 1998; 51: 363–70.

20 Iranzo A, Molinuevo JL, Santamaria J, *et al.* Sixty-four percent of patients with idiopathic REM sleep behavior disorder developed a neurological disorder after a mean clinical follow-up of seven years. Sleep 2008; 31(Suppl): A280.

21 Iranzo A, Serradell M, Molinuevo J, Santamaria J. Neuropsychological profile of mild cognitive impairment in patients with REM sleep behavior disorder. J Sleep Res 2008; 17(Suppl 1): 103.

22 Caviness, Driver-Dunckley E, Connor DJ, *et al.* Defining mild cognitive impairment in Parkinson's disease. Mov Disord 2007; 22: 1272–7.

23 Boeve BF, Ferman TJ, Smith GE, *et al.* Mild cognitive impairment preceding dementia with Lewy bodies. Neurology 2004; 62(Suppl 5): A86.

24 Gagnon JF, Vendette M, Postuma RB, *et al.* Mild cognitive impairment in rapid eye movement disorder and Parkinson. Ann Neurol; doi: 10.1002/ana.21680.

25 Plazzi G, Corsini R, Provini F, *et al.* REM sleep behavior disorders in multiple system atrophy. Neurology 1997; 48: 1094–7.

26 Iranzo A, Rye DB, Santamaria J, *et al.* Characteristics of idiopathic REM sleep behavior disorder and that associated with MSA and PD. Neurology 2005; 65: 247–52.

27 De Cock VC, Vidailhet M, Leu S, *et al.* Restoration of normal muscle control in Parkinson's disease during REM sleep. Brain 2007; 130: 450–6.

28 Wetter TC, Trenkwalder C, Gershanik O, Högl B. Polysomnographic measures in Parkinson's disease: a comparison between patients with and without REM sleep disturbances. Wien Klin Wochenschr 2001; 113: 249–53.

29 Gagnon JF, Bédard MA, Fantini ML, *et al.* REM sleep behavior disorder and REM sleep without atonia in Parkinson's disease. Neurology 2002; 59: 585–9.

30 Olson EJ, Boeve BF, Silber MH. Rapid eye movement sleep behavior disorder: demographic, clinical and laboratory findings in 93 cases. Brain 2000; 123: 331–9.

31 Gagnon F, Petit F, Fantini ML, *et al.* REM sleep behavior and REM sleep without atonia in probable Alzheimer disease. Sleep 2006; 29: 1321–5.

32 Kumru H, Santamaria J, Tolosa E, *et al.* Rapid eye movement disorder in parkinsonism with PARKIN mutations. Ann Neurol 2004; 56: 599–603.

33 Kumru H, Santamaria J, Tolosa E, Iranzo A. Relation between subtype of Parkinson's disease and REM sleep behavior disorder. Sleep Med 2007; 8: 779–83.

34 Sinforiani E, Zangaglia R, Manni R, *et al*. REM sleep behavior disorder, hallucinations, and cognitive impairment in Parkinson's disease. Mov Disord 2006; 21: 462–6.

35 Gagnon JF, Fantini ML, Bédard MA, *et al*. Association between waking EEG slowing and REM sleep behavior in PD without dementia. Neurology 2004; 62: 401–6.

36 Postuma RB, Gagnon JF, Vendette M, Charland K, Montplaisir J. REM sleep behavior disorder in Parkinson's disease is associated with specific motor features. J Neurol Neurosurg Psychiatry 2008; 79: 1117–21.

37 Postuma RB, Gagnon JF, Vendette M, Charland K, Montplaisir J. Manifestations of Parkinson disease differ in association with REM sleep behavior disorder. Mov Disord 2008; 15: 1665–72.

38 Marion MH, Quarashi M, Marshall G, Foster O. Is REM sleep behaviour disorder (RBD) a risk factor of dementia in idiopathic Parkinson's disease?. J Neurol 2008; 255: 192–6.

39 Yoritaka A, Ohizumi H, Tanaka S, Hattori N. Parkinson's disease with and without REM sleep behaviour disorder: are there any clinical differences?. Eur Neurol 2009; 61: 164–70.

40 Vendette M, Gagnon JF, Décary A, *et al*. REM sleep behavior disorder predicts cognitive impairment in Parkinson disease without dementia. Neurology 2007; 69: 1843–9.

41 Benninger D, Waldvogel D, Bassetti CL. REM sleep behavior disorder predicts cognitive impairment in Parkinson disease without dementia. Neurology 2008; 71: 955–6.

42 Rye D, Iranzo A. The nocturnal manifestations of waking movement disorders: focus on Parkinson's disease. In: Guilleminault C (ed.). Handbook of clinical neurophysiology, vol. 6. Sleep and its disorders. Philadelphia: Elsevier, 2005; pp. 263–72.

43 Abbott RD, Ross GW, White LR, *et al*. Excessive daytime sleepiness and subsequent development of Parkinson disease. Neurology 2005; 65: 1442–6.

44 Gjerstad MD, Aarsland D, Larsen JP. Development of daytime somnolence over time in Parkinson's disease. Neurology 2002; 58: 1544–6.

45 Fabbrini G, Barbanti P, Aurilia C, Pauletti C, Vanacore N, Meco G. Excessive daytime somnolence in Parkinson's disease. Follow-up after 1 year of treatment. Neurol Sci 2003; 24: 178–9.

46 Tan EK, Lum SY, Fook-Chong SMC, *et al*. Evaluation of somnolence in Parkinson's disease: comparison with age- and sex-matched controls. Neurology 2002; 58: 465–8.

47 Paus S, Brecht HM, Köster J, Seeger G, Klockgether T, Wüllner U. Sleep attacks, daytime sleepiness, and dopamine agonists in Parkinson's disease. Mov Disord 2003; 18: 659–67.

48 Körner Y, Meindorfner C, Möller JC, *et al*. Predictors of sudden onset of sleep in Parkinson's disease. Mov Disord 2004; 19: 1298–1305.

49 Rye DB, Bliwise DL, Dihenia B, Gurecki P. Daytime sleepiness in Parkinson's disease. J Sleep Res 2000; 9: 63–9.

50 Arnulf I, Konofal E, Merino-Andreu M, *et al*. Parkinson's disease and sleepiness. An integral part of PD. Neurology 2002; 58: 1019–24.

51 Boddy F, Rowan EN, Lett D, O'Brien JT, McKeith IG, Burn DJ. Subjectively reported sleep quality and excessive daytime somnolence in Parkinson's disease with and without dementia, dementia with Lewy bodies and Alzheimer's disease. Int J Geriatr Psychiatry 2007; 22: 529–35.

52 Tandberg E, Larsen JP, Karlsen K. Excessive daytime sleepiness and sleep benefit in Parkinson's disease: a community-based study. Mov Disord 1999; 14: 922–7.

53 Hobson DE, Lang AE, Martin WWR, Razmy A, Rivest J, Fleming J. Excessive daytime sleepiness and sudden-onset sleep in Parkinson disease. A survey by the Canadian movement disorder group. J Am Med Assoc 2002; 287: 455–63.

54 Kumar S, Bhatia M, Behari M. Sleep disorders in Parkinson's disease. Mov Disord 2002; 17: 775–81.

55 Matsui H, Nishinaka K, Oda M, *et al.* Excessive daytime sleepiness in Parkinson disease: a SPECT study. Sleep 2006; 29: 917–20.

56 Arnulf I, Bonnet AM, Damier P, *et al.* Hallucinations, REM sleep, and Parkinson's disease. A medical hypothesis. Neurology 2000; 55: 281–8.

57 Santamaria J, Compta Y, Marti M, *et al.* CSF hypocretin in Parkinson's disease with and without dementia. J Sleep Res 2008; 17(Suppl 1): 177.

58 Thannickal TC, Lai YY, Siegel JM. Hypocretin (orexin) cell loss in Parkinson's disease. Brain 2007; 130: 1586–95.

59 Fronczeck R, Overeem S, Lee SY, *et al.* Hypocretin (orexin) loss in Parkinson's disease. Brain 2007; 130: 1577–85.

60 Geraschencko D, Murillo-Rodriguez E, Lin L, *et al.* Relationship between CSF hypocretin levels and hypocretin neuronal loss. Exp Neurol 2003; 184: 1010–16.

61 Chaudhuri KR, Healy D, Schapira AHV. The non motor symptoms of Parkinson's disease. Diagnosis and management. Lancet Neurology 2006; 5: 235–45.

62 Tolosa E, Compta Y, Gaig C. The premotor phase of Parkinson's disease. Parkinsonism Relat Disord 2007; 13(Suppl): S2–S7.

63 Magerkurth C, Schnitzer R, Braune S. Symptoms of autonomic failure in Parkinson's disease: prevalence and impact on daily life. Clin Auton Res 2005; 15: 76–82.

64 Visser M, Marinus J, Stiggelbout AM, Van Hilten JJ. Assessment of autonomic dysfunction in Parkinson's disease: the SCOPA-AUT. Mov Disord 2004; 19: 1306–12.

65 Martinez-Martin P, Schapira AH, Stocchi F, *et al.* Prevalence of nonmotor symptoms in Parkinson's disease in an international setting; study using nonmotor symptoms questionnaire in 545 patients. Mov Disord 2007; 22: 1623–9.

66 Stocchi F, Badiali D, Vacca L, *et al.* Anorectal function in multiple system atrophy and Parkinson's disease. Mov Disord 2000; 15: 71–6.

67 Sakakibara R, Shinotoh H, Uchiyama T, *et al.* Questionnaire-based assessment of pelvic organ dysfunction in Parkinson's disease. Auton Neurosci 2001; 92: 76–85.

68 Senard JM, Rai S, Lapeyre-Mestre M, *et al.* Prevalence of orthostatic hypotension in Parkinson's disease. J Neurol Neurosurg Psychiatry 1997; 63: 584–9.

69 Verbaan D, Marinus J, Visser M, van Rooden SM, Stiggelbout AM, van Hilten JJ. Patient-reported autonomic symptoms in Parkinson disease. Neurology 2007; 69: 333–41.

70 Idiaquez J Benarroch E, Rosal H, *et al.* Autonomic and cognitive dysfunction in Parkinson's disease. Clin Auton Res 2007; 17: 93–8.

71 Peralta C, Stampfer-Kountchev M, Karner E, *et al.* Orthostatic hypotension and attention in Parkinson's disease with and without dementia. J Neural Transm 2007; 114: 585–8.

72 Allan LM, Ballard CG, Allen J, *et al.* Autonomic dysfunction in dementia. J Neurol Neurosurg Psychiatry 2007; 78: 671–7.

73 Graham JM, Sagar HJ. A data-driven approach to the study of heterogeneity in idiopathic Parkinson's disease: identification of three distinct subtypes. Mov Disord 1999; 14: 10–20.

74 Hely MA, Morris JG, Reid WG, Trafficante R. Sydney Multicenter Study of Parkinson's disease: non-L-dopa-responsive problems dominate at 15 years. Mov Disord 2005; 20: 190–9.

75 Hely, M, Reid, W Adena M, *et al.* Sydney Multicenter Study of Parkinson's Disease: the inevitability of dementia at 20 years. Mov Disord 2008; 23: 837–44.

76 Braak H, Sastre M, Bohl JR, de Vos RA, Del Tredici K. Parkinson's disease: lesions in dorsal horn layer. I. Involvement of parasympathetic and sympathetic pre and postganglionic neurons. Acta Neuropathol (Berl) 2007; 113: 421–9.

77 Calopa M, Tolosa E, Ferrer I, *et al.* Cortical Lewy bodies in Parkinson's disease with dementia. In: Tolosa E, Schulz JB, Mckeith IG, Ferrer I (eds). Neurodegenerative disorders associated with α-synuclein pathology. Barcelona: Ars Medica; 2002. pp. 127–34.

78 Apaydin H, Ahlskog JE, Parisi JE, *et al.* Parkinson's disease neuropathology. Later-developing dementia and loss of the levodopa response. Arch Neurol 2002; 59: 102–12.

79 Hurtig HI, Trojanowski JQ, Galvin J, *et al.* Alpha-synuclein cortical Lewy bodies correlate with dementia in Parkinson's disease. Neurology 2000; 54: 1916–21.

80 Braak H, Rüb U, Jansen Steur ENH, *et al.* Cognitive status correlates with neuropathologic stage in Parkinson disease. Neurology 2005; 64: 1404–10.

81 Blok BF. Central pathways controlling micturition and urinary continence. Urology 2002; 59(5 Suppl 1): 13–17.

82 Cersosimo MG, Benarroch E. Neural control of the gastrointestinal tract: implications for Parkinson disease. Mov Disord 2008; 23: 1065–75.

83 Winge K, Friberg L, Werdelin L, Nielsen KK, Stimpel H. Relationship between nigrostriatal dopaminergic degeneration, urinary symptoms, and bladder control in Parkinson's disease. Eur J Neurol 2005; 12: 842–50.

84 Winge K, Fowler CL. Bladder dysfunction in parkinsonism: mechanisms, prevalence, symptoms, and management. Mov Disord 2006; 21: 737–45.

85 Wakabayashi K, Takahashi H. The intermediolateral nucleus and Clarke's column in Parkinson's disease. Acta Neuropathol 1997; 94: 287–9.

86 Mathers SE, Kempster PA, Swash M, Lees AJ. Constipation and paradoxical puborectalis contraction in anismus and Parkinson's disease: a dystonic phenomenon?. J Neurol Neurosurg Psychiatry 1988; 51: 1503–7.

87 Allan L, McKeith I, Ballard C, Kenny RA. The prevalence of autonomic symptoms in dementia and their association with physical activity, activities of daily living and quality of life. Dement Geriatr Cogn Disord 2006; 22: 230–7.

88 Goetz C. Drugs to treat autonomic dysfunction in Parkinson's disease. Mov Disord 2002; 17(Suppl 4): S103–11.

Chapter 10

Neuroimaging in patients with Parkinson's disease dementia

Michael J. Firbank and John T. O'Brien

Introduction

Compared to other dementias, such as Alzheimer's disease (AD) and vascular dementia, relatively few imaging studies have investigated changes seen in Parkinson's disease with dementia (PD-D). Studies in PD without dementia have predominantly focused on imaging transmitter systems, especially dopaminergic changes, as the traditional view has been that structural brain changes are either absent or minimal. However, more recent studies have shown subtle structural changes even in non-demented PD, with more pronounced changes as cognitive impairment progresses. Imaging studies have attempted to define the structural and transmitter changes associated with PD-D and to compare these with those found in AD, and in the closely related dementia with Lewy bodies (DLB). The main goals of imaging are to identify early diagnostic markers or predictors of cognitive decline in PD, to define early neurobiological changes which underpin cognitive impairment, and to determine whether imaging can be a useful tool for monitoring disease progression, either from a clinical perspective or as an outcome measure in clinical trials. This chapter will summarize recent findings from structural and functional imaging studies in PD-D.

Structural imaging with MRI

Medial temporal lobe atrophy, especially affecting the hippocampus and entorhinal cortex, is characteristic of AD. A number of region-of-interest studies have investigated medial temporal lobe structures in PD-D to see if similar changes occur. They have mostly found some evidence of hippocampal and amygdala atrophy in PD without dementia [1–5], with the degree of atrophy being related to memory function, and being greater in PD subjects with dementia. The extent of medial temporal atrophy is, however, less in PD-D than in AD [3,5], very similar to findings in DLB. Figure 10.1 shows typical examples of structural magnetic resonance imaging (MRI) in PD-D and AD in comparison to a healthy subject.

Putamen atrophy has also been observed in PD [6,7] and DLB [8] and may be a result of increased striatal synuclein pathology. In these studies putamen atrophy was associated with severity of motor problems rather than cognitive ability.

The technique of voxel-based morphometry [9] has been used to investigate grey matter atrophy in an unbiased fashion throughout the brain. In this method, grey matter is

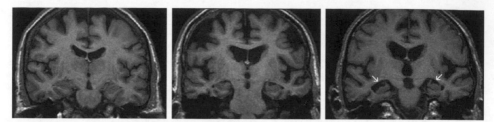

Fig. 10.1 Coronal T1 weighted MR images of (from left to right) control, PD dementia, AD. Atrophy of the medial temporal structures is severe on the AD (arrows) but mild on the PD-D.

identified from a T1-weighted MR image using an automated technique, and then grey matter from all subjects is transformed into a common coordinate system. Statistical comparisons of the amount of grey matter in each voxel are then performed. These studies have confirmed that in the medial temporal region, PD-D have more atrophy than age-matched controls [10–12], but less than Alzheimer's patients [13,14]. Other regions with focal atrophy include the anterior cingulate/prefrontal regions, superior temporal gyrus/insula region, and the thalamus. Atrophy in the occipital cortex has also been noted, more than that seen in AD [13–15]. In PD without dementia, atrophy in the occipital lobe and inferior parietal region has been associated with visual hallucinations [16].

There have been two direct comparisons of atrophy in DLB vs PD-D, with one study finding no difference [14] and one suggesting greater atrophy in DLB [13]. However, there were differences in the populations studied – in the one study [14], the duration of dementia between PD-D and DLB was comparable, and the duration of parkinsonism in PD-D was 7 years, whereas in the other [13], the PD-D had a longer duration of parkinsonism 12 years) but a shorter duration of dementia than their DLB group, who were also older.

In longitudinal studies rates of whole brain atrophy on serial MRI in PD-D are increased, and probably intermediate between healthy ageing and AD [17]. Increased rate of atrophy has been associated with cognitive decline in PD [18] and PD-D [15].

Unlike AD and vascular dementia, studies with T2-weighted MRI have not consistently found increased white matter lesions (WML) in PD or PD-D [19–22]. It is likely that any WML are due to concomitant vascular problems. As moderate associations have been found between WML and both cognitive decline [23,24] and gait disorder [25] it is likely that their presence will contribute to patients' symptoms.

In summary, there is some degree of widespread brain atrophy in PD-D, associated with cognitive decline, but the degree of hippocampal atrophy is not as marked as in AD.

Diffusion-weighted MRI

Diffusion-weighted imaging (DWI) is an MRI technique which produces images whose intensity varies according to the overall direction and magnitude of the diffusion of water in the brain. Changes to cellular structure affect water diffusion, and DWI is a sensitive indicator of changes in the integrity of axons [26,27]. Because of the highly structured

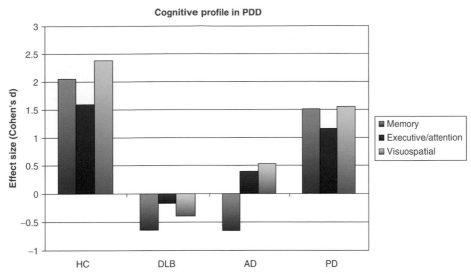

Plate 1 Overall cognitive profile in Parkinson's disease with dementia (PD-D) compared with Alzheimer's disease (AD), dementia with Lewy bodies (DLB) and Parkinson's disease without dementia (PD). The bars represent average effect-size (Cohen's d) of comparisons between PD-D and healthy controls (HC), DLB, AD and PD. A positive number indicates that the group performed better than PD-D patients, whereas negative numbers indicate poorer performance than in PD-D.

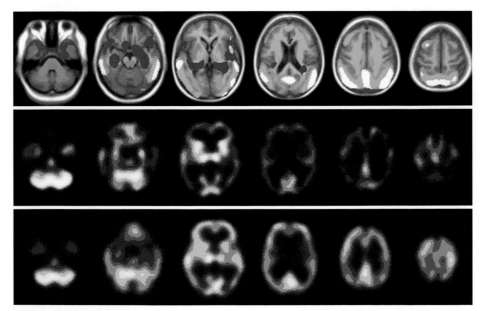

Plate 2 SPECT Perfusion in AD and PD-D. Top image (adapted from data in Firbank et al 2003) overlaid on an axial MRI are averaged perfusion deficits – PD-D in blue; AD in pink; both AD & PD-D in white. Second row, perfusion image from a typical subject with PD-D; third row, normal perfusion image.

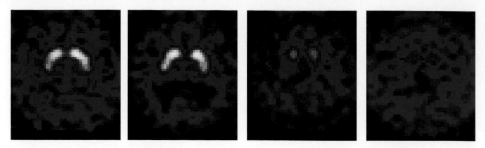

Plate 3 Typical FPCIT (dopamine transporter) images (from left to right) control, AD, PD, PD-D.

nature of axons, water tends to diffuse along the direction of white matter axons rather than perpendicular to them. Fractional anisotropy (FA) quantifies this tendency – decreases of FA may be caused by cellular damage, allowing water to diffuse perpendicular to the axon direction.

Using diffusion-weighted MRI, reduced fractional anisotropy has been found in the frontal lobe of PD [28], and widespread changes have been seen in PD-D [29] and DLB [30]. In PD-D [29] and DLB, [31] changes have been noted particularly in the posterior cingulate region. This white matter is immediately adjacent to the precuneus and inferior parietal lobes, both of which have profoundly reduced perfusion/glucose metabolism in PD-D. White matter integrity in this region has been associated with global atrophy in DLB [32], and both global [32] and hippocampal atrophy in AD [33], where it also correlates with posterior cingulate glucose metabolism. Further studies are needed to determine if the WM changes are cause or effect of the adjacent hypometabolism.

Functional activity imaging

Imaging studies of brain activation can be undertaken using positron emission tomography (PET) or functional MRI (fMRI). Both measure blood flow-related changes in one condition vs another, typically while the subject performs two or more alternating mental tasks over a 5–10-min period. Using fMRI, one study [34] in DLB found reduced activity in response to moving stimuli. Studies of Parkinson's disease with hallucinations have found reduced cortical responsiveness to visual stimuli [35,36].

Both functional MRI and PET blood flow studies (utilizing $H_2{}^{15}O$) have been used to investigate cognition in PD without dementia. These studies have mostly looked at executive function, and have typically found abnormal basal ganglia and prefrontal activations. Using working memory or executive function tasks, reduced basal ganglia and prefrontal task related activity has been found in several studies [37–40]. Monchi *et al.* [41,42], using a card-sorting task, have concluded that the caudate is involved in set-shifting (adjusting to new rules), and that activity in the prefrontal areas, which co-activate with the caudate in controls, is reduced along with caudate activity in tasks involving set-shifting, whereas frontal and parietal areas not related to caudate activity show hyperactivation in PD. Sawamoto *et al.* found caudate activity related to prefrontal activation with increasing task speed in control, but not in PD [43]. Uptake of ^{123}I-*N*-3-fluoropropyl-2-β-carbomethoxy-3-β-(4-iodophenyl)-nortropane (FP-CIT; dopamine transporter ligand) in the caudate has been correlated with task performance in PD, and with prefrontal perfusion during a sequence learning task in controls, but not in PD [44]. In executive tasks in PD patients with no impairment of performance, cortical hyperactivation has also been seen, suggestive of compensatory activity [45,46].

In normal subjects a number of regions (inferior parietal, cingulate, medial temporal) show relative activation during rest relative to a wide range of tasks [47]. This pattern of relative activation at rest is perhaps reduced in PD [45,48] and DLB [34]. Functional MRI and PET have also been used to investigate the cognitive effects of levodopa [49–52] where it has been found to modulate task-related activation in frontal and occipital regions, associated with improved response to executive tasks, but slightly worse performance on a motor sequence learning task [50].

Perfusion and metabolism

PET and single photon emission computed tomography (SPECT) both use intravenously injected radioactive ligands to form brain images. The ligand is taken up by the brain, and an image of the radioactive distribution is then made. Different ligands are used to investigate different aspects of brain function, e.g. perfusion or neurotransmitter systems.

Changes in brain perfusion and metabolism have been investigated in PD patients with cognitive impairment and also dementia. Glucose metabolism has been measured using ^{18}F-fluorodeoxyglucose (FDG) PET and perfusion imaging using SPECT with a variety of ligands: ^{99m}Tc-hexamethylpropylene amine oxime (HMPAO), N-isopropyl-p-^{123}I-iodoamphetamine (IMP) and ^{99m}Tc-ethyl cysteinate dimer (ECD). Using blood sampling, the FDG technique can be quantified in absolute units, but is often analysed relative to a reference region – either whole brain average or cerebellar uptake. Perfusion likewise is nearly always in relative units. The disadvantage of using the whole brain (or grey matter) average as a reference is that if there is a large area of hypoperfusion, unaffected areas will appear relatively hyperperfused (and the affected area will seem relatively less hypoperfused). The choice of a reference region is not completely standard – the

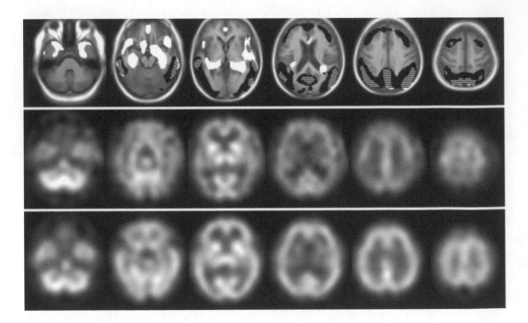

Fig. 10.2 SPECT Perfusion in AD and PD-D. Top image, (adapted from data in Firbank et al 2003) overlaid on a axial MRI are averaged perfusion deficits– PD-D in black; AD in white; both AD & PD-D in horizontal shading. Second row, perfusion image from a typical subject with PD-D; third row, normal perfusion image. See Plate 2.

cerebellum has been shown to be a good choice in AD, since it is relatively unaffected [53], but there are reports of increased cerebellar activity in PD. Borghammer *et al.* [54] have recently suggested using the white matter region as a reference, though this has not yet been widely adopted.

Using FDG and principal component analysis, Huang *et al.* identified patterns of relative regional metabolism which accounted for the variability in FDG scans across subjects. They then identified one of these component patterns in which FDG uptake correlated with cognition in PD [55]. This consisted of relatively reduced metabolism in the midline frontal, precuneus, inferior parietal and prefrontal regions, with increased metabolism in the cerebellum/pons region. They have shown this pattern of regional hypo/hypermetabolism to be associated in PD with mild cognitive impairment [56], and also that longitudinal changes in it are associated with decreasing cognitive ability [57]. A study of FDG in PD-D found that patients have extensive regions of reduced metabolism including the midline frontal and parietal regions, lateral frontal, lateral parieto-temporal and occipital cortex [58].

A number of studies have used SPECT to investigate perfusion in PD-D with findings similar to those of FDG PET, with particularly reduced perfusion in the midline and lateral parietal regions [59–63]; posterior parietal perfusion was found to correlate with cognitive ability [64]. Frontal and occipital cortex hypoperfusion has also been much reported [65–68]. By comparing structural MRI with perfusion SPECT, some degree of hypoperfusion has been shown still to be present after correcting for grey matter atrophy [63]. A few studies have directly compared DLB to PD-D and found very similar patterns [58,63,67], with perhaps lower overall metabolism in DLB compared to PD-D matched for dementia severity. Figure 10.2 shows regions of reduced perfusion in AD as compared to PD-D, as well as typical SPECT perfusion images.

Visual hallucinations, which are a prominent feature of PD-D, have been investigated in cognitively intact PD patients, though without much consensus between studies as to areas of hypo- or hyperperfusion/metabolism, with parietal [69,70], temporal [71] and frontal [72] regions implicated.

In summary, PD-D patients have marked reduction of perfusion/metabolism throughout the brain, particularly in parietal and frontal regions, with possibly increased perfusion in the cerebellum. The degree of perfusion reduction is linked to cognitive decline.

Dopaminergic imaging

The dopaminergic system has been investigated through both PET and SPECT. ^{18}F-6-Fluorodopa (FDOPA) PET is a marker of presynaptic nerve terminal function and has been used widely to investigate PD [73]. Analysis is usually by the graphical method of Patlak and Blasberg [74], which calculates the k_i or tracer influx constant, using a reference region, usually the occipital lobe. Decreased FDOPA uptake has been demonstrated in PD in the whole striatum, particularly the putamen relative to healthy controls. Both the putamen and caudate uptake correlate with measures of motor function (e.g. UPDRS) though the putamen generally has the stronger correlation [75–78]. The caudate FDOPA uptake has been shown to correlate with measures of executive functions [77,78].

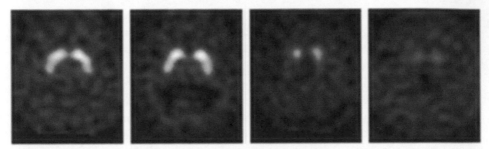

Fig. 10.3 Typical FPCIT (dopamine transporter) images (from left to right) control, AD, PD, PD-D. See Plate 3.

Ito *et al.* [79] used FDOPA to compare PD patients with controls and those with PD-D. They found that patients with PD-D had reduced striatal FDOPA compared both with controls and PD. Some studies have investigated cortical FDOPA uptake, with reports of both decreased [77] and increased [2] values. However, Cropley *et al.* [80] found a greater calculated FDOPA influx constant in the white vs grey matter, which is contrary to the expected distribution. They suggest that the Patlak method is unreliable for this tracer for cortical areas due to differences in perfusion in the reference occipital region.

PET has also been used to investigate postsynaptic dopamine receptors. Cropley *et al.* [80] found no difference between PD and controls with a D1 receptor ligand ^{11}C-NNC 112. Using ^{11}C-raclopride (RAC), a marker of D2 receptor availability, decreased binding potential (indicative of greater endogenous dopamine) was found in a working memory task relative to a visuomotor task in controls and PD, with a small region of the caudate having greater task-related decreases in controls vs PD.

The presynaptic dopamine transporter ligand FP-CIT has been extensively studied in PD-D/DLB. In normal subjects and AD, the ligand is taken up in the putamen and caudate, whereas in the parkinsonian disorders, uptake is almost absent in the putamen, and reduced in the caudate. The presence of abnormal FP-CIT uptake has very good diagnostic accuracy for DLB/PD-D with a sensitivity/specificity of ~80/90% [81–84]. Compared with cognitively intact PD subjects, where the putamen is affected more than the caudate, both DLB and PD-D have relatively uniform reduction in FP-CIT uptake throughout the striatum [85,86], implying that dopaminergic loss in the caudate is involved in dementia. This adds to the evidence from PET and fMRI studies implicating caudate dysfunction in cognitive impairment in PD. In addition, PD-D was associated with more pronounced overall striatal dopaminergic loss than DLB [85], consistent with the autopsy findings of greater underlying nigrostriatal dopaminergic cell loss.

In summary, profound deficits in the basal ganglia dopaminergic system of PD and PD-D can be demonstrated with PET and SPECT (Fig. 10.3).

Cholinergic imaging

The cholinergic system has been investigated with a number of radioligands in order to assess the integrity of the cortical cholinergic innervation. Hilker *et al.* [87] performed an imaging study in PD and PD-D using both FDOPA and N-^{11}C-methyl-4-piperidyl acetate (MP4A), an analogue of acetylcholine. They found MP4A binding to be moderately reduced in PD and severe widespread reductions (~30%) in PD-D, particularly in the parietal lobes. Cortical binding of MP4A in some regions showed a significant association with striatal FDOPA in both PD and PD-D, although there were no significant differences between PD and PD-D in striatal FDOPA. Another acetylcholine analogue, N-^{11}C-methyl-piperidin-4-yl propionate (^{11}C-PMP) is also moderately reduced in PD, and markedly reduced in PD-D (~20%) relative to controls [88] and AD [89]. Levels of PMP were reduced by about 10% in AD in all regions apart from the inferior temporal lobe, where the reduction was 20% and comparable to PD-D. Reductions in the PMP uptake correlated well with poor performance on executive and spatial tasks, which are typically impaired in PD-D, but not with verbal memory task or motor impairment [88]. Imaging of muscarinic receptors with SPECT using (R,R) ^{123}I-iodo-quinuclidinyl-benzilate (QNB) [90] and nicotinic receptors with ^{125}I-5-iodo-3-[2(S)-2-azetidinylmethoxy]pyridine (5IA-85380) has found decreases in the frontal and temporal lobes of PD-D and DLB, and relative increase in uptake of both ligands in the occipital lobe, with the nicotinic ligand uptake being higher in DLB subjects with recent hallucinations [91].

Amyloid imaging

Imaging of amyloid protein *in vivo* is possible using the PET tracer N-methyl-^{11}C-2-(4'-methylaminophenyl)-6-hydroxybenzothiazole (Pittsburgh Compound B, PIB). This substance binds to Aβ deposits, and there is increased uptake of PIB relative to cerebellum throughout the cortex of patients with AD [92], particularly in posterior cingulate, frontal, lateral temporal and parietal regions. Although increased uptake is a sensitive indicator of AD, 10–20% of subjects without any cognitive impairment also show increased PIB uptake [93,94]. In DLB, PIB uptake is also increased, comparable to AD [94–96]; however, in PD-D [94,95,97] there is no increase in cortical uptake relative to controls, with possibly increased uptake in the brainstem [97].

Cardiac imaging

There is loss of sympathetic innervation in the heart of patients with PD [98]. This has been demonstrated with cardiac scintigraphy using ^{123}I-metaiodobenzylguanidine ^{123}I-MIBG) an analogue of noradrenaline, with the ratio of uptake in heart to mediastinum calculated to quantify the images. This ratio has been found to be reduced in PD, particularly in advanced stages [99,100], and also in DLB and PD-D in comparison to AD and healthy subjects. Studies have found a diagnostic accuracy for DLB/PD-D vs AD of sensitivity and specificity of about 90% [101–103]. However, decreased uptake has also been reported in patients with AD and those with cardiovascular disease presenting with parkinsonian features [100]. Hence studies with larger group sizes are needed to confirm the diagnostic accuracy.

Conclusion

Using neuroimaging techniques, widespread changes throughout the brains of patients with PD-D in structure, metabolism and neurotransmitters can be demonstrated which appear similar to DLB, but distinct from AD. These include whole brain atrophy, atrophy in medial temporal, prefrontal, parieto-occipital, insula and putamen in structural imaging, and reduced metabolism in midline frontal, posterior cingulate & precuneus, inferior parietal and prefrontal regions in functional imaging. Imaging of neurotransmitter systems revealed reduction in cortical cholinergic binding, and diffuse and widespread reduction in dopaminergic binding in striatum. Although such differences can be shown when comparing groups of patients, there is no single pattern of imaging findings which can be used for routine diagnostic purposes. Relatively less atrophy in hippocampus/amygdala and relatively more atrophy in the parietal–occipital region is the common pattern in PD-D. Clinically, an FP-CIT scan can be helpful in differentiating PD-D/DLB from AD patients. Initial studies using amyloid imaging show differences between AD (and DLB) and PD-D, although larger validation studies are needed before this could be recommended as a clinically useful tool.

References

1 Bouchard TP, Malykhin N, Martin WRW, *et al*. Age and dementia associated atrophy predominates in the hippocampal head and amygdala. Neurobiol Aging 2008; 29: 1027–39.

2 Brück A, Aalto S, Nurmi E, Bergman J, Rinne JO. Cortical 6-[F-18]fluoro-L-dopa uptake and frontal cognitive functions in early Parkinson's disease. Neurobiol Aging 2005; 26: 891–8.

3 Camicioli R, Moore MM, Kinney A, Corbridge E, Glassberg K, Kaye JA. Parkinson's disease is associated with hippocampal atrophy. Mov Disord 2003; 18: 784–90.

4 Junque C, Ramirez-Ruiz B, Tolosa E, *et al*. Amygdalar and hippocampal MRI volumetric reductions in Parkinson's disease with dementia. Mov Disord 2005; 20: 540–4.

5 Tam CWC, Burton EJ, McKeith IG, Burn DJ, O'Brien JT. Temporal lobe atrophy on MRI in Parkinson disease with dementia – a comparison with Alzheimer disease and dementia with Lewy bodies. Neurology 2005; 64: 861–5.

6 Geng DY, Li YX, Zee CS. Magnetic resonance imaging-based volumetric analyses of basal ganglia nuclei and substantia nigra in patients with Parkinson's disease. Neurosurgery 2006; 58: 256–61.

7 Alegret M, Junque C, Pueyo R, *et al*. MRI atrophy parameters related to cognitive and motor impairment in Parkinson's disease. Neurologia 2001; 16: 63–9.

8 Cousins DA, Burton EJ, Burn D, Gholkar A, McKeith IG, O'Brien JT. Atrophy of the putamen in dementia Lewy bodies but not Alzheimer's disease – an MRI study. Neurology 2003; 61: 1191–5.

9 Good CD, Johnsrude IS, Ashburner J, Henson RN, Friston KJ, Frackowiak RS. A voxel based morphometric study of ageing in 465 normal adult human brains. NeuroImage 2001; 141: 21–36.

10 Nagano-Saito A, Washimi Y, Arahata Y, *et al*. Cerebral atrophy and its relation to cognitive impairment in Parkinson disease. Neurology 2005; 64: 224–9.

11 Beyer MK, Janvin CC, Larsen JP, Aarsland D. A magnetic resonance imaging study of patients with Parkinson's disease with mild cognitive impairment and dementia using voxel-based morphometry. J Neurol Neurosurg Psychiatry 2007; 78: 254–9.

12 Summerfield C, Junqué C, Tolosa E, *et al*. Structural brain changes in Parkinson's disease with dementia: a voxel-based morphometry study. Arch Neurol 2005; 62: 281–5.

13 Beyer MK, Larsen JP, Aarsland D. Gray matter atrophy in Parkinson disease with dementia and dementia with Lewy bodies. Neurology 2007; 69: 747–54.

14 Burton EJ, McKeith IG, Burn DJ, Williams ED, O'Brien JT. Cerebral atrophy in Parkinson's disease with and without dementia: a comparison with Alzheimer's disease, dementia with Lewy bodies and controls. Brain 2004; 127: 791–800.

15 Ramirez-Ruiz B, Marti MJ, Tolosa E, et al. Longitudinal evaluation of cerebral morphological changes in Parkinson's disease with and without dementia. J Neurol 2005; 252: 1345–52.

16 Ramirez-Ruiz B, Marti MJ, Tolosa E, et al. Cerebral atrophy in Parkinson's disease patients with visual hallucinations. Eur J Neurol 2007; 14: 750–6.

17 Burton EJ, McKeith IG, Burn DJ, O'Brien JT. Brain atrophy rates in Parkinson's disease with and without dementia using serial magnetic resonance imaging. Mov Disord 2005; 20: 1571–6.

18 Hu MTM, White SJ, Chaudhuri KR, et al. Correlating rates of cerebral atrophy in Parkinson's disease with measures of cognitive decline. J Neural Transm 2001; 108: 571–80.

19 Beyer MK, Aarsland D, Greve OJ, Larsen JP. Visual rating of white matter hyperintensities in Parkinson's disease. Mov Disord 2006; 21: 223–9.

20 Burton EJ, McKeith IG, Burn DJ, Firbank MJ, O'Brien JT. Progression of white matter hyperintensities in Alzheimer disease, dementia with Lewy bodies, and Parkinson disease dementia: a comparison with normal aging. Am J Geriatr Psychiatry 2006; 14: 842–9.

21 Acharya HJ, Bouchard TP, Emery DJ, Camicioli RM. Axial signs and magnetic resonance imaging correlates in Parkinson's disease. Can J Neurol Sci 2007; 34: 56–61.

22 Meyer JS, Huang JB, Chowdhury MH. MRI confirms mild cognitive impairments prodromal for Alzheimer's, vascular and Parkinson–Lewy body dementias. J Neurol Sci 2007; 257: 97–104.

23 Schmidt R, Ropele S, Enzinger C, et al. White matter lesion progression, brain atrophy, and cognitive decline: the Austrian stroke prevention study. Ann Neurol 2005; 58: 610–16.

24 van der Flier WM, van Straaten EC, Barkhof F, et al. Medial temporal lobe atrophy and white matter hyperintensities are associated with mild cognitive deficits in no-disabled elderly people: the LADIS study. J Neurol Neurosurg Psychiatry 2005; 76: 1497–1500.

25 Baezner H, Blahak C, Poggesi A, et al. Association of gait and balance disorders with age-related white matter changes: the LADIS study. Neurology 2008; 70: 935–42.

26 Le Bihan D. Looking into the functional architecture of the brain with diffusion MRI. Nat Rev Neurosci 2003; 4: 469–80.

27 Moseley M. Diffusion tensor imaging and aging – a review. NMR Biomed 2002; 15: 553–60.

28 Karagulle Kendi AT, Lehericy S, Luciana M, Ugurbil K, Tuite P. Altered diffusion in the frontal lobe in Parkinson disease. Am J Neuroradiol 2008; 29: 501–5.

29 Matsui H, Nishinaka K, Oda M, Niikawa H, Kubori T, Udaka F. Dementia in Parkinson's disease: diffusion tensor imaging. Acta Neurol Scand 2007; 116: 177–81.

30 Bozzali M, Falini A, Cercignani M, et al. Brain tissue damage in dementia with Lewy bodies: an in vivo diffusion tensor MRI study. Brain 2005; 128: 1595–604.

31 Firbank MJ, Blamire AM, Krishnan MS, et al. Diffusion tensor imaging in dementia with Lewy bodies and Alzheimer's disease. Psychiatry Res Neuroimag 2007; 155: 135–45.

32 Firbank MJ, Blamire AM, Krishnan MS, et al. Atrophy is associated with posterior cingulate white matter disruption in dementia with Lewy bodies and Alzheimer's disease. NeuroImage 2007; 36: 1–7.

33 Villain N, Desgranges B, Viader F, et al. Relationship between hippocampal atrophy, white matter disruption, and gray matter hypometabolism in Alzheimer's disease. J Neurosci 2008; 28: 6174–81.

34 Sauer J, Ffytche DH, Ballard C, Brown RG, Howard R. Differences between Alzheimer's disease and dementia with Lewy bodies: an fMRI study of task-related brain activity. Brain 2006; 129: 1780–8.

35 Stebbins GT, Goetz CG, Carrillo MC, et al. Altered cortical visual processing in PD with hallucinations – an fMRI study. Neurology 2004; 63: 1409–16.

36 Howard R, David A, Woodruff P, *et al.* Seeing visual hallucinations with functional magnetic resonance imaging. Dement Geriatr Cogn Disord 1997; 8: 73–7.

37 Owen AM, Doyon J, Dagher A, Sadikot A, Evans AC. Abnormal basal ganglia outflow in Parkinson's disease identified with PET – implications for higher cortical functions. Brain 1998; 121: 949–65.

38 Lewis SJG, Dove A, Robbins TW, Barker RA, Owen AM. Cognitive impairments in early Parkinson's disease are accompanied by reductions in activity in frontostriatal neural circuitry. J Neurosci 2003; 23: 6351–6.

39 Grossman M, Cooke A, DeVita C, *et al.* Grammatical and resource components of sentence processing in Parkinson's disease – an fMRI study. Neurology 2003; 60: 775–81.

40 Thiel AH, Kessler R, Habedank J, Herholz B, Heiss K. Activation of basal ganglia loops in idiopathic Parkinson's disease: a PET study. J Neural Transm 2003; 110: 1289–1301.

41 Monchi O, Petrides M, Mejia-Constain B, Strafella AP. Cortical activity in Parkinson's disease during executive processing depends on striatal involvement. Brain 2007; 130: 233–44.

42 Monchi O, Petrides M, Doyon J, Postuma RB, Worsley K, Dagher A. Neural bases of set-shifting deficits in Parkinson's disease. J Neurosci 2004; 24: 702–10.

43 Sawamoto N, Honda M, Hanakawa T, *et al.* Cognitive slowing in Parkinson disease is accompanied by hypofunctioning of the striatum. Neurology 2007; 68: 1062–8.

44 Carbon M, Ma YL, Barnes A, *et al.* Caudate nucleus: influence of dopaminergic input on sequence learning and brain activation in Parkinsonism. NeuroImage 2004; 21: 1497–1507.

45 Tinaz S, Schendan HE, Stern CE, Chantal E. Fronto-striatal deficit in Parkinson's disease during semantic event sequencing. Neurobiol Aging 2008; 29: 397–407.

46 Marie RM, Lozza C, Chavoix C, Defer GL, Baron JC. Functional imaging of working memory in Parkinson's disease: compensations and deficits. J Neuroimaging 2007; 17: 277–85.

47 Raichle ME, MacLeod AM, Snyder AZ, Powers WJ, Gusnard DA, Shulman GL. A default mode of brain function. Proc Natl Acad Sci USA 2001; 98: 676–82.

48 Dirnberger G, Frith CD, Jahanshahi M. Executive dysfunction in Parkinson's disease is associated with altered pallidal–frontal processing. NeuroImage 2005; 25: 588–99.

49 Fera F, Nicoletti G, Cerasa A, *et al.* Dopaminergic modulation of cognitive interference after pharmacological washout in Parkinson's disease. Brain Res Bull 2007; 74: 75–83.

50 Feigin A, Ghilardi MF, Carbon M, *et al.* Effects of levodopa on motor sequence learning in Parkinson's disease. Neurology 2003; 60: 1744–9.

51 Cools R, Stefanova E, Barker RA, Robbins TW, Owen AM. Dopaminergic modulation of high-level cognition in Parkinson's disease: the role of the prefrontal cortex revealed by PET. Brain 2002; 125: 584–94.

52 Mattay VST, Callicott A, Bertolino JH, *et al.* Dopaminergic modulation of cortical function in patients with Parkinson's disease. Ann Neurol 2002; 51: 156–64.

53 Soonawala D, Amin T, Ebmeier KP, *et al.* Statistical parametric mapping of 99mTc-HMPAO-SPECT images for the diagnosis of Alzheimer's disease: normalizing to cerebellar tracer uptake. Neuroimage 2002; 17: 1193–202.

54 Borghammer P, Jonsdottir KY, Cumming P, *et al.* Normalization in PET group comparison studies – the importance of a valid reference region. NeuroImage 2008; 40: 529–40.

55 Huang CR, Mattis P, Tang CK, Perrine K, Carbon M, Eidelberg D. Metabolic brain networks associated with cognitive function in Parkinson's disease. Neuroimage 2007; 34: 714–23.

56 Huang C, Mattis P, Perrine K, Brown N, Dhawan V, Eidelberg D. Metabolic abnormalities associated with mild cognitive impairment in Parkinson disease. Neurology 2008; 70: 1470–7.

57 Huang CR, Tang CK, Feigin A, *et al.* Changes in network activity with the progression of Parkinson's disease. Brain 2007; 130: 1864–6.

58 Yong SW, Yoon JK, An YS, Lee PH. A comparison of cerebral glucose metabolism in Parkinson's disease, Parkinson's disease dementia and dementia with Lewy bodies. Eur J Neurol 2007; 14: 1357–62.

59 Waragai M, Yamada T, Matsuda H. Evaluation of brain perfusion SPECT using an easy Z-score imaging system (eZIS) as an adjunct to early-diagnosis of neurodegenerative diseases. J Neurol Sci 2007; 260: 57–64.

60 Matsui H, Udaka F, Miyoshi T, Hara N, Tamura A. N-Isopropyl-p-I-123 iodoamphetamine single photon emission computed tomography study of Parkinson's disease with dementia. Intern Med 2005; 44: 1046–50.

61 Osaki Y, Morita Y, Fukumoto M, Akagi N, Yoshida S, Doi Y. Three-dimensional stereotactic surface projection SPECT analysis in Parkinson's disease with and without dementia. Mov Disord 2005; 20: 999–1005.

62 Derejko M, Slawek J, Wieczorek D, Brockhuis B, Dubaniewicz M, Lass P. 2006. Regional cerebral blood flow in Parkinson's disease as an indicator of cognitive impairment. Nucl Med Commun 27: 945–51.

63 Firbank M, Colloby ST, Burn D, McKeith IG, O'Brien JT. Regional cerebral blood flow in Parkinson's disease with and without dementia. Neuroimage 2003; 20: 1309–19.

64 van Laere K, Santens P, Bosman T, de Reuck J, Mortelmans L, Dierckx R. Statistical parametric mapping of 99mTc-ECD SPECT in idiopathic Parkinson's disease and multiple system atrophy with predominant parkinsonian features: correlation with clinical parameters. J Nucl Med 2004; 45: 933–42.

65 Chang CC, Liu JS, Chang YY, Chang WN, Chen SS, Lee CH. Tc-99m-ethyl cysteinate dimer brain SPECT findings in early stage of dementia with Lewy bodies and Parkinson's disease patients: a correlation with neuropsychological tests. Eur J Neurol 2008; 15: 57–61.

66 Wallin A, Ekberg S, Lind K, Milos V, Granerus AK, Granerus G. Posterior cortical brain dysfunction in cognitively impaired patients with Parkinson's disease – a rCBF scintigraphy study. Acta Neurol Scand 2007; 116: 347–54.

67 Mito Y, Yoshida K, Yabe I, et al. Brain 3D-SSP SPECT analysis in dementia with Lewy bodies, Parkinson's disease with and without dementia, and Alzheimer's disease. Clin Neurol Neurosurg 2005; 107: 396–403.

68 Antonini A, de Notaris R, Benti R, de Gaspari D, Pezzoli G. Perfusion ECD/SPECT in the characterisation of cognitive deficits in Parkinson's disease. Neurol Sci 2001; 22: 45–6.

69 Boecker H, Ceballos-Baumann AO, Volk D, Conrad B, Forstl H, Haussermann P. Metabolic alterations in patients with Parkinson disease and visual hallucinations. Arch Neurol 2007; 64: 984–88.

70 O'Brien JT, Firbank MJ, Mosimann UP, Burn DJ, McKeith IG. Change in perfusion, hallucinations and fluctuations in consciousness in dementia with Lewy Bodies. Psychiatry Res Neuroimag 2005; 139: 79–88.

71 Oishi N, Udaka F, Kameyama M, Sawamoto N, Hashikawa K, Fukuyama H. Regional cerebral blood flow in Parkinson's disease with nonpsychotic visual hallucinations. Neurology 2005; 65: 1708–15.

72 Nagano-Saito A, Washimi Y, Arahata Y, et al. Visual hallucination in Parkinson's disease with FDG PET. Mov Disord 2004; 19: 801–6.

73 Heiss WD, Hilker R. The sensitivity of 18-fluorodopa positron emission tomography and magnetic resonance imaging in Parkinson's disease. Eur J Neurol 2004; 11: 5–12.

74 Patlak CS, Blasberg RG. Graphical evaluation of blood-to-brain transfer constants from multiple-time uptake data – generalizations. J Cerebr Blood Flow Metab 1985; 5: 584–90.

75 Weder BJ, Leenders KL, Vontobel P, et al. Impaired somatosensory discrimination of shape in Parkinson's disease: association with caudate nucleus dopaminergic function. Hum Brain Mapp 1999; 8: 1–12.

76 Broussolle E, Dentresangle C, Landais P, *et al.* The relation of putamen and caudate nucleus F-18-Dopa uptake to motor and cognitive performances in Parkinson's disease. J Neurol Sci 1999; 166: 141–51.

77 Rinne JO, Portin R, Ruottinen H, *et al.* Cognitive impairment and the brain dopaminergic system in Parkinson disease – F18 fluorodopa positron emission tomographic study. Arch Neurol 2000; 57: 470–5.

78 van Beilen M, Portman AT, Kiers HAL, *et al.* Striatal FDOPA uptake and cognition in advanced non-demented Parkinson's disease: a clinical and FDOPA-PET study. Parkinsonism Relat Disord 2008; 14: 224–8.

79 Ito K, Nagano-Saito A, Kato T, *et al.* Striatal and extrastriatal dysfunction in Parkinson's disease with dementia: a 6-[F-18]fluoro-L-dopa PET study. Brain 2002; 125: 1358–65.

80 Cropley VL, Fujita M, Bara-Jimenez W, *et al.* Pre- and post-synaptic dopamine imaging and its relation with frontostriatal cognitive function in Parkinson disease: PET studyes with [C-11]NNC 112 and [F-18]FDOPA. Psychiatry Res Neuroimag 2008; 163: 171–82.

81 McKeith I, O'Brien J, Walker Z, *et al.* Sensitivity and specificity of dopamine transporter imaging with I-123-FP-CIT SPECT in dementia with Lewy bodies: a phase III, multicentre study. Lancet Neurology 2007; 6: 305–13.

82 Walker Z, Jaros E, Walker RWH, *et al.* Dementia with Lewy bodies: a comparison of clinical diagnosis, FP-CIT single photon emission computed tomography imaging and autopsy. J Neurol Neurosurg Psychiatry 2007; 78: 1176–81.

83 Marshall VL, Patterson J, Hadley DM, Grosset KA, Grosset DG. Two-year follow-up in 150 consecutive cases with normal dopamine transporter imaging. Nucl Med Commun 2006; 27: 933-937.

84 Ortega Lozano SJ, Martínez del Valle Torres MD, Jiménez-Hoyuela García JM, Gutiérrez Cardo AL, Campos Arillo V. Diagnostic accuracy of FP-CIT SPECT in patients with parkinsonism Revista. Esp Medicina Nucl 2007; 26: 277–85.

85 O'Brien JT, Colloby S, Fenwick J, *et al.* Dopamine transporter loss visualized with FP-CIT SPECT in the differential diagnosis of dementia with Lewy bodies. Arch Neurol 2004; 61: 919–25.

86 Walker Z, Costa DC, Walker RWH, *et al.* Striatal dopamine transporter in dementia with Lewy bodies and Parkinson disease – a comparison. Neurology 2004; 62: 1568–72.

87 Hilker R, Thomas AV, Klein JC, *et al.* Dementia in Parkinson disease – functional imaging of cholinergic and dopaminergic pathways. Neurology 2005; 65: 1716–22.

88 Bohnen NI, Kaufer DI, Hendrickson R, *et al.* Cognitive correlates of cortical cholinergic denervation in Parkinson's disease and parkinsonian dementia. J Neurol 2006; 253: 242–7.

89 Bohnen NI, Kaufer DI, Ivanco LS, *et al.* Cortical cholinergic function is more severely affected in Parkinsonian dementia than in Alzheimer disease. Arch Neurol 2003; 60: 1745–8.

90 Colloby SJ, Pakrasi S, Firbank MJ, *et al.* In vivo SPECT imaging of muscarinic acetylcholine receptors using (R,R) I-123-QNB in dementia with Lewy bodies and Parkinson's disease dementia. Neuroimage 2006; 33: 423–9.

91 O'Brien JT, Colloby SJ, Pakrasi S, *et al.* Nicotinic alpha4beta2 receptor binding in dementia with Lewy bodies using 123I-5IA-85380 SPECT demonstrates a link between occipital changes and visual hallucinations. NeuroImage 2008; 40: 1056–63.

92 Klunk WE, Engler H, Nordberg A, *et al.* Imaging brain amyloid in Alzheimer's disease with Pittsburgh Compound-B. Ann Neurol 2004; 55: 306–19.

93 Mintun MA, LaRossa GN, Sheline YI, *et al.* [11C]PIB in a nondemented population: potential antecendent marker of Alzheimer disease. Neurology 2006; 67: 446–52.

94 Gomperts SN, Rentz DM, Moran E, *et al.* Imaging amyloid deposition in Lewy body diseases. Neurology 2008; 71: 903–10.

95 Edison P, Rowe CC, Rinne J, *et al*. Amyloid load in Lewy body dementia (LBD), Parkinson's disease dementia (PDD) and Parkinson's disease (PD) measured with C-11-PIB PET. Neurology 2007; 68: A98–A98.

96 Rowe CC, Ng S, Ackermann U, *et al*. Imaging beta-amyloid burden in aging and dementia. Neurology 2007; 68: 1718–25.

97 Maetzler W, Reimold M, Liepelt I, *et al*. [11C]PIB binding in Parkinson's disease dementia. NeuroImage 2008; 39: 1027–33.

98 Goldstein DS. Dysautonomia in Parkinson's disease; neurocardiological abnormalities. Lancet Neurology 2003; 2: 669–676.

99 Hamada K, Hirayama M, Watanabe H, *et al*. Onset age and severity of motor impairment are associated with reduction of myocardial 123I-MIBG uptake in Parkinson's disease. J Neurol Neurosurg Psychiatry 2003; 74: 423–26.

100 Nagayama H, Hamamoto M, Ueda M, Nagashima J, Katayama Y. Reliability of MIBG myocaridal scintigraphy in the diagnosis of Parkinson's disease. J Neurol Neurosurg Psychiatry 2005; 76: 249–51.

101 Hanyu H, Shimizu S, Hirao K, *et al*. The role of I-123-metaiodobenzylguanidine myocardial scintigraphy in the diagnosis of Lewy body disease in patients with dementia in a memory clinic. Dement Geriatr Cogn Disord 2006; 22: 379–84.

102 Wada-Isoe K, Kitayama M, Nakaso K, Nakashima K. Diagnostic markers for diagnosing dementia with Lewy bodies: CSF and MIBG cardiac scintigraphy study. J Neurol Sci 2007; 260: 33–7.

103 Yoshita M, Taki J, Tamada M. A clinical role for [123I]MIBG myocardial scintigraphy in the distinction between dementia of the Alzheimer's type and dementia with Lewy bodies. J Neurol Neurosurg Psychiatry 2001; 71: 583–8.

Chapter 11

Electrophysiological and other auxiliary investigations in patients with Parkinson's disease dementia

Yasuyuki Okuma and Yoshikuni Mizuno

Introduction

Recent studies have revealed that patients with Parkinson's disease (PD) often show cognitive deficits. Impairments have been documented in almost all areas of cognition, including general intellectual functions, visuospatial functions, attention, memory and executive functions [1–4]. Various electrophysiological investigations have been used to study these cognitive dysfunctions in patients with PD. In this chapter, the results of electrophysiological investigations in demented and non-demented PD patients are reviewed. In addition, recent data on ^{123}I-metaiodobenzylguanidine (^{123}I-MIBG) myocardial scintigraphy, which has been found very useful for differentiating Lewy body diseases such as PD and dementia with Lewy bodies (DLB) from Alzheimer's disease (AD) [5,6], are also reviewed as other auxiliary investigations.

Electrophysiological methods

Electroencephalography (EEG)

Early studies have shown that EEG findings are abnormal in around 30–40% of PD patients. The slowing of alpha rhythms and generalized or focal increase in slow activities are the common findings [7,8]. Neufeld *et al.* found a correlation between EEG abnormality and the age, mental state, and motor disability of PD patients, and suggested that subcortical structures may influence background activity [9]. De Weed *et al.* showed that diffuse slow activity, reduced frequency of rhythmic background activity, and focal disturbances were the predictive factors of dementia after 3 years [10]. Neufeld *et al.* later performed EEG frequency analysis and demonstrated that the relative alpha amplitude was significantly decreased in demented PD patients, unrelated to motor disability [11]. They also showed a non-significant but consistent trend of increased amplitude in the delta and theta range in demented PD patients. Soikkeli *et al.* also found increased theta and delta activities in demented PD patients by EEG spectral analysis, whereas only theta activities were increased in non-demented patients [12]. Domitrz and Friedman reported that demented PD patients more often showed no response to eye-opening (no arousal reaction) and presented slower wave activity in comparison with non-demented patients and healthy controls [13]. They hypothesized that the absence of arousal reaction may be the first EEG abnormality in patients who will develop dementia in the future. Tanaka *et al.* conducted EEG power spectral analysis and their results agreed with the previous findings that in demented PD patients delta and theta power increased, but they did not see a decreased alpha power as compared with controls [14]. The underlying pathophysiology of EEG changes in PD is very difficult to elucidate. Both subcortical and cortical involvements may account for the EEG slowing, but Soikkeli *et al.* suggested that the deficit in the cholinergic system could in part explain the slowing of the EEG, particularly in demented PD patients [12].

To explore whether EEG abnormalities can discriminate between DLB, AD, and PD with dementia (PD-D) in the earliest stages of dementia, Bonanni *et al.* studied EEG on 50 DLB, 50 AD, and 40 PD-D patients with slight cognitive impairment at first visit [15]. Dominant mean frequencies were 8.3 Hz for the AD group and 7.4 Hz for the DLB group. The dominant frequency variability also differed between the AD (1.1 Hz) and DLB groups (1.8 Hz). By comparison, fewer than half of the patients with PD-D exhibited the EEG abnormalities seen in those with DLB. The authors concluded that if revised consensus criteria for DLB diagnosis [16] are properly applied, EEG may be helpful to discriminate between AD and DLB at the earliest stages of dementia.

Evoked potentials

Auditory evoked potentials (AEP)

There are several reports regarding AEP in PD. Gawel *et al.* reported prolongation of wave V latency [17], whereas Prasher and Bannister described normal AEP findings [18]. This difference may be due to the selection of the patients. Tachibana *et al.* showed normal latencies in non-demented PD patients. By contrast, demented patients revealed significant prolongation of wave I–V (particularly wave III–V) interpeak latencies compared to patients without dementia and healthy subjects [19]. These results show that auditory brainstem pathways are involved in PD patients with dementia and could be explained by the more general involvements in the brainstem pathways of the disease process and/or other concomitant pathology in such patients. Green *et al.* reported that the P1 (50 ms) of the middle latency AEP was lacking in 39% of AD and 58% of demented PD patients and suggested that abnormalities of P1 in dementia may be due to cholinergic dysfunction [20,21].

Visual evoked potentials (VEP)

There have been contradictory results on the changes in VEP in patients with PD. Bodis-Wollner and Yahr reported that the average latency was prolonged but became less prolonged on levodopa therapy, suggesting that both extrapyramidal connections of the visual cortex and retinal dopaminergic neurons can be affected in PD [22]. Dinner *et al.* and Nightingale *et al.* did not show prolonged VEP latencies [23,24]. Calzetti *et al.* compared VEP and electroretinogram and concluded that VEP changes are not entirely dependent on alterations at the retinal level [25]. Okuda *et al.* have found that prolonged P100 latency was revealed only in demented PD patients and speculated that dysfunction in the central visual system plays a role in the abnormal pattern of VEP in PD [26]. In conclusion, the disturbance of both retinal and basal ganglionic dopaminergic systems may contribute to the delayed VEP latency.

Somatosensory evoked potentials (SEP)

Short-latency SEPs were reported to be normal when recorded from the parietal region regardless of cognitive functions [18,27,28], although Potolicchio and O'Doherty reported that interwave latencies were prolonged in some patients [29]. In contrast to parietal SEPs, Rossini *et al.* found reduced frontal N30 amplitude in PD patients [28]. They suggest that dysfunctions of the thalamo-basal ganglia–frontal cortex circuit or supplementary motor cortex would play a role in reducing the frontal N30 amplitude.

Event-related potentials (ERP)

P300 (P3, target P3)

The P300 (P3) ERP can be elicited whenever one stimulus is discriminated from another [30]. The subject is instructed to respond to the infrequent (oddball) or target stimulus and not to respond to the frequently presented or standard stimulus. Goodin *et al.* showed that the peak latency of the P3 becomes longer as age increases [31]. In addition, P3 latency was found to be longer in dementing illness than the normal values for a given age [31,32]. It is sensitive to the cognitive changes associated with ageing and the mental decline associated with various diseases including PD.

There have been a number of studies examining P3 in PD patients. The results of P3 latencies in non-demented PD patients are contradictory, whereas P3 latency in demented PD patients is prolonged. Table 11.1 shows the summary of reports of auditory oddball P3 latency and amplitude in non-demented PD patients [14,33–43]. Interestingly, the effects of levodopa therapy were variable. Amabile *et al.* reported that the basal P3 latency was delayed but became normalized after levodopa therapy [36]. Starkstein *et al.* examined PD patients with severe motor fluctuation and reported a significant improvement of the P300 latency of the ERP in 'on' phase [37]. In contrast, Prasher and Findley showed that P3 was normal before treatment but that after treatment P3 latency was significantly prolonged with the reduction of reaction time [38]. Dopamine replacement is followed by a significantly reduced motor processing time despite increased cognitive processing time. They suggest that dopaminergic overstimulation of other regions may adversely affect cognitive processing. Yamada and Hirayama also observed a similar effect and speculated that it may be due to a hyper-arousal state provoked by levodopa [44]. Regarding the relationship between P3 latency and neuropsychological testings, Hansch *et al.* reported that the Symbol Digit Modalities Test, but not the Mini-Mental State Examination (MMSE) showed correlation with P3 latency [33]. O'Brien *et al.* showed that P3 latency was correlated with MMSE score and other psychological measures, indicating that cognitive decline influences P3 latency [45].

Table 11.1 Auditory oddball P300 latency and amplitude in non-demented Parkinson's disease patients

Study	Medication	Latency	Amplitude
Hansch et al. (1982) [33]	+	↑	N
Goodin and Aminoff (1987) [35]	+	N	N
Amabile et al. (1990) [36]	+	N	N
	–	↑	N
Prasher and Findlay (1991) [38]	+	↑	N
	–	N	N
Ebmeier et al. (1992) [39]	+	N	N
Vieregge et al. (1994) [40]	+	N	N
Green et al. (1996) [41]	+	N	↑
Lagopoulos et al. (1998) [42]	+/–	N	N
Iijima et al. (2000) [43]	+	↑	N
Tanaka et al. (2000) [14]	+	N	↑

Medication: +, on levodopa treatment; –, off levodopa treatment.

N: normal; ↑: prolonged (latency) or increased (amplitude).

ERP during the performance of visual discrimination tasks was also studied. Tachibana et al. reported that P3 latency was normal in non-demented PD, but it was significantly prolonged in demented PD patients [46]. However, they observed that during semantic discrimination tasks, P3 latency was significantly prolonged even in non-demented PD patients as compared with the controls [47]. Wang et al. used the same methods as those of Tachibana et al., and showed that P3 latency was delayed in non-demented PD patients only when long interstimulus intervals (5100 ms) were used [48,49]. Some of these discrepancies may appear to be task specific, depending on both stimulus modality and response requirements. Bodis-Wollner et al. studied auditory and visual ERP in non-demented PD patients and found that visual P3 was prolonged but auditory P3 was not [50]. It is possible that early non-demented PD patients performed normally in the more simple decision tasks, but had a significant slowing of decision process in complicated tasks with higher cognitive load. Somatosensory ERP were less well studied. Ito showed that P3 latency was significantly prolonged compared with that in controls in PD patients with dementia, AD, and vascular dementia [51].

P3 amplitude has mostly been reported to be normal with auditory oddball paradigm, but some investigators showed an increased amplitude in non-demented PD patients. Green et al. showed enlarged P3 amplitude in unmedicated mild PD patients, and speculated that it reflects abnormality in the use of attentional resources to compensate for brain dysfunction [41]. Tanaka et al. reported increased P3 amplitude and resting EEG total power in non-demented PD, but both of them decreased with increasing dementia [14]. Future prospective studies will determine whether increased P3 and EEG amplitude in intellectually normal PD patients is a predictor of later intellectual changes. Iijima et al.

reported that topographical mapping (TM) of P300 demonstrated abnormal distribution in four of 20 non-demented PD patients and three of them showed frontal shift [43]. Its significance is difficult to determine, since their P300 latencies were normal. P3 latency has been considered to be the index of the time for controlled information processing, whereas P3 TM and amplitude are the indices of selective attention to stimulation and allocation of information resources. Wang *et al.* used a visual oddball and an S1–S2 paradigm to evoke ERP and showed decreased P3 amplitude only in S1–S2 paradigm, but not in the usual oddball paradigm in non-demented PD patients [48].

Non-target P3 (P3a, novelty P3, no-go P3)

Two types of P3 have been reported in normal subjects; one is a parietal maximal P3 component designated as P3b and the other is a fronto-central or sometimes parietal maximal P3 component named P3a [53,54]. P3a is elicited by unexpected neutral stimuli under conditions of passive attention. Tachibana *et al.* studied actively and passively evoked P3 components (P3a and P3b) using visual discrimination tasks [53]. P3a and P3b were identified as responses to infrequent target stimuli and infrequent non-target stimuli. Although P3b latency was prolonged in demented PD patients, P3a latency was normal. In AD, however, both P3a and P3b latencies were prolonged. They suggested that the automatic processing stage associated with P3a may be less impaired than the attention-controlled processing reflected by P3b in patients with PD [53].

Hozumi *et al.* studied auditory ERP topography in 15 non-demented PD patients, using two kinds of novelty tones (10% each) added to target tones (20%) [55]. Patients had shorter P3a latencies to the novel stimuli and a more frontal distribution on the P3 map. These findings suggest that decreased mental switching causes lack of novelty P3 habituation in PD and that it is related to learning disabilities due to dysfunction of the frontal lobe and basal ganglia.

No-go ERPs are known to reflect the process of inhibition of motor responses. Iijima *et al.* studied push/wait paradigm no-go P3 using two Japanese Kanji words: 'push' as the go stimulus and 'wait' as the no-go stimulus [52]. The latency of go P3 did not differ significantly between PD and controls, but the no-go P3 had a longer latency in non-demented PD patients than in controls. They concluded that the process of inhibition of motor response declines earlier than does its production process, and no-go P3 might be a useful tool for evaluating inhibitory cognitive function in PD.

N100, P200, N200 (N1, P2, N2)

Although Goodin and Aminoff reported that N1 latency was prolonged in the demented group of PD as compared with the non-demented PD and control subjects, subsequent reports showed normal N1 and P2 latencies even in demented PD patients [46,56]. Ebmeier *et al.* reported increased P2 and N2 latencies in non-demented PD patients, and particularly increased peak latencies of N2 were moderately associated with Parkinsonian motor impairment and Benton Multiple Choice Visual Retention Test [39]. N2 response can be divided into two components, NA and N2, and they reflect stages of processing associated with pattern recognition and stimulus classification, respectively [57].

Tachibana *et al.* also obtained NA and N2 components by subtraction methods and applied these to non-demented PD patients [46]. They found that N2 latency was significantly longer than that of controls although NA latency was normal. These results suggest that the automatic processing stage associated with NA may be less impaired than the attention-controlled processing reflected by N2 in patients with PD [46]. Wang *et al.* also found delayed N200 latency with visual S1–S2 paradigm [48].

Mismatch negativity (MMN) (N2a)

The MMN reflects the automatic aspect of attention and it is elicited by deviant stimuli when compared with standard stimuli. Vieregge *et al.* studied MMN during their two-channel selective auditory attention task. They measured MMN by subtracting the average of ignored standard tones from the average of the ignored deviant tones. MMN was not different between PD patients and controls, indicating that there is no gross preattentive deficit in PD [40]. Karayanidis *et al.* also found that MMN in PD showed little further disruption with ageing [58].

Processing negativity (PN)

Selective attention refers to the ability to focus on one channel of information in the presence of other distracting channels [59]. The auditory ERP evoked by the attended tones are negatively shifted in relation to those of unattended tones. The shift often begins before the peak of the N1 wave and may last for several hundred milliseconds. It is called processing negativity (PN) and is attributed to the subjects' maintenance of a vivid internal template of the attended stimulus. PN was significantly smaller in the PD patients than in the controls, providing evidence for an impairment of auditory selective attention in PD patients (59).

Contingent negative variation (CNV)

Changes in attention and response preparation are reflected by CNV. Analysis of components in the cue–target interval permits an assessment of cue processing and response preparation that occurs prior to an anticipated target stimulus. Wright *et al.* showed greatly reduced CNV for the PD group during a task involving covert orientation of visual attention [59]. Oishi *et al.* examined CNV and movement-related cortical potentials using S1 (click)–S2 (flash)–key press paradigm [60]. The amplitude of early CNV was smaller in the PD group than in the control group. However, the amplitude increased significantly after levodopa infusion, indicating that a small amplitude of the early CNV is related to decreased levels of dopaminergic activity [60,61].

MIBG myocardial scintigraphy

Metaiodobenzylguanidine (MIBG) is a physiological analogue of noradrenaline (norepinephrine), and ^{123}I-MIBG myocardial scintigraphy is used to evaluate postganglionic cardiac sympathetic innervation [62]. This method has been briefly mentioned in Chapter 10 and will be described more in detail here. Recent studies have shown that reduction of myocardial MIBG uptake is associated with Lewy body diseases such as PD and DLB regardless of the presence of autonomic failure [63–65]. In PD, cardiac uptake tends to decrease as the disease progresses and it decreases more in DLB than in PD [63,66,67]. MIBG myocardial scintigraphy is particularly useful in differentiating PD from atypical parkinsonism such as progressive supranuclear palsy and multiple system atrophy [63,68–70]. It has also been reported to be useful to differentiate DLB from AD; MIBG uptake is markedly reduced in DLB, whereas it is normal in AD [5,6] (Fig. 1). MIBG myocardial scintigraphy is a sensitive tool for discriminating DLB from AD even in patients without parkinsonism [71]. MIBG myocardial scintigraphy is more useful than medial occipital hypoperfusion measurement using SPECT in diagnosing DLB [72]. Likewise Wada-Isoe *et al.* found that the value of MIBG scintigraphy is superior to that of CSF markers such as Aβ42 and p-tau in differentiating AD from DLB [73]. The same group found that the presence of visual hallucinations independently predicted decreased cardiac MIBG uptake [74]. Since its importance has been increasingly recognized, the low MIBG uptake has been included as a supportive feature in the revised criteria for the clinical diagnosis of DLB [16].

Conclusions

EEG abnormalities in patients with PD consist of slowing of the background activities, particularly in demented patients. P3 latency is prolonged in patients with PD-D, but conflicting results are obtained in non-demented PD patients. The conflicting results may be due to both patient selection and methodological differences. P3 amplitude is largely normal or even increased in non-demented PD patients, but it decreases as dementia emerges. N1, P2, and NA components and mismatch negativity are normal, whereas N2, contingent negative variation, and processing negativity are abnormal. These results suggest that the automatic processing stage may be less affected than the attention-controlled processing and that both the speed of cognitive processing and amount of processed

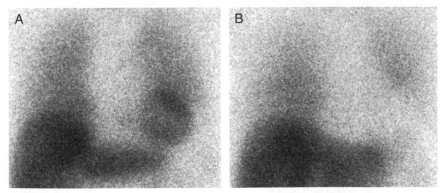

Fig. 11.1 Examples of myocardial ^{123}I-MIBG uptake in a patient with Alzheimer's disease (AD) (left) and a patient with dementia with Lewy bodies (DLB) (right). The myocardial uptake of MIBG is normal in AD, but cardiac accumulation is markedly reduced in DLB.

information decrease as cognitive dysfunction develops in PD. MIBG myocardial scintigraphy is a sensitive tool for discriminating DLB and PD-D from AD.

References

1 Raskin SA, Borod JC, Tweedy J. Neuropsychological aspects of Parkinson's disease. Neuropsychol Rev 1990; 1: 185–221.

2 Biggins CA, Boyd JL, Harrop FM, et al. A controlled, longitudinal study of dementia in Parkinson's disease. J Neurol Neurosurg Psychiatry 1992; 55: 566–71.

3 Bayles KA, Tomoeda CK, Wood JA, et al. Change in cognitive function in idiopathic Parkinson's disease. Arch Neurol 1996; 53: 1140–6.

4 Jacobs DM, Marder K, Cote LJ, Sano M, Stern R, Mayeaux R. Neuropsychological characteristics of preclinical dementia in Parkinson's disease. Neurology 1995; 45: 1691–6.

5 Watanabe H, Iida T, Katayama T, et al. Cardiac ^{123}I-meta-iodobenzylguanidine (MIBG) uptake in dementia with Lewy bodies: comparison with Alzheimer's disease. J Neurol Neurosurg Psychiatry 2001; 70: 781–3.

6 Yoshita M, Taki J, Yamada M. A clinical role for [123I] MIBG myocardial scintigraphy in the distinction between dementia of the Alzheimer's type and dementia with Lewy bodies. J Neurol Neurosurg Psychiatry 2001; 71: 583–8.

7 Sirakov AA, Mezan IS. EEG findings in parkinsonism. Electroencephalogr Clin Neurophysiol 1963; 15: 321–2.

8 Yeager CL, Alberts WW, Delattre LD. Effect of stereotaxic surgery upon electroencephalographic status of parkinsonian patients. Neurology 1966; 16: 904–10.

9 Neufeld MY, Inzelberg R, Korczyn AD. EEG in demented and non-demented parkinsonian patients. Acta Neurol Scand 1988; 78: 1–5.

10 de Weed AW, Perquin WVM, Jonkman EJ. Role of the EEG in the prediction of dementia in Parkinson's disease. Dementia 1990; 1: 115–18.

11 Neufeld MY, Blumen S, Aitkin I, Parmet Y, Korczyn AD. EEG frequency analysis in demented and nondemented Parkinsonian patients. Dementia 1994; 5: 23–8.

12 Soikkeli R, Partanen J, Soininen H, Paakkonen A, Piekkinen P. Slowing of EEG in Parkinson's disease. Electroencehaph Clin Neurophysiol 1991; 79: 159–65.

13 Domitrz I, Friedman A. Electroencephalography of demented and non-demented Parkinson's disease patients. Parkinsonism Relat Disord 1999; 5: 37–41.

14 Tanaka H, Koenig T, Pascual-Marqui RD, Hirata K, Kochi K, Lehmann D. Event-related potential and EEG measures in Parkinson's disease without and with dementia. Dement Geriatr Cogn Disord 2000; 11: 39–45.

15 Bonanni L, Thomas A, Tiraboschi P, Perfetti B, Varanese S, Onofrj M. EEG comparisons in early Alzheimer's disease, dementia with Lewy disease and Parkinson's disease with dementia patients with a 2-year follow-up. Brain 2008; 131: 690–705.

16 McKeith IG, Dickson DW, Lowe J, et al. Diagnosis and management of dementia with Lewy bodies: third report of the DLB Consortium. Neurology 2005; 65: 1863–72.

17 Gawel MJ, Das P, Vincent S, Rose FC. Visual and auditory evoked responses in patients with Parkinson's disease. J Neurol Neurosurg Psychiatry 1981; 44: 227–32.

18 Prasher D, Bannister R. Brain stem auditory evoked potentials in patients with multiple system atrophy with progressive autonomic failure (Shy–Drager syndrome). J Neurol Neurosurg Psychiatry 1986; 49: 278–89.

19 Tachibana H, Takeda M, Sugita M. Short-latency somatosensory and brainstem auditory evoked potentials in patients with Parkinson's disease. Int J Neurosci 1989; 44: 321–6.

20 Green JB, Flagg L, Freed DM, Schwankhaus JD. The middle latency auditory evoked potential may be abnormal in dementia. Neurology 1992; 42: 1034–6.

21 Buchwald JS, Erwin S, Read D, *et al.* Midlatency auditory evoked responses: differential abnormality of P1 in Alzheimer's disease. Electroenchephalogr Clin Neurophysiol 1989; 74: 378–84.

22 Bodis-Wollner I, Yahr MD. Measurements of visual evoked potentials in Parkinson's disease. Brain 1978; 101: 661–71.

23 Dinner DS, Luders H, Hanson M, Lesser RP. Pattern evoked potentials (PEPs) in Parkinson's disease. Neurology 1985; 35: 610–13.

24 Nightingale S, Mitchell KW, Howe JW. Visual evoked cortical potentials and pattern electroretinograms in Parkinson's disease and control subjects. J Neurol Neurosurg Psychiatry 1986; 49: 1280–7.

25 Calzetti S, Franchi A, Taratufolo G, Groppi E. Simultaneous VEP and PERG investigations in early Parkinson's disease. J Neurol Neurosurg Psychiatry 1990; 53: 114–17.

26 Okuda B, Tachibana H, Kawabata M, Takeda K, Toda K, Sugita M. Correlation of visual evoked potentials with dementia in Parkinson's disease. Jpn J Geriat 1992; 29: 475–9.

27 Koller WC. Sensory symptoms in Parkinson's disease. Neurology 1984; 34: 957–9.

28 Rossini PM, Babiloni F, Bernardi G, *et al.* Abnormalities of short-latency somatosensory evoked potentials in parkinsonian patients. Electroencephalogr Clin Neurophysiol 1989; 74: 277–89.

29 Potolicchio SJ Jr, O'Doherty DS. Somatosensory evoked potentials in subcortical and cortical lesions. In: Nodar RH, Barber C (eds). Evoked potentials II. Second International Evoked Potentials Symposium. London: Butterworth, 1984; pp. 423–31.

30 Polich J. P300 in clinical applications: meaning, method, and management. Am J EEG Technol 1991; 31: 201–31.

31 Goodin DS, Squires KC, Starr A. Long latency event-related components of the auditory evoked potential in dementia. Brain 1978; 101: 635–48.

32 Goodin DS, Squires K, Henderson B, Starr A. Age-related variations in evoked potentials to auditory stimuli in normal human subjects. Electroencephalogr Clin Neurophysiol 1978; 44: 447–458.

33 Hansch EC, Syndulko K, Cohen SN, *et al.* Cognition in Parkinson disease: an event-related potential perspective. Ann Neurol 1982; 11: 599–607.

34 Goodin DS, Aminoff MJ. Electrophysiological differences between subtypes of dementia. Brain 1986; 109: 1103–1113.

35 Goodin DS, Aminoff MJ. Electrophysiological differences between demented and nondemented patients with Parkinson's disease. Ann Neurol 1987; 21: 90–4.

36 Amabile G, Fattapposta F, Pierelli F. Evoked potentials in Parkinson's disease: sensory and cognitive aspects. A review. J Psychophysiol 1990; 4: 115–22.

37 Starkstein SE, Esteguy M, Berthier ML, Garcia H, Leiguarda R. Evoked potentials, reaction time and cognitive performance in on and off phases of Parkinson's disease. J Neurol Neurosurg Psychiatry 1989; 52: 338–40.

38 Prasher D, Findley L. Dopaminergic induced changes in cognitive and motor processing in Parkinson's disease: an electrophysiological investigation. J Neurol Neurosurg Psychiatry 1991; 54: 603–9.

39 Ebmeier KP, Potter DD, Cochrane RHB, *et al.* Event related potentials, reaction time, and cognitive performance in idiopathic Parkinson's disease. Biol Psychol 1992; 33: 73–89.

40 Vieregge P, Verleger R, Wascher E, Stuven F, Kompf D. Auditory selective attention is impaired in Parkinson's disease – event-related evidence from EEG potentials. Cogn Brain Res 1994; 2: 117–29.

41 Green J, Woodard JL, Sirockman BE, *et al.* Event-related potential P3 change in mild Parkinson's disease. Mov Disord 1996; 11: 33–42.

42 Lagopoulos J, Clouston P, Barhamali H, *et al.* Late components of the event-related potentials and their topography in Parkinson's disease. Mov Disord 1998; 2: 262–7.

43 Iijima M, Osawa M, Ushijima R, Iwata M. Nogo event-related potentials in Parkinson's disease. Electoroencephalogr Clin Neurophysiol 1999; 49(Suppl): 199–203.

44 Yamada T, Hirayama K. Effect of L-dopa on P300 component – study in patients with juvenile parkinsonism having wearing off phenomena. Clin Neurol 1987; 27: 53–7.

45 O'Donnell BF, Squires NK. Evoked potentials changes and neuropsychological performance in Parkinson's disease. Biol Psychol 1987; 24: 23–7.

46 Tachibana H, Aragane K, Miyata Y, Sugita M. Electrophysiological analysis of cognitive slowing in Parkinson's disease. J Neurol Sci 1997; 149: 47–56.

47 Tachibana H, Aragane K, Kawabata K, Sugita M. P3 latency change in aging and Parkinson's disease. Arch Neurol 1997; 54: 296–302.

48 Wang L, Kuroiwa Y, Kamitani T. Visual event-related potential changes at two different tasks in nondemented Parkinson's disease. J Neurol Sci 1999; 164: 139–47.

49 Wang L, Kuroiwa Y, Kamitani T, Takahashi T, Suzuki Y, Hasegawa O. Effect of interstimulus interval on visual P300 in Parkinson's disease. J Neurol Neurosurg Psychiatry 1999; 67: 497–503.

50 Bodis-Wollner I, Borod JC, Cicero B, *et al.* Modality dependent changes in event-related potentials correlate with specific cognitive functions in nondemented patients with Parkinson's disease. J Neural Transm 1995; 9: 197–209.

51 Ito J. Somatosensory event-related potentials (ERPs) in patients with different types of dementia. J Neurol Sci 1994; 121: 139–46.

52 Iijima M, Osawa M, Iwata M, Miyazaki A, Tei H. Topographic mapping of P300 and frontal cognitive function in Parkinson's disease. Behav Neurol 2000; 12: 143–8.

53 Tachibana H, Toda K, Sugita M. Actively and passively evoked P3 latency of event-related potentials in Parkinson's disease. J Neurol Sci 1992; 111: 134–42.

54 Squires NK, Squires KC, Hillyard SA. Two varieties of long-latency positive waves evoked by unpredictable auditory stimuli. Electroencephalogr Clin Neurophysiol 1975; 38: 387–401.

55 Hozumi A, Hirata K, Tanaka H, Yamazaki K. Perseveration for novel stimuli in Parkinson's disease: an evaluation based on event-related potentials topography. Mov Disord, 2000; 15: 835–42.

56 Filipovic S, Kostic VS, Sternic N, Marinkovic Z, Ocic G. Auditory event-related potentials in different types of dementia. Eur Neurol 1990; 30: 189–93.

57 Ritter W, Simson R, Vaughan HG. Event-related potentials correlates of two stages of information processing in physical and semantic discrimination tasks. Psychophysiology 1983; 20: 168–79.

58 Karayanidis F, Andrews S, Ward PB, Michie PT. ERP indices of auditory selective attention in aging and Parkinson's disease. Psychophysiology 1995; 32: 335–50.

59 Wright MJ, Geffen GM, Geffen LB. Event-related potentials associated with covert orientation of visual attention in Parkinson's disease. Neuropsychologia 1993; 31: 1283–97.

60 Oishi M, Mochizuki Y, Du C, Takasu T. Contingent negative variation and movement-related cortical potentials in parkinsonism. Electroencephalogr Clin Neurophysiol 1995; 95: 346–9.

61 Amabile G, Fattapposta F, Pozzessere G, *et al.* Parkinson disease: electrophysiological (CNV) analysis related to pharmacological treatment. Electroencephalogr Clin Neurophysiol 1986; 64: 521–4.

62 Wieland DM, Brown LE, Rogers WL, *et al.* Myocardial imaging with a radioiodinated norepinephrine storage analog. J Nucl Med 1981; 22: 22–31.

63 Orimo S, Ozawa E, Nakade S, Sugimoto T, Mizusawa H. ^{123}I-metaiodobenzylguanidine myocardial scintigraphy in Parkinson's disease. J Neurol Neurosurg Psychiatry 1999; 67: 189–94.

64 Braune S, Reinhardt M, Schnitzer R, Riedel A, Lucking CH. Cardiac uptake of MIBG separates Parkinson's disease from multiple system atrophy. Neurology 1999; 53: 1020–5.

65 Taki J, Nakajima K, Hwang E-H, *et al.* Peripheral sympathetic dysfunction in patients with Parkinson's disease without autonomic failure is heart selective and disease specific. Eur J Nucl Med 2000; 27: 566–73.

66 Saiki S, Hirose G, Sakai K, *et al.* Cardiac ^{123}I-MIBG scintigraphy can assess the disease severity and phenotype of PD. J Neurol Sci, 2004; 220: 105–11.

67 Suzuki M, Kurita A, Hashimoto M, *et al.* Impaired myocardial ^{123}I-metaiodobenzylguanidine uptake in Lewy body disese: comparison between dementia with Lewy bodies and Parkinson's disease. J Neurol Sci 2006; 240: 15–19.

68 Yoshita M. Differentiation of idiopathic Parkinson's disease from striatonigral degeneration and progressive supranuclear palsy using iodine-123 meta-iodobenzylguanidine myocardial scintigraphy. J Neurol Sci 1998; 155: 60–7.

69 Druschky A, Hilz MJ, Platsch G, *et al.* Differentiation of Parkinson's disease and multiple system atrophy in early disease stages by means of I-123-MIBG-SPECT. J Neurol Sci 2000; 175: 3–12.

70 Nagayama H, Hamamoto M, Ueda M, Nagashima J, Katayama Y. Reliability of MIBG myocardial scintigraphy in the diagnosis of Parkinson's disease. J Neurol Neurosurg Psychiatry 2005; 76: 249–51.

71 Yoshita M, Taki J, Yokoyama K, *et al.* Value of [123]I -MIBG radioactivity in the differential diagnosis of DLB from AD. Neurology 2006; 66: 1850–4.

72 Hanyu H, Shimizu S, Hirao K, *et al.* Comparative value of brain perfusion SPECT and [^{123}I]-MIBG myocardial scintigraphy in distinguishing between dementia with Lewy bodies and Alzheimer's disease. Eur J Nucl Med Mol Imaging 2006; 33: 248–53.

73 Wada-Isoe K, Kitayama M, Nakaso K, Nakashima K. Diagnostic markers for diagnosing dementia with Lewy bodies: CSF and MIBG cardiac scintigraphy study. J Neurol Sci 2007; 260: 33–7.

74 Kitayama M, Wada-Isoe K, Irizawa Y, Nakashima K. Association of visual hallucinations with reduction of MIBG cardiac uptake in Parkinson's disease. J Neurol Sci 2008; 264: 22–6.

Chapter 12

Genetic basis of dementia in Parkinson's disease

Rita Guerreiro and Andrew Singleton

Introduction

Parkinson's disease (PD) is a heterogeneous disease both genetically and arguably also clinically. A simple goal, with complicated means, is to dissect out the role of genetics in the clinical heterogeneity of PD. The occurrence of dementia in PD, in particular, has been a target of this type of genotype–phenotype research. In the last 10 years genetics has taken a major role in the understanding of the pathobiological underpinnings of PD. However, the role of genetics in PD with dementia (PD-D) is still poorly understood. In this chapter we examine the evidence for a genetic component of PD-D, first by reviewing studies of familial PD-D and reporting on the genes and mutations involved, then by discussing the role of genetic risk factors such as ApoE, the best-known genetic risk factor for Alzheimer's disease (AD). Finally, we examine the expected next steps in the genetics research that are likely to yield insight into the basis of PD-D, in light of the new technologies currently available.

Finding genes that underlie disease

Disease genetics is a discipline that aims to detect a signal in the background of an extremely large amount of noise, the proverbial 'needle in a haystack'. We can be most sure of the results and most confident in success, when a systematic genome-wide approach is taken to define a risk or causative locus; this approach does not rely on a perceived understanding of the processes underlying disease to nominate genes of interest for interrogation. As a consequence the most successful genetic approaches in PD have been those centred on, or founded on evidence from, family-based studies, where genome-wide linkage (a method that surveys the whole genome to define segregation between DNA segments and disease) and positional cloning (analysis of those segments for mutations) are used.

Family-based genetic work has led to the identification of several genes that contain mutations that cause PD, and some of the patients with these mutations progress to, or even present with, dementia. Because dementia is a relatively common occurrence in the ageing population, a critical question is whether the co-occurring dementia observed in these PD families is related to the underlying PD aetiology or just a random coincidence. This is not necessarily an easy question to answer; although one can compare age-matched incidence rates between the population and patients within families that harbour particular mutations, the number of people in the latter group affected by these mutations is relatively low (with some exceptions discussed later). With this in mind, the next section will discuss the incidence of dementia in monogenic forms of PD. Herein we will concentrate on the two autosomal dominant forms of PD. Whereas mutation in three genes has been linked to young-onset autosomal recessive forms of PD [1–3], patients with PD caused by mutations in these genes are rarely reported to show signs of dementia.

Gene mutations known to cause PD associated with dementia

SNCA (PARK1, PARK4; encoding the protein α-synuclein)

The first key advance that occurred in the genetics of PD is closely related with PD-D. This happened when a large kindred with early-onset, Lewy-body-positive autosomal dominant PD was studied [4] and a missense mutation (A53T) in the gene encoding α-synuclein identified [5].

Although mutations in *SNCA* have been found to be very rare in patients with PD, they did provide the first clue that this protein is involved in the molecular pathway leading to this disease. The utility of studying rare familial forms of a disease in understanding the more common, apparently sporadic, forms became evident when Lewy bodies and Lewy neuritis present in sporadic PD were found to contain aggregates of α-synuclein [6]. This work neatly demonstrated a commonality between familial and sporadic disease and placed α-synuclein at the centre of scientific research into PD. Three missense mutations have been identified in α-synuclein to date (A53T, A30P and E46K) [5,7,8]; further, several families have now been described where the cause of PD lies in the genetic burden of α-synuclein: patients presenting with one or two extra copies of this gene (locus duplication and triplication respectively) [9]. PD-D and dementia with Lewy bodies (DLB) were explicitly described as the presenting diseases in the family carrying the E46K mutation; however, it is clear that dementia occurs as a common feature of families linked to α-synuclein mutation, both missense and copy number (Table 12.1).

It is also worth noting that within the families where disease is caused by α-synuclein locus multiplication, the genetic load appears to be correlated with both the severity of disease and the presence/absence of dementia. Thus, patients who carry two additional copies of α-synuclein tend to present in their thirties and the disease progresses to include severe dementia, whereas patients who carry only one additional copy of α-synuclein tend to get disease a decade or so later and dementia is not as frequent a feature (although it does still occur) [9,17,18]. The prevalence of dementia in these families argues strongly that this is truly a facet of the disease process and not simply coincidental. This notion is supported by neuropathological examination of patients that carry these mutations, which reveals a widespread and severe α-synuclein pathology involving neocortical as well as archecortical systems [19].

Table 12.1 Kindreds for Parkinson's disease with dementia where a genetic lesion in *SNCA* has been associated with the disease

Gene	Mutation	Study	No. of affected individuals	Neuropathology		
				Autopsy	AD	Lewy bodies
SNCA	A53T	Globe *et al.* (1990) [10] Globe *et al.* (1996) [11] Duda *et al.* (2002) [12]	60	2	0	2 (SN + NC)
		Spira *et al.* (2001) [13]	5	2	0	1 (SN + NC) 1 (SN)
	Triplication	Waters and Miller (1994) [14] Muenter *et al.* (1998) [15] Farrer *et al.* (1999) [16] Singleton *et al.* (2003) [9]	22	6	0	6 (SN + NC)
	E46K	Zarranz *et al.* (2004) [8]	5	1	0	1 (SN + NC)

SN, substantia nigra; NC, neocortex; AD, Alzheimer-type pathology.

LRRK2 (PARK8; encoding the protein Lrrk2/dardarin)

The *LRRK2* (Leucine-rich repeat kinase 2) gene, located in chromosome 12 (12q12), encodes the protein dardarin. This contains both GTPase and kinase domains, as well as two protein–protein interaction domains (leucine-rich and WD40 repeats) [20]. In 2004, mutations in this gene were associated with the development of PD in several kindreds [21,22]. Since then, pathogenic *LRRK2* substitutions have become recognized as one of the most important causes of both familial and sporadic forms of PD [23–25].

While the majority of patients with *LRRK2*-linked disease present with a phenotype that is clinically indistinguishable from typical PD, there are several case reports of patients who present with clinically and neuropathologically atypical forms of disease [22]. Two members of family A (one of the families where mutations in *LRRK2* were first described as associated with PD) [22] presented with dementia in the absence of parkinsonian symptoms and carried the Y1699C amino acid change [26]. More recently, a novel mutation (L1165P) was found in a PD patient who developed severe neuropsychological symptoms and dementia [27], although in this instance the pathogenicity of this mutation is not proven.

The most common *LRRK2* mutation in Caucasian populations is the G2019S variant, which affects a key residue in the kinase domain of this large complex protein. This variant appears to underlie disease in about 2% of all North American cases of PD and a higher proportion in Portuguese PD patients (~8%) [24], Ashkenazi Jewish PD patients (~20%) [28], and North African Berber Arab PD patients (~40%) [29]. Overall, the prevalence of cognitive dysfunction and dementia among *LRRK2* G2019S patients is low [30,31]. This is an important finding since *LRRK2* is located on chromosome 12q12 and this locus has previously been associated with late-onset AD [32] and there was some speculation that variability at this locus could underlie both diseases. While dementia is not necessarily a common feature of G2019S linked disease it is not clear whether the co-occurrence of dementia takes place more often that one would expect by chance. In this regard, the high frequency of G2019S mutations in the PD population offers a unique opportunity to examine prevalence rates of dementia in a genetic form of PD, and this type of work is a clear aim of the many groups worldwide working on prospective study of *LRRK2*-linked patients and their relatives.

Other dementias with parkinsonism

Synucleinopathies

The clinical expression of mutations in genes proven to be associated with different dementias is variable. Some of these mutations may give rise to parkinsonian syndromes and thus these genes may be of potential importance in the development of dementia in PD. For example, mutations of *PSEN1* and *PSEN2* cause a familial form of young-onset AD. In *PSEN1* the G217D mutation was found in a Japanese family affected by a disease characterized by dementia, parkinsonism, a stooped posture and an antiflexion gait with an onset in the fourth decade of life. Neuropathologically, the disease was characterized by the presence of 'cotton wool' plaques, senile plaques, severe amyloid angiopathy, neurofibrillary tangles, neuronal rarefaction and gliosis [33]. In *PSEN2*, the A85V mutation was found in an Italian family in which the proband was diagnosed with DLB. All the other affected members exhibited a clinical phenotype of AD. Neuropathologically, the proband presented with unusually abundant and widespread cortical Lewy bodies in addition to the hallmark lesions of AD [34]. These cases further emphasize the overlap existing between PD, PD-D and DLB.

DLB is a pathology mainly characterized by dementia and parkinsonism, among other distinguishing features. The question whether PD-D and DLB are different entities or different demonstrations of the same pathological spectrum has been extensively discussed (including elsewhere in this book); however, it is important to stress that even fully penetrant, autosomal dominant mutations may lead to different clinical phenotypes across the spectrum of PD-D, DLB and beyond. Families with mutations in *SNCA* emphasize this premise: (1) the family described by Zarranz *et al.* includes individuals carrying the same mutation (E46K) with PD-D and DLB phenotypes within the same cohort [8]; (2) multiplications of the *SNCA* locus may lead to either PD-D or DLB [17,35,9]. Neuropathological examination of brain tissue from dominantly inherited forms of AD and from Down's syndrome patients frequently reveals Lewy body pathology. Mutations in *LRRK2* may lead to α-synuclein, tau or ubiquitin pathology with or without Lewy bodies. Clearly there are multiple genetic factors that can trigger the formation of Lewy bodies, irrespective of the disease phenotype, and this implicitly links the underlying molecular aetiology of these diseases to that of PD.

Multiple system atrophy (MSA) is the second most common parkinsonian syndrome after idiopathic PD, presenting clinically with various combinations of parkinsonism, cerebellar ataxia and autonomic failure. Even though cognitive dysfunction appears to be minimal, the majority of patients have frontal system impairment and some develop dementia late in the course of the disease. Pathologically, it is characterized by glial cytoplasmic inclusions mainly composed by α-synuclein. MSA is usually a sporadic disease, but the fact that several MSA patients have relatives with PD led to the study of various genes. Clearly, from a molecular pathology point of view, the most plausible gene responsible for MSA pathogenesis is *SNCA*. Although genetic analysis of pathologically confirmed MSA cases has failed to find any pathogenic mutations in *SNCA* [36] it is clear that common genetic variability at this locus confers risk for MSA [37].

Tauopathies

Tauopathies are a heterogeneous group of neurodegenerative diseases that share the presence of aberrant tau aggregates [38]. Tau is a microtubule-associated protein that binds to tubulin and works to stabilize microtubules and promote microtubule assembly [39]. The *MAPT* gene is located in an atypical genomic region of chromosome 17 and produces six isoforms of the tau protein by alternative splicing of exons 2, 3 and 10 [40]. The interaction of tau with the microtubules occurs through three (3R) or four (4R) imperfect repeat sequences in the carboxyl terminal of the protein. One of these four domains is encoded by exon 10; hence, the alternative splicing of this exon determines the number of microtubule-binding domains. In the adult human brain, 3R and 4R tau are present in approximately equal quantities [41].

Several pathogenic mutations in the *MAPT* gene have been associated with different clinical phenotypes. These mutations appear clustered between exons 9 and 13 of the gene and may be roughly divided into two categories, depending on the pathogenic mechanism involved: protein function and splicing regulation mutations. The first group of mutations impairs the ability of tau to interact with microtubules or to promote microtubule assembly; the second corresponds to mutations located in exon 10 (with the exception of those occurring in codon 301) and in flanking intronic regions that affect the alternative splicing of this exon and consequently increase the 4R/3R tau ratio. 4R tau appears to aggregate more readily than 3R tau, thus overproduction of 4R tau may lead to an excess of free 4R and consequently promote tau aggregation [42].

The most frequent phenotype associated with *MAPT* mutations is frontotemporal dementia with parkinsonism linked to chromosome 17 (FTDP-17). This is a familial disorder mainly characterized by behavioural and cognitive disturbances with progression to dementia followed by parkinsonism. The clinical spectrum associated with *MAPT* mutations is, however, extensive. The same mutation may cause different clinical expressions in different families and even within the same family. This is the case with the most frequent *MAPT* mutation: P301L that has been associated with cases resembling Pick's disease, corticobasal degeneration, and progressive supranuclear palsy [43,44]. Whereas it can be clearly argued that FTDP and PD-D are undoubtedly distinct entities, recent evidence implicating genetic variability in *MAPT* to lifetime risk for PD suggests that expression of this protein is a critical factor in PD, despite the general lack of tau pathology in this disease (discussed further below).

Genetic risk factors for PD-D

The identification of rare causal mutations for PD and PD-D has been extremely success-ful over the previous decade, yet the search for genetic variants that alter risk for disease has been more difficult. The primary work in this area has been done in PD cohorts that include patients both with and without dementia; this is primarily because such cohorts are easier to collect and more readily available. In the instances where PD-D has been separated out as a distinct entity, the sample size tends to be quite low. As the genetics field is now appreciating, to discover novel genetic loci that exert an effect in complex diseases, cohorts of several thousand cases are required, and thus success for PD-D in this area will require a concerted effort to collect larger sample sizes.

ApoE

The ApoE ε4 allele is probably the best-known genetic risk factor in adult onset human disease. This variant confers substantial risk for AD, heterozygous carriers being approx-imately three times more likely to develop the disease and homozygous carriers eight times more likely to develop AD. Apolipoprotein E (ApoE) is a glycoprotein involved in the transport of lipoproteins, fat-soluble vitamins and cholesterol into the lymph system and then into the blood. ApoE is synthesized and secreted by many tissues, primarily liver, brain, skin, and tissue macrophages throughout the body, sites where it plays criti-cally important roles [45]. The gene coding for ApoE resides on the long arm of chromo-some 19 in a cluster with Apolipoprotein C1 and Apolipoprotein C2. It is a polymorphic gene with three major alleles, ApoE2, ApoE3 and ApoE4, which translate into three isoforms of the protein: ApoE-ε3; ApoE-ε2 and ApoE-ε4. These isoforms differ from each other by amino acid substitutions at positions 112 and 158 [46].

Although APOE is neither necessary nor sufficient for the development of AD, its risk has been shown to be dose dependent and correlated with the age at onset of the disease [47]. Given the robust association between ApoE and AD it has been hypothesized that a similar relationship exists with PD-D and DLB. Several studies have evaluated the role of ApoE in dementia associated with PD with contradictory results [48–51]. As noted above, however, these studies are individually of quite limited sample size. A meta-analysis of the studies published between 1966 and 2004 concluded that the ApoE E4 allele appears to be associated with a higher prevalence of dementia in PD (with an increased odds ratio of 1.6). The ApoE-ε4 variant has been clearly associated with DLB [52], lending further support for the idea that PD-D, DLB and AD are, at least in part, members of an aetiological spectrum of disorders.

Other genetic risk factors for PD-D

The primary catalyst for the investigation of genetic risk factors associated with PD-D comes from previous association with AD, PD or DLB. Given sample size requirements mentioned above and the numerous confounds in candidate gene association studies, robust genetic associations in these diseases have been relatively few and far between. In PD probably the most consistent genetic risk associations are with common variants in

SNCA and *MAPT*, although even these associations have not been without controversy [53–55]. Nonetheless, the overall results tend towards an association with PD for both *SNCA* and *MAPT*.

Most of the studies evaluating the role of genetic variants in MAPT and SNCA in the risk of developing PD-D failed to find significant association [53,56,57]. Divergent results suggesting that the tau inversion influences the development of cognitive impairment and dementia in patients with idiopathic PD were reported by Goris *et al.* when studying 659 PD patients, 109 of which were followed up for 3.5 years from diagnosis, and 2176 control subjects. Although only 11 of the incident cohort of 109 PD patients experienced the development of new-onset dementia during the 3.5 years of follow-up, H1 homozygotes presented a greater rate of cognitive decline than H2 carriers, assessed by the changes observed in Mini-Mental State Examination per year. Similarly, a case–control study investigating the role of genetic variability in *SNCA* showed no associations with PD-D. Six polymorphic loci (including the Rep1 microsatellite) in the promoter of the *SNCA* gene were examined in 114 demented patients and 114 non-demented patients with sporadic PD [58]. In this case the absence of evidence does not imply evidence of absence; without exception these studies comprise relatively small case numbers, particularly when considering the number of patients with cognitive decline or dementia. It is therefore difficult to rule out variability at *SNCA* or *MAPT* as a risk factor for PD-D until well-powered comprehensive studies have been performed. Given the association between the *MAPT* haplotype and other dementing illnesses, parsimony would suggest an association with PD-D; however, time and well-structured analyses will tell.

Additionally, case–control analysis of variants in *COMT* [59], *CYPD6* [60], *MAOB* [61], *GSK3B* [62], *BCHE* [63] and *ESR1* [64] suggest that these loci present no significant risk in the development of PD-D. Contrarily, the interaction between a DCP1 insertion polymorphism and ApoE4 was reported to increase the risk of PD with coexisting AD pathology [63]. A possible role for gene–toxin interactions in PD-D was also revealed when a high predicted probability for developing PD-D was established in PD patients carrying a particular CYP2D6 allele that were exposed to pesticides [61]. Again, these results should be considered preliminary until they have been replicated in further well-powered series.

Next steps in gene identification for dementia in PD

As we discussed at the beginning of this chapter, identification of genetic factors for disease appears to be most successful when a relatively unbiased genome-wide approach can be taken, rather than a focused candidate gene analysis. Technological limitations have previously made it unfeasible to take this kind of approach in association mapping (as opposed to linkage mapping), revealing candidate gene association work the primary tenable alternative. The development of high throughput genotyping platforms in the past 3 years has now made genome-wide association a realistic possibility. Such platforms are capable of accurately genotyping hundreds of thousands of SNPs in parallel and this method has now been successfully applied to identify risk loci in many complex diseases [65].

Successful identification of genetic variability that confers risk for disease by Genome Wide Association Studies depends on many factors, including sample size, population homogeneity and effect size (described comprehensively elsewhere) [66]. Nevertheless, the primary limitation for PD-D will be one of sample size and agreement on diagnostic criteria for this disorder. Even as common genetic risk loci for PD-D are identified, many challenges will exist; most immediate will be fine mapping of these loci (i.e. a better understanding of the actual alleles that confer risk within the risk region) and mapping out the immediate effects of risk variants: which transcripts do they effect, do they alter expression, if so in which way, or do they alter splicing? There is also room for further genetic exploration of complex diseases such as PD-D [66], including deep resequencing to identify rare risk variants, analysis of genomic copy number variation as a risk factor for disease, epigenetic assays to detect a role for this type of variation in disease and deep sequence analysis to define whether somatic mutation may play a role in the development and progression of PD-D. All of these approaches offer unique insights and challenges; however, if the past is a predictor of the future, the availability of techniques to address these issues will occur sooner rather than later, workers in this field should be preparing for the tasks ahead. The most obvious preparation would be collection of large cohorts of well-characterized patients.

Conclusions

SNCA and *LRRK2* mutations are associated with familial forms of PD and patients with these mutations may also exhibit dementia. The genetic basis of dementia occurring in apparently sporadic PD is less well understood, with variability in *APOE* being the only suggested genetic risk factor. The primary goal of disease genetics is to shed light onto the molecular aetiology of disease with an eye toward defining potential points of therapeutic intervention. Clearly there has been substantial progress in the genetics of PD (and implicitly PD-D); however, there is still a long way to go. The tools are now at hand to achieve a more complete understanding of the genetic basis of common complex diseases, including PD-D. Not only will a more complete genetic understanding of these diseases inform from an aetiological basis, but it is also likely to add more clarity to the idea that this disease is aetiologically similar to DLB and AD. There will certainly be challenges to a successful dissection of the genetic basis of PD-D, perhaps the most immediate of which is that of achieving sufficient sample size to detect and confirm genuine genetic association; however, for the first time the route to success is relatively clear.

References

1 Kitada T, Asakawa S, Hattori N, *et al.* Mutations in the parkin gene cause autosomal recessive juvenile parkinsonism. Nature 1998; 392: 605–8.

2 Valente EM, Abou-Sleiman PM, Caputo V, *et al.* Hereditary early-onset Parkinson's disease caused by mutations in PINK1. Science 2004; 304: 1158–60.

3 Bonifati V, Rizzu P, van Baren MJ, *et al.* Mutations in the DJ-1 gene associated with autosomal recessive early-onset parkinsonism. Science 2003; 299: 256–9.

4 Polymeropoulos MH, Higgins JJ, Golbe LI, *et al.* Mapping of a gene for Parkinson's disease to chromosome 4q21-q23. Science 1996; 274: 1197–9.

5 Polymeropoulos MH, Lavedan C, Leroy E, *et al.* Mutation in the alpha-synuclein gene identified in families with Parkinson's disease. Science 1997; 276: 2045–7.

6 Spillantini MG, Schmidt ML, Lee VM, Trojanowski JQ, Jakes R, Goedert M. Alpha-synuclein in Lewy bodies. Nature 1997; 388: 839–40.

7 Krüger R, Kuhn W, Müller T, *et al.* Ala30Pro mutation in the gene encoding alpha-synuclein in Parkinson's disease. Nat Genet 1998; 18: 106-8.

8 Zarranz JJ, Alegre J, Gómez-Esteban JC, *et al.* The new mutation, E46K, of alpha-synuclein causes Parkinson and Lewy body dementia. Ann Neurol 2004; 55: 164–73.

9 Singleton AB, Farrer M, Johnson J, *et al.* alpha-Synuclein locus triplication causes Parkinson's disease. Science 2003; 302: 841.

10 Golbe LI, Di Iorio G, Bonavita V, *et al.* A large kindred with autosomal dominant Parkinson's disease. Ann Neurol 1990; 27: 276–82.

11 Golbe LI, Di Iorio G, Sanges G, *et al.* Clinical genetic analysis of Parkinson's disease in the Contursi kindred. Ann Neurol 1996; 40: 767–75.

12 Duda JE, Giasson BI, Mabon ME, *et al.* Concurrence of alpha-synuclein and tau brain pathology in the Contursi kindred. Acta Neuropathol 2002; 104: 7–11.

13 Spira PJ, Sharpe DM, Halliday G, *et al.* Clinical and pathological features of a Parkinsonian syndrome in a family with an Ala53Thr alpha-synuclein mutation. Ann Neurol 2001; 49: 313–9.

14 Waters CH, Miller CA. Autosomal dominant Lewy body parkinsonism in a four-generation family. Ann Neurol 1994; 35: 59–64.

15 Muenter MD, Forno LS, Hornykiewicz O, *et al.* Hereditary form of parkinsonism – dementia. Ann Neurol 1998; 43: 768–81.

16 Farrer M, Gwinn-Hardy K, Muenter M, *et al.* A chromosome 4p haplotype segregating with Parkinson's disease and postural tremor. Hum Mol Genet 1999; 8: 81–5.

17 Chartier-Harlin M, Kachergus J, Roumier C, *et al.* Alpha-synuclein locus duplication as a cause of familial Parkinson's disease. Lancet 2004; 364: 1167–9.

18 Farrer M, Kachergus J, Forno L, *et al.* Comparison of kindreds with parkinsonism and alpha-synuclein genomic multiplications. Ann Neurol 2004; 55: 174–9.

19 Gwinn-Hardy K, Mehta ND, Farrer M, *et al.* Distinctive neuropathology revealed by alpha-synuclein antibodies in hereditary parkinsonism and dementia linked to chromosome 4p. Acta Neuropathol 2000; 99: 663–72.

20 Cookson MR, Dauer W, Dawson T, Fon EA, Guo M, Shen J. *et al.* The roles of kinases in familial Parkinson's disease. J Neurosci 2007; 27: 11865–8.

21 Paisán-Ruíz C, Jain S, Evans EW, *et al.* Cloning of the gene containing mutations that cause PARK8-linked Parkinson's disease. Neuron 2004; 44: 595–600.

22 Zimprich A, Biskup S, Leitner P, *et al.* Mutations in LRRK2 cause autosomal-dominant parkinsonism with pleomorphic pathology. Neuron 2004; 44: 601–7.

23 Farrer M, Stone J, Mata IF, *et al.* LRRK2 mutations in Parkinson disease. Neurology 2005; 65: 738–40.

24 Bras JM, Guerreiro RJ, Ribeiro MH, *et al.* G2019S dardarin substitution is a common cause of Parkinson's disease in a Portuguese cohort. Mov Disord 2005; 20: 1653-5.

25 Mata IF, Taylor JP, Kachergus J, *et al.* LRRK2 R1441G in Spanish patients with Parkinson's disease. Neurosci Lett 2005; 382: 309–11.

26 Wszolek ZK, Vieregge P, Uitti RJ, *et al.* German-Canadian family (family A) with parkinsonism, amyotrophy, and dementia – longitudinal observations. Parkinsonism Relat Disord 1997; 3: 125–39.

27 Covy JP, Yuan W, Waxman EA, *et al.* Clinical and pathological characteristics of patients with leucine-rich repeat kinase-2 mutations. Mov Disord 2009; 24: 32–9.

28 Ozelius LJ, Senthil G, Saunders-Pullman R, *et al.* LRRK2 G2019S as a cause of Parkinson's disease in Ashkenazi Jews. N Engl J Med 2006; 354: 424–5.

29 Lesage S, Dürr A, Tazir M, *et al.* LRRK2 G2019S as a cause of Parkinson's disease in North African Arabs. N Engl J Med 2006; 354: 422–3.

30 Di Fonzo A, Rohé CF, Ferreira J, *et al.* A frequent LRRK2 gene mutation associated with autosomal dominant Parkinson's disease. Lancet 2005; 365: 412–5.

31 Aasly JO, Toft M, Fernandez-Mata I, *et al.* Clinical features of LRRK2-associated Parkinson's disease in central Norway. Ann Neurol 2005; 57: 762–5.

32 Scott WK, Grubber JM, Conneally PM, *et al.* Fine mapping of the chromosome 12 late-onset Alzheimer disease locus: potential genetic and phenotypic heterogeneity. Am J Hum Genet 2000; 66: 922–32.

33 Takao M, Ghetti B, Hayakawa I, *et al.* A novel mutation (G217D) in the Presenilin 1 gene (PSEN1) in a Japanese family: presenile dementia and parkinsonism are associated with cotton wool plaques in the cortex and striatum. Acta Neuropathol 2002; 104: 155–70.

34 Piscopo P, Marcon G, Piras MR, *et al.* A novel PSEN2 mutation associated with a peculiar phenotype. Neurology 2008; 70: 1549–54.

35 Nishioka K, Hayashi S, Farrer MJ, *et al.* Clinical heterogeneity of alpha-synuclein gene duplication in Parkinson's disease. Ann Neurol 2006; 59: 298–309.

36 Ozawa T, Takano H, Onodera O, *et al.* No mutation in the entire coding region of the alpha-synuclein gene in pathologically confirmed cases of multiple system atrophy. Neurosci Lett 1999; 270: 110–2.

37 Scholz SW, Houlden H, Schulte C, *et al.* SNCA variants are associated with increased risk of multiple system atrophy. Ann Neurol 2009; 65: 610–14.

38 Robert M, Mathuranath PS. Tau and tauopathies. Neurol India 2007; 55: 11–6.

39 Hirokawa, N. Microtubule organization and dynamics dependent on microtubule-associated proteins. Curr Opin Cell Biol 1994; 6: 74–81.

40 Goedert M, Spillantini MG, Potier MC, Ulrich J, Crowther RA. Cloning and sequencing of the cDNA encoding an isoform of microtubule-associated protein tau containing four tandem repeats: differential expression of tau protein mRNAs in human brain. EMBO J 1989; 8: 393–9.

41 Gustke N, Trinczek B, Biernat J, Mandelkow EM, Mandelkow E. Domains of tau protein and interactions with microtubules. Biochemistry 1994; 33: 9511-22.

42 Rademakers, R, Hutton, M. The genetics of frontotemporal lobar degeneration. Curr Neurol Neurosci Rep 2007; 7: 434–42.

43 Mirra SS, Murrell JR, Gearing M, *et al.* Tau pathology in a family with dementia and a P301L mutation in tau. J Neuropathol Exp Neurol 1999; 58: 335–45.

44 Nasreddine ZS, Loginov M, Clark LN. From genotype to phenotype: a clinical pathological, and biochemical investigation of frontotemporal dementia and parkinsonism (FTDP-17) caused by the P301L tau mutation. Ann Neurol 1999; 45: 704–15.

45 Mahley, R.W, Rall, S.C. Apolipoprotein E: far more than a lipid transport protein. Annu Rev Genomics Hum Genet 2000; 1: 507–37.

46 Saunders AM, Strittmatter WJ, Schmechel D, *et al.* Association of apolipoprotein E allele epsilon 4 with late-onset familial and sporadic Alzheimer's disease. Neurology 1993; 43: 1467–72.

47 van Duijn CM, de Knijff P, Cruts M, *et al.* Apolipoprotein E4 allele in a population-based study of early-onset Alzheimer's disease. Nat Genet 1994; 7: 74–8.

48 Parsian A, Racette B, Goldsmith LJ, Perlmutter JS. Parkinson's disease and apolipoprotein E: possible association with dementia but not age at onset. Genomics 2002; 79: 458–61.

49 Marder K, Maestre G, Cote L, *et al.* The apolipoprotein epsilon 4 allele in Parkinson's disease with and without dementia. Neurology 1994; 44: 1330–1.

50 Inzelberg R, Chapman J, Treves TA, *et al.* Apolipoprotein E4 in Parkinson disease and dementia: new data and meta-analysis of published studies. Alzheimer Dis Assoc Disord 1998; 12: 45–8.

51 Pankratz N, Byder L, Halter C, *et al.* Presence of an APOE4 allele results in significantly earlier onset of Parkinson's disease and a higher risk with dementia. Mov Disord 2006; 21: 45–9.

52 Huang X, Chen P, Kaufer DI, Tröster AI, Poole C. *et al.* Apolipoprotein E and dementia in Parkinson disease: a meta-analysis. Arch Neurol 2006; 63: 189–93.

53 Zhang J, Song Y, Chen H, Fan D. The tau gene haplotype h1 confers a susceptibility to Parkinson's disease. Eur Neurol 2005; 53: 15–21.

54 Farrer M, Maraganore DM, Lockhart P, *et al.* alpha-Synuclein gene haplotypes are associated with Parkinson's disease. Hum Mol Genet 2001; 10: 1847–51.

55 Spadafora P, Annesi G, Pasqua AA, *et al.* NACP-REP1 polymorphism is not involved in Parkinson's disease: a case–control study in a population sample from southern Italy. Neurosci Lett 2003; 351: 75–8.

56 Zappia M, Annesi G, Nicoletti G, *et al.* Association of tau gene polymorphism with Parkinson's disease. Neurol Sci 2003; 24: 223-4.

57 Ezquerra M, Campdelacreu J, Gaig C, *et al.* Lack of association of APOE and tau polymorphisms with dementia in Parkinson's disease. Neurosci Lett 2008; 448: 20–3.

58 De Marco EV, Tarantino P, Rocca FE, *et al.* Alpha-synuclein promoter haplotypes and dementia in Parkinson's disease. Am J Med Genet B Neuropsychiatr Genet 2008; 147: 403–7.

59 Camicioli R, Rajput A, Rajput M, *et al.* Apolipoprotein E epsilon4 and catechol-O-methyltransferase alleles in autopsy-proven Parkinson's disease: relationship to dementia and hallucinations. Mov Disord 2005; 20: 989–94.

60 Gołab-Janowska M, Honczarenko K, Gawrońska-Szklarz B, *et al.* CYP2D6 gene polymorphism as a probable risk factor for Alzheimer's disease and Parkinson's disease with dementia. Neurol Neurochir Pol 2008; 41: 113–21.

61 Hubble JP, Kurth JH, Glatt SL, *et al.* Gene-toxin interaction as a putative risk factor for Parkinson's disease with dementia. Neuroepidemiology 1998; 17: 96–104.

62 Goris A, Williams-Gray CH, Clark GR, *et al.* Tau and alpha-synuclein in susceptibility to, and dementia in, Parkinson's disease. Ann Neurol 2007; 62: 145–53.

63 Mattila KM, Rinne JO, Röyttä M, *et al.* Dipeptidyl carboxypeptidase 1 (DCP1) and butyrylcholinesterase (BCHE) gene interactions with the apolipoprotein E epsilon4 allele as risk factors in Alzheimer's disease and in Parkinson's disease with coexisting Alzheimer pathology. J Med Genet 2000; 37: 766–70.

64 Isoe-Wada K, Maeda M, Yong J, *et al.* Positive association between an estrogen receptor gene polymorphism and Parkinson's disease with dementia. Eur J Neurol 1999; 6: 431-5.

65 Hindorff LA, Junkins HA, Mehta JP, Manolio TA. A catalog of published genome-wide association studies. Available at: http://www.genome.gov/26525384 (accessed 03/23/09).

66 Hardy J, Singleton AB. Toward a complete resolution of the genetic architecture of disease. N Engl J Med (in press).

Chapter 13

Neurochemical pathology of Parkinson's disease dementia

Margaret Ann Piggott and Elaine K. Perry

Introduction

Whether neurotransmitter deficits and changes in Parkinson's disease dementia (PD-D) differ in kind or degree compared with idiopathic Parkinson's disease is an important question when considering the clinical manifestations they underlie. A detailed understanding of neurotransmitter function and consequences of their deficits can lead to rational drug design and treatment strategies appropriate for PD-D patients. In this chapter neurochemical pathologies in transmitter systems in PD-D and their potential association with clinical symptoms will be reviewed.

In terms of guiding therapy, information on neurotransmitter make-up and receptors is gleaned most usefully from *in vivo* imaging; but it is obtained in greater detail and with information on several parameters together from postmortem investigation.

The original finding of Hornykiewicz and Ehringer of reduced dopamine concentration in postmortem striatal tissue from parkinsonism patients (first reported early in the 1960s [1] and republished in English in 1998 [2]) and its replacement therapy [3,4] were revolutionary developments. Neurochemists have sought with hope to find similar, apparently simple, relationships between other disorders or symptoms and single transmitter systems, but have often found that combinations of neurotransmitter changes are responsible. PD-D by definition evolves from levodopa-responsive PD, but even PD is more than a disorder of movement and a deficiency of dopamine [5].

Changes in neurotransmitter systems in PD-D

Dopamine

Presynaptic dopaminergic measures

Concentrations of dopamine and homovanillic acid (HVA) [1,2] continue to decline and are consequently even more pronounced in PD-D than in PD. The loss of dopamine follows a pattern which reflects neuron loss in the substantia nigra (SN) [6] progressively affecting areas of low calbindin immunostaining first. The ratio of homovanillic acid to dopamine (each measured as pmol/mg protein) is an index of dopamine turnover, which is elevated in PD to an average of 45 times normal in putamen (but is not increased significantly over controls in dementia with Lewy bodies) [7]. Although this 1999 study was not prospective, within the PD cases analysed those cases who had cognitive problems recorded in their case notes ($n = 6$) had lower HVA/dopamine ratios than those without ($n = 9$) (8 ± 6 vs 50 ± 44; two-tailed t-test: $P = 0.04$). Increased turnover is one of the compensatory changes that occur in PD and begin to fail in PD-D.

Reduced dopamine concentration is mirrored by dopamine transporter (DAT) density. These have been measured *in vitro* and *in vivo* in PD-D, and are reliably shown to be reduced beyond PD levels, and also lower compared to dementia with Lewy bodies (DLB). By [123]I-*N*-3-fluoropropyl-2-β-carbomethoxy-3-β-(4-iodophenyl)-nortropane (FP-CIT) single photon emission computed tomography (SPECT), DAT density in PD-D is more than 50% reduced compared with DLB or PD [8]; while *in vitro* with [125]I-*N*-(3-iodopro-2E-enyl)-2β-carbomethoxy-3β-(4'-methylphenyl) nortropane (PE2I), DAT are also lower than DLB or PD (Piggott, unpublished, see Fig. 13.1)

SN and DAT loss may not initially be symmetrical between hemispheres, and this is reflected by unilateral expression of symptoms, especially rigidity [9,10], although there is still significant loss bilaterally. Evolution to PD-D shows dopamine markers reduced to similar extents bilaterally [8].

Given the huge reduction in dopamine transmission in PD-D, affecting extrastriatal areas (thalamus, nucleus accumbens, and probably cortical areas which are more difficult to investigate) there are consequent effects on more than motor function. The thalamus receives dopamine via nigrostriatal collaterals, which have been shown to have depleted dopamine transporter immunoreactivity in the 1-methyl-4-phenyl-1,2,3,6-tetrahydropyridine (MPTP)-treated monkey model of PD [11]. Nigrothalamic dopamine is likely to be reduced in PD-D. Using ^{125}I-PE2I autoradiography, tracts from the SN bifurcating to course both through the globus pallidus and along the margin of the reticular nucleus of the thalamus can be visualized, and these tracts are at least 50% lower density in PD-D, DLB, and PD compared with controls. At these most posterior striatal levels, DAT were more extensively reduced in PD-D compared to PD and DLB in the caudate, especially in the ventromedial section. At these caudal levels clinical correlations were, not surprisingly, with extrapyramidal symptoms, with greater reductions associated with more severe

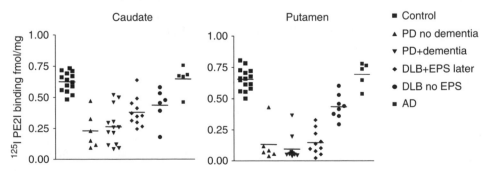

Fig. 13.1 Dopamine transporter density as measured by [125]I- PE2I (M.A. Piggott, unpublished data). PD, Parkinson's diease; DLB, dementia with Lewy bodies; EPS, extrapyramidal symptoms; AD, Alzheimer's disease.

Hoehn and Yahr (HY) and Unified Parkinson's Disease Rating Scale (UPDRS) scores in putamen and the tract along the reticular nucleus. Comparing PD-D to DLB with similar severity of movement disability (HY stage 3 only) there was greater loss of DAT in ventromedial putamen and medial caudate in PD-D, perhaps showing some residual efficacy of compensatory mechanisms in PD (which are not invoked in DLB). Reduced DAT was found in PD-D and DLB cases with auditory hallucinations (but not in relation to other typical neuropsychiatric symptoms of PD-D) in lateral putamen particularly (however, PD-D cases were more likely than DLB to have auditory hallucinations), and this was a significant finding in both anterior and posterior striatum in separate studies (Piggott, unpublished). There was a tendency for reduced cognition (lower MMSE) with lower DAT, reaching significance in the nucleus accumbens. A report using F-dopa positron emission tomography (PET) imaging also suggests that striatal dopaminergic depletion in caudate contributes to cognitive impairment in PD patients [12], and a study of progressive decline in DAT in PD-D, PD and DLB showed correlation with cognitive decline [13].

Postsynaptic dopaminergic measures

In postmortem analysis, dopamine D2 receptor density is upregulated in PD without dementia, in the striatum by more than 70% [7], a compensatory change tending to 'damp down' overactivity of striatopallidal neurons. Although this study did not include prospective assessment, PD cases which had cognitive problems recorded in their case notes had lower striatal D2 binding (particularly dorsally) than PD cases with unimpaired cognition. In the thalamus, D2 receptors were upregulated twofold in all regions examined in PD compared with controls [14], but in PD-D D2 receptors showed up-regulation compared to controls only in the motor thalamic ventrointermedius nucleus, which, although significant, was relatively modest [14]. Although there is some difficulty imaging D2 receptors *in vivo* due to the presence of intrinsic dopamine, PET and SPECT have shown upregulation of striatal D2 receptors to be a very early event in PD [15,16], with the levels falling over the years as disease progresses and with pro-dopaminergic therapy [17], until D2 density falls back to control levels.

After the striatum and thalamus, the highest brain D2 densities are in cortex, particularly temporal. In temporal cortex in PD-D and DLB, D2 receptors were significantly reduced by more than 40% [though not reduced in Alzheimer's disease (AD)] [14]. In PD, D2 were double control levels in insular cortex, but in PD-D the density was no different from controls (while being slightly, but not quite significantly, lower in DLB) (Piggott, unpublished data).

D2 receptor changes have an impact on clinical symptoms. Reduced temporal cortical D2 density correlated with cognitive decline (Fig. 13.2), but not with hallucinations or delusions, giving theoretical grounds for the deleterious effect neuroleptics have on cognition in PD-D [18].

Dopaminergic medications are usually reported to have limited benefit in DLB, with low likelihood of motor improvement and risk of exacerbating psychosis [19], but conversely levodopa challenge was found not have clinically significant adverse cognitive effects in PD-D and may improve neuropsychiatric symptoms [20]. Expert opinion is nevertheless to withdraw dopamine agonists in PD-D.

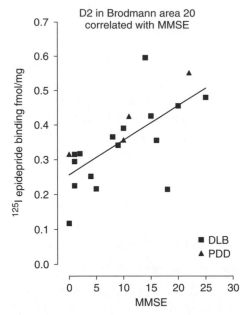

Fig. 13.2 Reduced temporal cortical D2 density correlated with cognitive decline. MMSE, Mini-Mental State Examination; DLB, dementia with Lewy bodies; PD-D, Parkinson's disease with dementia.

In DLB, D2 striatal density was lowest in cases which had severe neuroleptic sensitivity and was slightly higher in cases which were tolerant of neuroleptic treatment [21,22]; it may be that cases with lower D2 density are more at risk of sudden catastrophic blockade due to the D2 antagonist action of neuroleptics. By this token, in PD-D risk of neuroleptic blockade of D2 receptors must increase as disease progresses, and severe reactions to neuroleptics were found to occur as often in PD-D as in DLB [23].

D1 receptors in the caudate are reported to be reduced with cognitive impairment in PD, unrelated to the degree of AD pathology, in a postmortem analysis [24].

Although somewhat complicated by neuroleptic use, in PD-D and DLB there was higher thalamic D2 binding in cases with disturbances of consciousness (DOC) particularly in nuclei with a role in the maintenance of consciousness, including the reticular nucleus [14] and also in insular cortex, with significance of $P = 0.0013$ and 0.016, respectively. Among these cases there were roughly equal numbers of PD-D and DLB cases (reticular nucleus, +DOC: 6 PD-D, 7 DLB; −DOC: 2 PD-D, 3 DLB; insular cortex, +DOC: 7 PD-D, 6 DLB; −DOC: 2 PD-D, 4 DLB) ([14] and Piggott, unpublished data, Fig. 13.3).

D2 receptors located on reticular nucleus GABA-ergic neurons will, being inhibitory, help maintain thalamic and cortical activity, thus enabling fluctuations. In an environment of reduced transmitter concentration, relatively higher D2 receptors may amplify small transmitter changes, leading to variations in consciousness and attention. Similarly, nicotinic receptors were higher in some thalamic nuclei in cases with variations in consciousness [25] (see below), possibly suggesting cholinergic and dopaminergic

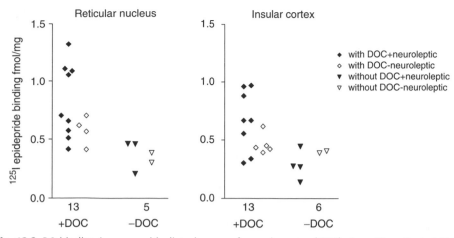

Fig. 13.3 D2 binding in cases with disturbances of consciousness (DOC). From Piggott *et al.* [14] and M.A. Piggott, unpublished data.

substrates for fluctuations, and that combined cholinergic and dopaminergic therapy is required to treat disturbed consciousness in PD-D and DLB.

Acetylcholine

The other major transmitter system associated with the symptoms of PD-D is the cholinergic system. Arising from the basal forebrain (including septal, diagonal band and Meynert nuclei which constitute the cholinergic projections to the neocortex) the cholinergic system innervates all areas of the cerebral cortex including hippocampus, and also the reticular nucleus of the thalamus. Cholinergic brainstem neurons (from the pedunculopontine and laterodorsal tegmental nuclei) innervate the thalamus and cerebellum. By contrast, the highly cholinergic putamen and caudate nucleus do not receive inputs, but have their own intrinsic cholinergic neurons (large striatal interneurons).

The importance of acetylcholine (ACh) and cholinergic deficits in cognitive impairment and dementia in general was recognized more than 30 years ago [26], and a few years later also in PD [27,28]. In PD, initial reports indicated no deficit in cholinergic parameters [29] and anticholinergic treatment to promote movement was recommended [30], although there were some near contemporaneous reports warning against the use of anticholinergics in PD [31]. Gradually the loss of other transmitters besides dopamine was recognized as contributing to PD-D [32], with several early reports highlighting the significant reduction in both cholinergic basal forebrain neurons [33] and cortical choline acetyltransferase (ChAT) (the enzyme that synthesizes acetylcholine) and acetylcholinesterase (AChE) activities [28,34]. A seminal paper by Perry *et al.* [35] reported that dementia in PD, which had up until then generally been attributed to the presence of AD-type cortical pathology, actually usually occurs in the absence of substantial AD-type changes and is rather related to abnormalities in the cortical cholinergic system. In PD-D there were extensive reductions of ChAT and less extensive reductions of AChE in all four cortical lobes [35]. ChAT reductions in temporal cortex in PD-D correlated with degree of mental impairment, but not with the extent of plaque or tangle formation. In PD but not AD the decrease in neocortical (particularly temporal) ChAT correlated with the number of neurons in the nucleus of Meynert, suggesting that primary degeneration of these cholinergic neurons may be related to declining cognitive function in PD [35]. A further study confirmed these findings, showing that cognitive impairment in PD correlated with ChAT activity in temporal and prefrontal cortex and hippocampus, unrelated to AD pathology and additionally showing a correlation with the numbers of cortical Lewy bodies [24]. *In vivo* PET measurement of AChE showed remarkable reductions in the entire cortex in PD-D [36].

In the thalamus in PD-D (but not in DLB) there were significant reductions in ChAT in the reticular, mediodorsal and centromedian nuclei, associated with long duration of parkinsonism and dementia [37]. It is now recognized that cholinergic losses are generally greater in PD-D than in AD, both in terms of presynaptic cortical activities but also in the striatum and in the projection from the pedunculopontine nucleus to the thalamus. As in AD, there is consistent involvement of the nucleus basalis of Meynert, but with Lewy body pathology and more extensive cell loss [38]. In DLB too, in the cerebral cortex, ChAT and AChE losses determined postmortem exceed those in AD (except in the hippocampus) and are apparent early in the disease course [39].

While studies of neurochemical pathology of PD-D were pursued in Newcastle for several years before 1989, investigations of the originally named senile dementia of Lewy body type were based on cases identified in retrospective pathological studies as 'atypical Alzheimer's'. Since they had come to autopsy through psychiatry services, they included mainly individuals with few apparent extrapyramidal features [40] and became designated DLB at the 1995 International Workshop – Consortium on DLB [41]. By the later 1990s prospectively assessed clinical cohorts included cases with DLB similar to those in the previous pathological studies, as well as dementia cases with concurrent, or subsequently developed extrapyramidal symptoms, or diagnosed levodopa-responsive Parkinson's disease of several to many years standing, allowing comparison of DLB with and without extrapyramidal symptoms and PD-D. Although DLB and PD-D may be very similar there are documented subtle differences clinically and pathologically, and it should not be assumed that significant findings in one will be replicated in the other.

In PD-D *in vivo* SPECT imaging of the vesicular ACh transporter has shown considerable losses throughout the cortex, whereas in PD there was some reduction only in parietal and occipital cortex [42]. Similarly, a PET study of AChE activity showed greater reduction in PD-D compared to AD [43], with cortical AChE activity down 21% in PD-D compared to 13% in PD, correlating with measures of working memory, attention and executive function, but not correlating with severity of motor symptoms [44]. The strong correlation of declining cholinergic measures with cognitive function was not the only clinical consequence; there was also increased depression with greater reduction in cortical AChE by PET in PD and PD-D [45].

In PD-D and DLB, cases with the greatest reductions in cholinergic measures are those most likely to have visual hallucinations. ChAT deficits are greater in some visual cortical areas in DLB cases with visual hallucinations compared to those without, for example in Brodmann area 36 of the temporal cortex [46], and it may be that propensity to visual hallucinations is increased when much-reduced acetylcholine is combined with a relatively active serotonergic system [47].

Nicotinic receptor changes

Loss of nicotinic acetylcholine receptors (nAChR) in DLB is likely to reflect reduced cholinergic innervation (cortex and thalamus), dopaminergic innervation (striatum), and also attenuation of glutamatergic, GABA-ergic and serotonergic neurons in cortex, thalamus and basal ganglia. Neocortical binding to nAChR containing $\alpha4$ and $\beta2$ subunits is reduced in PD, PD-D, and DLB [48,49], and there is an apparent correlation between this nAChR deficit and cortical ChAT reduction [50].

In the striatum nAChRs are more reduced in DLB and PD than is the case in AD, notably of the $\alpha6$-, $\alpha4$-, $\beta2$- and $\beta3$-containing subtypes [49]. Reduced nAChR binding in this region, which is at least in part on dopaminergic terminals, is as severe in DLB as PD [49,51] perhaps indicating that loss of these receptors occurs at a relatively early stage of nigrostriatal degeneration [51].

By contrast, $\alpha4\beta2$-containing nAChRs visualized *in vitro* with ^{125}I-5-IA85380 were not reduced in the thalamus in DLB (although there were reductions in PD) [25], but significant deficits were observed in cases without disturbances in consciousness [52]. Also in the temporal cortex nAChR binding was relatively preserved in DLB cases with disturbed consciousness [53]. Since patients with disturbances of consciousness are able, some of the time, to be more alert than at other times, the neurotransmitter systems must be capable of supporting the higher level of awareness. In an analogous way to the suggested mechanism involving D2 receptors in thalamic nuclei with a role in maintaining consciousness (above), when the cholinergic system is very low, a higher density of nicotinic receptors may enable small transmitter fluctuations to lead to variations in consciousness and attention.

By *in vivo* SPECT with ^{123}I-5-IA85380 to show $\alpha4\beta2$ nicotinic receptors in DLB, there were reductions in frontal, temporal and cingulate cortex and striatal regions, but elevations in occipital cortex which were greater in cases with a recent history of visual hallucinations [54]. Muscarinic receptors M1 and M2/4 are particularly highly expressed in visual cortex, as shown by autoradiography [55], and M1/M4 were elevated bilaterally *in vivo* in PD-D by ^{123}I-iodo-quinuclidinyl-benzilate (QNB) SPECT in occipital cortex [56] which may contribute to visual disturbances in PD-D.

Whether cortical $\alpha7$-containing receptors are reduced generally in DLB is equivocal [49,50], but it is perhaps most likely to occur in DLB cases with hallucinations [57]. Reduced $\alpha7$ receptor binding has also been noted in the reticular nucleus of the thalamus in DLB (in common with AD), a region innervated by cholinergic neurons from the basal forebrain [58].

Muscarinic receptor changes

Multiple muscarinic, G-protein-linked acetylcholine receptors (mAChRs) are expressed in human brain (M1–5), the most prevalent being M1 (in cortical regions) and M2 (widely distributed). Postsynaptically, there is less neuronal damage in PD-D and DLB than in AD [38]. Muscarinic M1 receptor modulation differs between DLB and AD. Although unchanged or slightly reduced and with defective coupling in the cortex in severe AD, in DLB M1 receptors have been reported to be upregulated in temporal and parietal cortex [48] especially in cases with delusional symptoms [59], and higher in frontal cortex in PD-D and DLB compared to AD [60]. Similarly, immunohistochemistry indicates higher proportions of M1 in 'diffuse Lewy body disease' [61]. Additionally, coupling to G-protein second messenger systems is found to be preserved in DLB compared to AD, in temporal cortex [62], and in frontal cortex in both PD-D and DLB [60]. In contrast to the neocortex, in PD-D and DLB striatal M1 receptor binding is reduced, in parallel with D2 receptors (M1 and D2 are distributed together mainly on the same population of projection neurons from striatum to external globus pallidus) (Fig. 13.4) [63].

This is possibly why cholinesterase inhibitor therapy tends not to provoke worsening of Parkinsonism in PD-D and DLB patients.

In PD-D and DLB, M2 receptors were elevated in insular cortex compared to controls, and were significantly higher in PD-D compared to DLB [64] and this was significantly related to severity and duration of extrapyramidal symptoms (Piggott, unpublished data). M2 and M4 binding were higher in cingulate cortex in PD-D and DLB compared to controls, and these increases were associated with visual hallucinations [65]. Raised M4 receptor density in cingulate cortex was related to impaired consciousness [65], and in the insular cortex with the symptom of delusions. By contrast, M4 receptors were reduced in PD-D and DLB in the mediodorsal thalamic nucleus [66].

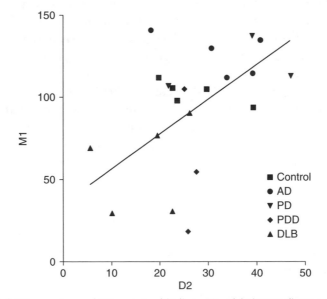

Fig. 13.4 Striatal M1 receptor and D2 receptor binding. AD, Alzheimer's disease; PD, Parkinson's diease; PD-D, Parkinson's disease with dementia; DLB, dementia with Lewy bodies. From Piggott *et al.* [63].

Relationship between cholinergic medication and AD-type pathology

In Parkinson's disease long-term administration of drugs with anticholinergic actions is associated with increased AD-type pathology, with increased plaques and tangles [67]. Conversely, it has also been demonstrated that long-term exposure to nicotine (tobacco use) is associated with reduced AD pathology (Aβ deposition) [68] and also, in normal elderly, to greater preservation of neuron numbers in SN. There is potential for the development of drugs acting selectively at muscarinic receptors both neuroprotectively (anti-AD pathology) by M1 agonists [69] and therapeutically at other muscarinic receptor subtypes [70].

Elaine Perry predicted in 1990 'that the cholinergic correlates of mental impairment in senile dementia of Lewy body type (and PD-D) together with the relative absence of cortical neurofibrillary tangles and evidence for postsynaptic cholinergic receptor compensation raise the question of whether this type of dementia may be more amenable to cholinotherapy than classical AD' [71]. She also recognized that the presence of visual hallucinations in the symptom profile would be diagnostic of greater cholinergic compromise [46,47], and predicted reliable response to cholinergic medication in these patients [72]. Activation of cholinergic receptors was recognized to be pro-cognitive, especially by improving attention [73,74].

Glutamate

Excitatory amino acid transmission occurs between several components of the basal ganglia circuitry which are affected in PD-D, and excitotoxic mechanisms have been implicated in the progression of the disease. In PD there is increased output from the subthalamic nucleus, and glutamatergic drive from the subthalamic nucleus may be part of the compensatory mechanisms which begin to fail with disease progression to PD-D. Investigations of glutamate markers in Lewy body dementias have been few. No change was shown in glutamate transporter protein in cortex in two DLB cases [75], no change in N-methyl-D-aspartate receptor immunoreactivity in entorhinal cortex and hippocampus [76], and no reduction in glutamate in cerebrospinal fluid (CSF) [77]. In another study in DLB, GluR2/3 α-amino-3-hydroxy-5-methyl-4-isoxazolepropionic acid receptor (AMPA) receptor immunoreactivity was, however, decreased in entorhinal cortex and hippocampus [76], and metabotropic mGluR1 and mGluR5 were reduced [78]. The mGluR5 receptor is increased in animal models of PD with dyskinesia [79] and seems to be reduced in striatum and cortex in PD cases without dyskinesia compared to both PD with dyskinesia and controls, and reduced further in PD-D (Piggott, Chazot, unpublished data). Further studies are needed to determine the extent of glutamate receptor changes in PD-D.

Gamma-aminobutyric acid (GABA)

Anxiety, insomnia and excessive daytime sleepiness are common complaints in PD-D and DLB, which may respond to treatment with benzodiazepines or modafinil which have GABA-ergic mechanisms. GABA-ergic components of the basal ganglia circuitry are probably affected in PD-D but there are few published reports of GABA-ergic changes. Selective dendritic derangement of GABA-ergic medium spiny neurons in the striatum in late PD have been reported, and suggested to be linked to disrupted executive function [80,81]. No difference in GABA CSF concentration was reported between DLB patients and a control group [77].

Serotonin

Depression is a frequent symptom in PD-D and DLB, but a possible link between serotonin loss and depression remains to be clarified. The raphe nucleus is affected early in the course of PD [82], and Lewy body pathology and neuron loss have been reported in the raphe nucleus in DLB [83], although no significant neuron loss was found in another study [84]. Raphe neuron loss and reduced serotonin concentration in the striatum, pallidum and cortex did not differ in PD with or without dementia [85], and similarly Perry *et al.* found no correlation with dementia [86]. Reduced serotonin has been reported in striatum and cortex in DLB [83,87,88], but not in another study in the putamen [89]. Serotonin transporter binding is reduced by about 70% in temporal and parietal cortex in DLB, and 5-HT$_{2A}$ receptors are reduced by 50% in putamen in PD (Piggott, unpublished data), with 5-HT$_{2A}$ receptors also reduced in temporal cortex in DLB and PD-D [90]. There is little evidence that selective serotonin reuptake inhibitors are effective in depression in PD [91], and untreated PD patients with depression showed no differences in CSF serotonin metabolites compared to patients without depression [92]. DLB patients with a history of major depression actually had relatively higher serotonin transporter binding in parietal cortex than cases without [93], though serotonin transporters were at slightly lower density in PD-D/DLB than controls.

PET imaging of 5-HT$_{1A}$ receptors, which are inhibitory autoreceptors, in the median raphe in PD showed a reduction (25%) in signal related to the presence of tremor but not to depression [94]. However *in vitro* in temporal cortex 5-HT$_{1A}$ receptors showed a significant increase (more than 80%) in numbers in temporal cortex (Brodmann area 36) in PD-D [95], and a significant 68% elevation in cortical 5-HT$_{1A}$ receptors was found in PD-D/DLB patients with, as compared to those without, depression [95]. In PD in a postmortem autoradiographic study (where cognitive function was not prospectively assessed) 5-HT$_{1A}$ receptors were increased in frontal and temporal cortex compared to controls (although any relationship to depression was not assessed in this study) [96]. Hence, treatment of depression in DLB and PD-D may be more efficacious with incorporation of a 5-HT$_{1A}$ antagonist, to increase the efficacy of serotonin reuptake inhibitors.

Greater preservation of serotonergic function may be related to more behavioural and psychological symptoms such as aggression, anxiety, depressed mood and agitation, whereas reduction of markers of serotonin activity may be related to cognitive impairment [97], and the balance between various transmitter systems is probably important [98]. Patients with visual hallucinations show a relative preservation of 5-HT markers along with markedly reduced cholinergic parameters [47,88,90].

Noradrenaline

Degeneration of the locus coeruleus has been reported in PD, and suggested to be linked to symptoms of mood disorder and subtle cognitive changes [85,99]. Using ^{11}C-RTI-32 PET imaging to indicate dopamine and noradrenaline terminals, reduced signal in cingulate cortex, amygdala, thalamus and locus coeruleus correlated with depression in PD compared to those with equal motor disability but without depression [100]. Noradrenergic loss is more extensive in PD-D than PD [32,99,101] and there are reductions in DLB [102,103]. Noradrenergic losses correlate with cognitive decline, morphological alteration of synapses in the locus coeruleus was more pronounced in PD-D than PD [104], and locus coeruleus neuron loss correlated with cognitive decline [103]. Szot *et al.* [103] found evidence of compensation for the neuron loss in the remaining locus coeruleus neurons in AD and DLB, but in both disorders there was reduced α_{1D} and α_{2C} adrenergic receptor mRNA in hippocampus. Alpha-2 adrenergic receptor density was reported to be increased slightly in DLB in frontal cortex [102]. Treatment with drugs active at α_1 or α_2 receptors has been suggested to improve spatial memory [105] or attention in PD [106] or PD-D [107].

Changes in noradrenergic system in limbic areas may contribute to depression and to behavioural symptoms such as aggression and pacing, to cognitive decline in cortical areas, and to movement disorder in basal ganglia, but in the main these relationships are still to be investigated. In DLB, noradrenaline is much reduced in putamen [83], which could mitigate symptoms of parkinsonism.

Calcium

Several lines of evidence indicate the importance of calcium homeostasis in mechanisms of symptom generation and disease progression in PD and PD-D. In cortex, neurons expressing calcium-binding proteins are more likely to be spared in DLB [108]. In the substantia nigra too the most vulnerable neurons are those with lowest expression of calbindin [6]. In the SN, pacemaking activity is dependent on L-type calcium channels, while in the ventral tegmental area it depends on sodium channels [109]. It may be that calcium homeostasis is the key to selective vulnerability among SN neurons (and as compared to ventral tegmental area neurons), since calcium concentration (via L-type calcium channels) together with cytosolic dopamine concentration and α-synuclein expression seem to be the three factors leading to neurotoxicity [110]. This is consistent with the observation that use of calcium channel antagonists to treat hypertension may confer diminished risk of developing PD [111].

Fast oscillations in the gamma frequency in cortex and thalamus have been implicated in attention, sensory processing and memory, modulated by noradrenaline, dopamine, acetylcholine and serotonin [112,113]. In PD-D there is greater slowing of resting state brain oscillatory activity compared to PD, as detected by magneto-encephalography [112]. Calcium t-channels have a physiological function in thalamic oscillations [114,115].

The status of calcium channels in PDD in SN or cortex is largely unknown; however, in a study carried out in the 1980s, nitrendipine binding to L-type calcium channels in temporal cortex was reported to be reduced in AD, but the greatest reduction (70%) was in cases which would today be more likely to be classified as DLB/PDD [116].

Conclusions

The best-documented neurotransmitter changes in PD-D include loss of cholinergic markers, and the progressive loss of dopamine. These deficits are associated with various changes in the related pre- and postsynaptic receptors. Alterations in serotonin, noradrenaline and to a lesser extent in other neurotransmitter systems have been reported; these are, however, less pronounced and need to be better elucidated. Neuropsychiatric and cognitive symptoms in PD-D are likely to be due to a combination of neurotransmitter deficits, particularly cholinergic and dopaminergic for cognitive dysfunction [117] (possibly with some noradrenergic influence); dopaminergic, noradrenergic and serotonergic for depression [118]; and dopaminergic/serotonergic and cholinergic for visual hallucinations [47]. Clinical trials with treatment modalities such as mixed transmitter reuptake inhibitors for symptoms including depression and psychosis in PD-D are warranted [118,119]. New possibilities for treatment targeting calcium channels are also emerging [110].

References

1 Ehringer H, Hornykiewicz O. [Distribution of noradrenaline and dopamine (3-hydroxytyramine) in the human brain and their behavior in diseases of the extrapyramidal system.]. Klin Wochenschr 1960; 38: 1236–9.

2 Ehringer H, Hornykiewicz O. Distribution of noradrenaline and dopamine (3-hydroxytyramine) in the human brain and their behavior in diseases of the extrapyramidal system. Parkinsonism Relat Disord 1998; 4: 53–7.

3 McGeer PL, Zeldowicz LR. Administration of Dihydroxyphenylalanine to Parkinsonian Patients. Can Med Assoc J 1964; 90: 463–6.

4 Cotzias GC, Van Woert MH, Schiffer LM. Aromatic amino acids and modification of parkinsonism. N Engl J Med 1967; 276: 374–9.

5 Archibald N, Burn D. Parkinson's disease. Medicine 2008; 36: 630–5.

6 Damier P, Hirsch EC, Agid Y, Graybiel AM. The substantia nigra of the human brain – II. Patterns of loss of dopamine-containing neurons in Parkinson's disease. Brain 1999; 122: 1437–48.

7 Piggott MA, Marshall EF, Thomas N, et al. Striatal dopaminergic markers in dementia with Lewy bodies, Alzheimer's and Parkinson's diseases: rostrocaudal distribution. Brain 1999; 122(Pt 8): 1449–68.

8 O'Brien JTDMM, Colloby SM, Fenwick JP, et al. Dopamine transporter loss visualized with FP-CIT SPECT in the differential diagnosis of dementia with Lewy bodies. Arch Neurol 2004; 61: 919–25.

9 Wenning GK, Donnemiller E, Granata R, Riccabona G, Poewe W. 123I-beta-CIT and 123I-IBZM-SPECT scanning in levodopa-naive Parkinson's disease. Mov Disord 1998; 13: 438–45.

10 Tissingh G, Bergmans P, Booij J, et al. Drug-naive patients with Parkinson's disease in Hoehn and Yahr stages I and II show a bilateral decrease in striatal dopamine transporters as revealed by [123I] beta-CIT SPECT. J Neurol 1998; 245: 14–20.

11 Freeman A, Ciliax B, Bakay R, et al. Nigrostriatal collaterals to thalamus degenerate in parkinsonian animal models. Ann Neurol 2001; 50: 321–9.

12 Jokinen P, Brück A, Aalto S, Forsback S, Parkkola R, Rinne JO. Impaired cognitive performance in Parkinson's disease is related to caudate dopaminergic hypofunction and hippocampal atrophy. Parkinsonism Relat Disord 2009; 15: 88–93.

13 Colloby SJ, Williams ED, Burn DJ, Lloyd JJ, McKeith IG, O'Brien JT. Progression of dopaminergic degeneration in dementia with Lewy bodies and Parkinson's disease with and without dementia assessed using 123I-FP-CIT SPECT. Eur J Nucl Med Molec Imag 2005; 32: 1176–85.

14 Piggott MA, Ballard CG, Dickinson HO, McKeith IG, Perry RH, Perry EK. Thalamic D2 receptors in dementia with Lewy bodies, Parkinson's disease, and Parkinson's disease dementia. Int J Neuropsychopharmacol 2007; 10: 231–44.

15 Giobbe D, Castellano GC, Podio V. Dopamine D2 receptor imaging with SPECT using IBZM in 16 patients with Parkinson disease. Ital J Neurol Sci 1993; 14: 165–9.

16 Antonini A, Schwarz J, Oertel WH, Beer HF, Madeja UD, Leenders KL. [11C]raclopride and positron emission tomography in previously untreated patients with Parkinson's disease: influence of L-dopa and lisuride therapy on striatal dopamine D2-receptors. Neurology 1994; 44: 1325–9.

17 Antonini A, Schwarz J, Oertel WH, Pogarell O, Leenders KL. Long-term changes of striatal dopamine D2 receptors in patients with Parkinson's disease: a study with positron emission tomography and [11C]raclopride. Mov Disord 1997; 12: 33–8.

18 Piggott MA, Ballard CG, Rowan E, et al. Selective loss of dopamine D2 receptors in temporal cortex in dementia with Lewy bodies, association with cognitive decline. Synapse 2007; 61: 903–11.

19 Goldman JG, Goetz CG, Brandabur M, Sanfilippo M, Stebbins GT. Effects of dopaminergic medications on psychosis and motor function in dementia with Lewy bodies. Mov Disord 2008; 23: 2248–50.

20 Molloy SA, Rowan EN, O'Brien JT, McKeith IG, Wesnes K, Burn DJ. Effect of levodopa on cognitive function in Parkinson's disease with and without dementia and dementia with Lewy bodies. J Neurol Neurosurg Psychiatry 2006; 77: 1323–8.

21 Piggott MA, Perry EK, Marshall EF, et al. Nigrostriatal dopaminergic activities in dementia with Lewy bodies in relation to neuroleptic sensitivity: comparisons with Parkinson's disease. Biol Psychiatry 1998; 44: 765–74.

22 Piggott MA, Perry EK, McKeith IG, Marshall E, Perry RH. Dopamine D2 receptors in demented patients with severe neuroleptic sensitivity [letter] [corrected] [published erratum appears in Lancet 1994; 343(8906): 1170]. Lancet 1994; 343(8904): 1044–5.

23 Aarsland D, Perry R, Larsen JP, et al. Neuroleptic sensitivity in Parkinson's disease and Parkinsonian dementias. J Clin Psychiatry 2005; 66: 633–7.

24 Mattila PM, Roytta M, Lonnberg P, Marjamaki P, Helenius H, Rinne JO. Choline acetytransferase activity and striatal dopamine receptors in Parkinson's disease in relation to cognitive impairment. Acta Neuropath 2001; 102: 160–6.

25 Pimlott SL, Piggott M, Owens J, et al. Nicotinic acetylcholine receptor distribution in Alzheimer's disease, dementia with Lewy bodies, Parkinson's disease, and vascular dementia: in vitro binding study using 5-[(125)i]-a-85380. Neuropsychopharmacology 2004; 29: 108–16.

26 Perry EK, Gibson PH, Blessed G, Perry RH, Tomlinson BE. Neurotransmitter enzyme abnormalities in senile dementia. Choline acetyltransferase and glutamic acid decarboxylase activities in necropsy brain tissue. J Neurol Sci 1977; 34: 247–65.

27 Ruberg M, Ploska A, Javoy-Agid F, Agid Y. Muscarinic binding and choline acetyltransferase activity in Parkinsonian subjects with reference to dementia. Brain Res 1982; 232: 129–39.

28 Perry RH, Tomlinson BE, Candy JM, et al. Cortical cholinergic deficit in mentally impaired Parkinsonian patients. Lancet 1983; 2(8353): 789–90.

29 Aquilonius SM, Nystrom B, Schuberth J, Sundwall A. Cerebrospinal fluid choline in extrapyramidal disorders. J Neurol Neurosurg Psychiatry 1972; 35: 720–5.

30 Sears ES. Therapeutics of disordered movement. American family physician 1977; 16: 145–54.

31 de Smet Y, Ruberg M, Serdaru M, Dubois B, Lhermitte F, Agid Y. Confusion, dementia and anticholinergics in Parkinson's disease. J Neurol Neurosurg Psychiatry 1982; 45: 1161–4.

32 Mann DM, Yates PO. Pathological basis for neurotransmitter changes in Parkinson's disease. Neuropathol Appl Neurobiol 1983; 9: 3–19.

33 Whitehouse PJ, Hedreen JC, White CL, 3rd, Price DL. Basal forebrain neurons in the dementia of Parkinson disease. Ann Neurol 1983; 13: 243–8.

34 Dubois B, Ruberg M, Javoy-Agid F, Ploska A, Agid Y. A subcortico-cortical cholinergic system is affected in Parkinson's disease. Brain Res 1983; 288: 213–8.

35 Perry EK, Curtis M, Dick DJ, et al. Cholinergic correlates of cognitive impairment in Parkinson's disease: comparisons with Alzheimer's disease. J Neurol Neurosurg Psych 1985; 48: 413–21.

36 Shinotoh H. [Imaging of brain acetylcholinesterase activity in dementias and extrapyramidal disorders]. Rinsho shinkeigaku [Clinical neurology] 2007; 47: 822–5.

37 Ziabreva I, Ballard CG, Aarsland D, et al. Lewy body disease: thalamic cholinergic activity related to dementia and parkinsonism. Neurobiol Aging 2006; 27: 433–8.

38 Tiraboschi P, Hansen LA, Alford M, et al. Cholinergic dysfunction in diseases with Lewy bodies. Neurology 2000; 54: 407–11.

39 Tiraboschi P, Hansen LA, Alford M, et al. Early and widespread cholinergic losses differentiate dementia with Lewy bodies from Alzheimer disease. Arch Gen Psych 2002; 59: 946–51.

40 Perry RH, Irving D, Blessed G, Fairbairn A, Perry EK. Senile dementia of Lewy body type. A clinically and neuropathologically distinct form of Lewy body dementia in the elderly. J Neurol Sci 1990; 95: 119–39.

41 McKeith IG, Galasko D, Kosaka K, et al. Consensus guidelines for the clinical and pathologic diagnosis of dementia with Lewy bodies (DLB): report of the consortium on DLB international workshop. Neurology 1996; 47: 1113–24.

42 Kuhl DE, Minoshima S, Fessler JA, et al. In vivo mapping of cholinergic terminals in normal aging, Alzheimer's disease, and Parkinson's disease. Ann Neurol 1996; 40: 399–410.

43 Bohnen NI, Kaufer DI, Ivanco LS, et al. Cortical cholinergic function is more severely affected in parkinsonian dementia than in Alzheimer disease: an in vivo positron emission tomographic study. Arch Neurol 2003; 60: 1745–8.

44 Bohnen NI, Kaufer DI, Hendrickson R, et al. Cognitive correlates of cortical cholinergic denervation in Parkinson's disease and parkinsonian dementia. J Neurol 2006; 253: 242–7.

45 Bohnen NI, Kaufer DI, Hendrickson R, Constantine GM, Mathis CA, Moore RY. Cortical cholinergic denervation is associated with depressive symptoms in Parkinson's disease and parkinsonian dementia. J Neurol Neurosurg Psychiatry 2007; 78: 641–3.

46 Perry EK, Kerwin J, Perry RH, Irving D, Blessed G, Fairbairn A. Cerebral cholinergic activity is related to the incidence of visual hallucinations in senile dementia of Lewy body type. Dementia 1990; 1: 2–4.

47 Perry EK, Marshall E, Kerwin J, et al. Evidence of a monoaminergic-cholinergic imbalance related to visual hallucinations in Lewy body dementia. J Neurochem 1990; 55: 1454–6.

48 Perry EK, Smith CJ, Court JA, Perry RH. Cholinergic nicotinic and muscarinic receptors in dementia of Alzheimer, Parkinson and Lewy body types. J Neural Transm 1990; 2: 149–58.

49 Gotti C, Moretti M, Bohr I, et al. Selective nicotinic acetylcholine receptor subunit deficits identified in Alzheimer's disease, Parkinson's disease and dementia with Lewy bodies by immunoprecipitation. Neurobiol Dis 2006; 23: 481–9.

50 Reid RT, Sabbagh MN, Corey-Bloom J, Tiraboschi P, Thal LJ. Nicotinic receptor losses in dementia with Lewy bodies: comparisons with Alzheimer's disease. Neurobiol Aging 2000; 21: 741–6.

51 Perry EK, Morris CM, Court JA, et al. Alteration in nicotine binding sites in Parkinson's disease, Lewy body dementia and Alzheimer's disease: possible index of early neuropathology. Neuroscience 1995; 64: 385–95.

52 Pimlott SL, Piggott M, Ballard C, *et al.* Thalamic nicotinic receptors implicated in disturbed consciousness in dementia with Lewy bodies. Neurobiol Dis 2006; 21: 50–6.

53 Ballard CG, Court JA, Piggott M, *et al.* Disturbances of consciousness in dementia with Lewy bodies associated with alteration in nicotinic receptor binding in the temporal cortex. Consciousness Cogn 2002; 11: 461–74.

54 O'Brien JT, Colloby SJ, Pakrasi S, *et al.* Nicotinic alpha4beta2 receptor binding in dementia with Lewy bodies using 123I-5IA-85380 SPECT demonstrates a link between occipital changes and visual hallucinations. Neuroimage 2008 15; 40: 1056–63.

55 Piggott M, Owens J, O'Brien J, *et al.* Comparative distribution of binding of the muscarinic receptor ligands pirenzepine, AF-DX 384, (R,R)-I-QNB and (R,S)-I-QNB to human brain. J Chem Neuroanat 2002; 24: 211–23.

56 Colloby SJ, Pakrasi S, Firbank MJ, *et al.* In vivo SPECT imaging of muscarinic acetylcholine receptors using (R,R) 123I-QNB in dementia with Lewy bodies and Parkinson's disease dementia. Neuroimage 2006; 33: 423–9.

57 Court JA, Ballard CG, Piggott MA, *et al.* Visual hallucinations are associated with lower alpha bungarotoxin binding in dementia with Lewy bodies. Pharmacol biochem behav 2001; 70: 571–9.

58 Court J, Spurden D, Lloyd S, *et al.* Neuronal nicotinic receptors in dementia with Lewy bodies and schizophrenia: alpha-bungarotoxin and nicotine binding in the thalamus. J Neurochem 1999; 73: 1590–7.

59 Ballard C, Piggott M, Johnson M, *et al.* Delusions associated with elevated muscarinic M1 receptor binding in dementia with Lewy bodies. Ann Neurol 2000; 48: 868–76.

60 Warren NM, Piggott MA, Lees AJ, Perry EK, Burn DJ. Intact coupling of M1 receptors and preserved M2 and M4 receptors in the cortex in progressive supranuclear palsy: contrast with other dementias. J Chem Neuroanat 2008; 35: 268–74.

61 Shiozaki K, Iseki E, Uchiyama H, *et al.* Alterations of muscarinic acetylcholine receptor subtypes in diffuse lewy body disease: relation to Alzheimer's disease. J Neurol Neurosurg Psychiatry 1999; 67: 209–13.

62 Perry E, Court J, Goodchild R, *et al.* Clinical neurochemistry: developments in dementia research based on brain bank material. J Neural Transm (Budapest) 1998; 105: 915–33.

63 Piggott MA, Owens J, O'Brien J, *et al.* Muscarinic receptors in basal ganglia in dementia with Lewy bodies, Parkinson's disease and Alzheimer's disease. J Chem Neuroanat 2003; 25: 161–73.

64 Warren NM, Piggott MA, Lees AJ, Burn DJ. The basal ganglia cholinergic neurochemistry of progressive supranuclear palsy and other neurodegenerative diseases. J Neurol Neurosurg Psychiatry 2007; 78: 571–5.

65 Teaktong T, Piggott MA, McKeith IG, Perry RH, Ballard CG, Perry EK. Muscarinic M2 and M4 receptors in anterior cingulate cortex: relation to neuropsychiatric symptoms in dementia with Lewy bodies. Behav Brain Res 2005; 161: 299–305.

66 Warren NM, Piggott MA, Lees AJ, Burn DJ. Muscarinic receptors in the thalamus in progressive supranuclear palsy and other neurodegenerative disorders. J Neuropathol Exp Neurol 2007; 66: 399–404.

67 Perry EK, Kilford L, Lees AJ, Burn DJ, Perry RH. Increased Alzheimer pathology in Parkinson's disease related to antimuscarinic drugs. [See comment]. Ann Neurology 2003; 54: 235–8.

68 Court JA, Johnson M, Religa D, *et al.* Attenuation of Abeta deposition in the entorhinal cortex of normal elderly individuals associated with tobacco smoking. Neuropathol appl neurobiol 2005; 31: 522–35.

69 Fisher A. Cholinergic treatments with emphasis on m1 muscarinic agonists as potential disease-modifying agents for Alzheimer's disease. Neurotherapeutics 2008; 5: 433–42.

70 Jakubik J, Michal P, Machova E, et al. Importance and prospects for design of selective muscarinic agonists. Physiol Res 2008; 57(Suppl 3): S39–47.

71 Perry EK, Marshall E, Perry RH, et al. Cholinergic and dopaminergic activities in senile dementia of Lewy body type. Alzh Dis Assoc Disord 1990; 4: 87–95.

72 Perry EK, Haroutunian V, Davis KL, et al. Neocortical cholinergic activities differentiate Lewy body dementia from classical Alzheimer's disease. Neuroreport 1994; 5: 747–9.

73 Perry E, Walker M, Grace J, Perry R. Acetylcholine in mind: a neurotransmitter correlate of consciousness? [see comment]. Trends Neurosci 1999; 22: 273–80.

74 Voytko ML. Cognitive functions of the basal forebrain cholinergic system in monkeys: memory or attention?. Behav Brain Res 1996; 75: 13–25.

75 Scott HL, Pow DV, Tannenberg AE, Dodd PR. Aberrant expression of the glutamate transporter excitatory amino acid transporter 1 (EAAT1) in Alzheimer's disease. J Neurosci 2002; 22: RC206.

76 Thorns V, Mallory M, Hansen L, Masliah E. Alterations in glutamate receptor 2/3 subunits and amyloid precursor protein expression during the course of Alzheimer's disease and Lewy body variant. Acta Neuropath 1997; 94: 539–48.

77 Molina JA, Gomez P, Vargas C, et al. Neurotransmitter amino acid in cerebrospinal fluid of patients with dementia with Lewy bodies. J Neural Transm 2005; 112: 557–63.

78 Albasanz JL, Dalfo E, Ferrer I, Martin M. Impaired metabotropic glutamate receptor/phospholipase C signaling pathway in the cerebral cortex in Alzheimer's disease and dementia with Lewy bodies correlates with stage of Alzheimer's-disease-related changes. Neurobiol Dis 2005; 20: 685–93.

79 Samadi P, Gregoire L, Morissette M, et al. mGluR5 metabotropic glutamate receptors and dyskinesias in MPTP monkeys. Neurobiol Aging 2008; 29: 1040–51.

80 Zaja-Milatovic S, Keene CD, Montine KS, Leverenz JB, Tsuang D, Montine TJ. Selective dendritic degeneration of medium spiny neurons in dementia with Lewy bodies. Neurology 2006; 66: 1591–3.

81 Zaja-Milatovic S, Milatovic D, Schantz AM, et al. Dendritic degeneration in neostriatal medium spiny neurons in Parkinson disease. Neurology 2005; 64: 545–7.

82 Braak H, Ghebremedhin E, Rub U, Bratzke H, Del Tredici K. Stages in the development of Parkinson's disease-related pathology. Cell and tissue research 2004; 318: 121–34.

83 Langlais PJ, Thal L, Hansen L, Galasko D, Alford M, Masliah E. Neurotransmitters in basal ganglia and cortex of Alzheimer's disease with and without Lewy bodies. Neurology 1993; 43: 1927–34.

84 Benarroch EE, Schmeichel AM, Low PA, Boeve BF, Sandroni P, Parisi JE. Involvement of medullary regions controlling sympathetic output in Lewy body disease. Brain 2005; 128: 338–44.

85 Scatton B, Javoy-Agid F, Rouquier L, Dubois B, Agid Y. Reduction of cortical dopamine, noradrenaline, serotonin and their metabolites in Parkinson's disease. Brain Res 1983; 275: 321–8.

86 Perry EK, McKeith I, Thompson P, et al. Topography, extent, and clinical relevance of neurochemical deficits in dementia of Lewy body type, Parkinson's disease, and Alzheimer's disease. Ann NY Acad Sci 1991; 640: 197–202.

87 Ohara K, Kondo N, Ohara K. Changes of monoamines in post-mortem brains from patients with diffuse lewy body disease. Prog Neuro-Psychopharmacol Biol Psychiatry 1998; 22: 311–7.

88 Perry EK, Marshall E, Thompson P, et al. Monoaminergic activities in Lewy body dementia: relation to hallucinosis and extrapyramidal features. J Neural Transm 1993; 6: 167–77.

89 Piggott MA, Marshall EF. Neurochemical correlates of pathological and iatrogenic extrapyramidal symptoms. In: Perry RH, McKeith IG, Perry EK, editors. Dementia with Lewy bodies: clinical, pathological, and treatment issues. Cambridge: Cambridge University Press, 1996; pp. 449–67.

90 Cheng AV, Ferrier IN, Morris CM, et al. Cortical serotonin-S2 receptor binding in Lewy body dementia, Alzheimer's and Parkinson's diseases. J Neurol Sci 1991; 106: 50–5.

91 Ghazi-Noori S, Chung TH, Deane K, Rickards H, Clarke CE. Therapies for depression in Parkinson's disease. Cochrane Database Syst Rev 2003; (3): CD003465.

92 Kuhn W, Muller T, Gerlach M, *et al*. Depression in Parkinson's disease: biogenic amines in CSF of "de novo" patients. J Neural Transm 1996; 103: 1441–5.

93 Ballard C, Johnson M, Piggott M, *et al*. A positive association between 5HT re-uptake binding sites and depression in dementia with Lewy bodies. J Affective Disord 2002; 69: 219–23.

94 Doder M, Rabiner EA, Turjanski N, Lees AJ, Brooks DJ. Tremor in Parkinson's disease and serotonergic dysfunction: an 11C-WAY 100635 PET study. Neurology 2003; 60: 601–5.

95 Sharp SI, Ballard CG, Ziabreva I, *et al*. Cortical serotonin 1A receptor levels are associated with depression in patients with dementia with Lewy bodies and Parkinson's disease dementia. Dementia Geriatr Cogn Dis 2008; 26: 330–8.

96 Chen CP, Alder JT, Bray L, Kingsbury AE, Francis PT, Foster OJ. Post-synaptic 5-HT1A and 5-HT2A receptors are increased in Parkinson's disease neocortex. Ann NY Acad Sci 1998; 861: 288–9.

97 Halliday GM, McCann HL, Pamphlett R, *et al*. Brain stem serotonin-synthesizing neurons in Alzheimer's disease: a clinicopathological correlation. Acta Neuropathol (Berl) 1992; 84: 638–50.

98 Lanari A, Amenta F, Silvestrelli G, Tomassoni D, Parnetti L. Neurotransmitter deficits in behavioural and psychological symptoms of Alzheimer's disease. Mechanisms Ageing Dev 2006; 127: 158–65.

99 Cash R, Dennis T, R LH, Raisman R, Javoy-Agid F, Scatton B. Parkinson's disease and dementia: norepinephrine and dopamine in locus ceruleus. Neurology 1987; 37: 42–6.

100 Remy P, Doder M, Lees A, Turjanski N, Brooks D. Depression in Parkinson's disease: loss of dopamine and noradrenaline innervation in the limbic system. Brain 2005; 128(Pt 6): 1314–22.

101 Zweig RM, Cardillo JE, Cohen M, Giere S, Hedreen JC. The locus ceruleus and dementia in Parkinson's disease. Neurology 1993; 43: 986–91.

102 Leverenz JB, Miller MA, Dobie DJ, Peskind ER, Raskind MA. Increased alpha 2-adrenergic receptor binding in locus coeruleus projection areas in dementia with Lewy bodies. Neurobiol Aging 2001; 22: 555–61.

103 Szot P, White SS, Greenup JL, Leverenz JB, Peskind ER, Raskind MA. Compensatory changes in the noradrenergic nervous system in the locus ceruleus and hippocampus of postmortem subjects with Alzheimer's disease and dementia with Lewy bodies. J Neurosci 2006; 26: 467–78.

104 Baloyannis SJ, Costa V, Baloyannis IS. Morphological alterations of the synapses in the locus coeruleus in Parkinson's disease. J Neurol Sci 2006; 248: 35–41.

105 Riekkinen M, Jakala P, Kejonen K, Riekkinen P, Jr. The alpha2 agonist, clonidine, improves spatial working performance in Parkinson's disease. Neuroscience 1999; 92: 983–9.

106 Bedard MA, el Massioui F, Malapani C, *et al*. Attentional deficits in Parkinson's disease: partial reversibility with naphtoxazine (SDZ NVI-085), a selective noradrenergic alpha 1 agonist. Clin Neuropharmacol 1998; 21: 108–17.

107 Coull JT. α-Adrenoceptors in the treatment of dementia: an attentional mechanism?. J Psychopharmacol 1996; 10(Suppl 3): 43–8.

108 Gomez-Tortosa E, Sanders JL, Newell K, Hyman BT. Cortical neurons expressing calcium binding proteins are spared in dementia with Lewy bodies. Acta Neuropath 2001; 101: 36–42.

109 Chan CS, Guzman JN, Ilijic E, *et al*. 'Rejuvenation' protects neurons in mouse models of Parkinson's disease. Nature 2007; 447(7148): 1081–6.

110 Mosharov EV, Larsen KE, Kanter E, *et al*. Interplay between cytosolic dopamine, calcium, and alpha-synuclein causes selective death of substantia nigra neurons.[see comment]. Neuron 2009; 62: 218–29.

111 Becker C, Jick SS, Meier CR. Use of antihypertensives and the risk of Parkinson disease. Neurology 2008; 70(16 Part 2): 1438–44.

112 Bosboom JL, Stoffers D, Stam CJ, *et al.* Resting state oscillatory brain dynamics in Parkinson's disease: an MEG study. Clin Neurophysiol 2006; 117: 2521–31.

113 Bosboom JL, Stoffers D, Stam CJ, Berendse HW, Wolters EC. Cholinergic modulation of MEG resting-state oscillatory activity in Parkinson's disease related dementia. Clin Neurophysiol 2009; 120: 910–5.

114 Jones EG. Synchrony in the interconnected circuitry of the thalamus and cerebral cortex. Ann NY Acad Sci 2009; 1157: 10–23.

115 Alexander GM, Carden WB, Mu J, *et al.* The native T-type calcium current in relay neurons of the primate thalamus. Neuroscience 2006; 141: 453–61.

116 Piggott MA, Candy JM, Perry RH. [3H]Nitrendipine binding in temporal cortex in Alzheimer's and Huntington's diseases. Brain Res 1991; 565: 42–7.

117 Calabresi P, Picconi B, Parnetti L, Di Filippo M. A convergent model for cognitive dysfunctions in Parkinson's disease: the critical dopamine–acetylcholine synaptic balance. Lancet neurology 2006; 5: 974–83.

118 Poewe W. Depression in Parkinson's disease. J Neurol 2007; 254(Suppl 5): 49–55.

119 Ballard C, Day S, Sharp S, Wing G, Sorensen S. Neuropsychiatric symptoms in dementia: importance and treatment considerations. Int Rev Psychiatry 2008; 20: 396–404.

Chapter 14

Pathological correlates of dementia in Parkinson's disease

Gonzalo J. Revuelta and Carol Lippa

Introduction

The time-honoured original work by James Parkinson has been proven to be quite insightful in its ability to integrate a constellation of symptoms into a cohesive syndrome, when observing a small group of patients. Dr Parkinson understood that this disease affected more than just the motor system; however, he did not feel that pathological change extended to the encephalon, henceforth, sparing the intellect [1]. With the advent of modern measures for cognitive assessment, and detailed pathological examination of brains affected by Parkinson's disease (PD), it is now clear that pathological change does extend to the encephalon, and subsequent cognitive dysfunction is not only common but of great consequence in this disease.

The definitions of cognitive dysfunction or dementia are not uniform, nor are the methods for its assessment. Adding to this complexity are patient populations which differ in terms of the pathology affecting them, comorbidities, and age. For these reasons, investigations to decipher the frequency of dementia in PD have yielded a broad range of results, with reports of prevalence ranging from 3% to 78% [2]. Average prevalence is estimated at 30–40% [3–5]. Dementia is not only more prevalent in ageing populations, but also more severe, and can be the presenting symptom. Furthermore, dementia in PD is associated with worse outcomes, including a more rapid progression, leading to earlier nursing home placement, reduced quality of life, and increased mortality [2].

Dementia in PD has been categorized clinically as PD dementia (PD-D) or dementia with Lewy bodies (DLB) depending on whether motor or cognitive symptoms dominated the early stages of disease, respectively. It is becoming more apparent to us that there is a spectrum of clinical syndromes which, when correlated pathologically, has been found to range from pure forms related exclusively to Lewy-body-related pathology (LRP), as in diffuse Lewy body disease (DLBD) to more heterogeneous forms with prominent Alzheimer's disease (AD)-related pathology (ARP), as in the Lewy body variant of AD (LBV).

The pathological changes responsible for cognitive dysfunction in PD are heterogeneous and complex. The principal pathological change is that of neuronal loss, or neurodegeneration; however, which areas are actually degenerating, and whether neurodegeneration in these areas is actually responsible for clinical findings, is not entirely clear. Moreover, the underlying causative agents for these pathological changes are multiple, including LRP,

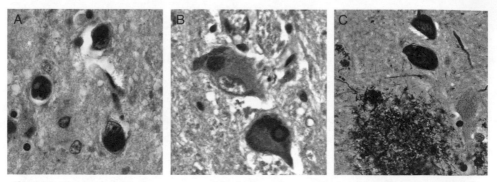

Fig. 14.1 Histopathological appearance of brain tissue from patients with Parkinson's disease and dementia (PD-D). (A) Several cortical neurones at high power containing cortical Lewy bodies. Cortical Lewy bodies typically lack a halo, and they are the strongest pathological feature associated with dementia in Parkinson's disease. Their density also correlates with specific clinical features in some studies. (B) Nigral Lewy bodies in the cytoplasm of brainstem neurones. These are associated more closely with the motor features of Parkinson's disease. Nigral Lewy bodies usually contain a 'halo' that stains strongly for α-synuclein (images A and B are stained with antibodies directed against α-synuclein). (C) Modified silver stain to demonstrate Alzheimer's neurofibrillary tangles (top) and a senile plaque (bottom) in cortical brain tissue from the medial temporal lobe of a PD patient. Alzheimer's pathological features are not uncommon in PD-D patients, but do not correlate with dementia as closely as synuclein pathology (Lewy bodies and Lewy neurites).

ARP, vascular pathology, or a combination. Of further dispute are contributions of neurochemical, neurophysiological, and 'normal' changes related with ageing. In this chapter we will review the current literature regarding these pathological changes and how they are thought to contribute to the clinical syndromes related to cognitive dysfunction in PD.

Lewy body pathology

Our knowledge of the underlying pathology in PD begins with Frederic H. Lewy's discovery of inclusion bodies in patients with PD in 1912 [6]. These spherical filamentous inclusions, now known as Lewy bodies (LBs), have been at the epicentre of discussions of the pathology of this disease for almost 100 years. In 1997, Polymeropoulos *et al.* reported the discovery of a mutation in the gene coding for a presynaptic protein called α-synuclein in one Italian kindred and three unrelated Greek families with autosomal dominant PD [7]. Following this finding Spillantini *et al.* found that LBs as well as dystrophic processes with equal immunohistochemical properties called Lewy neurites (LNs) found in patients with idiopathic PD and DLB stained strongly for this protein, yielding clues as to the composition of these inclusions [8]. Soon after, Baba *et al.* revealed that α-synuclein in LBs was aggregated into fibrils in both sporadic and genetic forms of PD [9]. More than 40 proteins have since been found to compose LBs including ubiquitin, tau, heat shock proteins (HSPs), neurofilaments, aggresomal proteins and mitochondrial proteins, but α-synuclein is by far the most prominent [10].

Several neurodegenerative diseases have also been found to have inclusions which are immunoreactive for α-synuclein including: multiple system atrophy (MSA), pure autonomic failure (PAF), and neurodegeneration with brain iron accumulation type 1 (NBIA-1). These and others have joined the ranks of PD and DLB to form a new class of disease now referred to as the synucleinopathies [11].

In PD-D, LBs are abundant in cortical structures. Cortical LBs (CLBs) have been described as having less distinct morphology particularly when using haematoxylin and eosin staining, and they typically lack a distinctive halo which is classically found in LBs in the substantia nigra (SN) [10]. CLBs are the most specific pathological finding in PD-D and they have been found to correlate with dementia consistently [12–14].

Alzheimer's disease-related pathology

Since Alois Alzheimer's discovery in 1907 of neuritic plaques and neurofibrillary tangles (NFTs) as the principal pathological change in AD, much has been learned of these entities. Notable discoveries in this pathological category include the understanding of the ultrastructure of NFTs and neuritic plaques and their correlation with dementia in AD. Equally important has been the discovery of the hyperphosphorylated tau protein as the major constituent of paired helical filaments and the discovery of Aβ peptide as the major component of amyloid plaques [15]. These findings have led to the classification of diseases in terms of their immunoreactivity for these proteins and has changed the way we think about these entities clinically. We now use the term amyloidopathy to refer to AD (of both familial and sporadic forms), Down's syndrome and others. Similarly, we use the term tauopathy to refer to frontotemporal dementia (FTD), progressive supranuclear palsy (PSP), corticobasal degeneration (CBD), and others. Other proteins have also been implicated in these neurodegenerative diseases which include progranulin (PGRN), transactive response DNA-binding protein 43 (TDP-43), and others [16].

Plaques and tangles are clearly present relatively frequently in PD-D, but they are less often significant contributors to the clinical dementia phenotype. Multiple cases have been reported of a clinical and pathological picture of PD-D without any ARP. Furthermore, multiple studies have found them weak correlates for dementia in PD-D, as opposed to LRP [12].

Distribution of pathology and clinico-pathological correlation

Although previous reports point to the substantia nigra (SN) as the primary site of neurodegeneration in PD, Tretiakoff in 1919 has been credited with this finding [17]. Since then, our understanding of the pathological changes in the SN has grown significantly. LRP is first found ventrally in the SN pars compacta (SNc), and then spreads to paranigral, medial and dorsal areas. There is neuronal loss in conjunction with LRP, specifically of melanized and dopaminergic neurones in area A9 of the SNc [18]. These pathological changes in A9, which result in decrease in dopamine, tyrosine hydroxylase (TH) and dopamine transporter (DAT) immunoreactivity in the striatum, correlate with duration and severity of motor symptoms [19]. It is not clear, however, whether these neurochemical changes are directly related to LRP.

It has become evident that neurodegeneration in PD goes well beyond the SN, and, in fact, affects not only subcortical dopaminergic nuclei, but basal cholinergic structures, dorsal motor nucleus of the vagus nerve, olfactory structures, raphe nuclei, locus ceruleus, pedunculo-pontine nuclei, hypothalamic nuclei, spinal nuclei and cortical structures as well. LRP, ARP and vascular change are the principal pathologies thought to result in neuronal loss in these structures. Specifically, LRP has been documented in the striatum of patients with a variety of synucleinopathies [20]. It has been suggested that greater LRP burden in the SN is indicative of a predominant motor syndrome as in PD or PD-D, and conversely, greater LRP burden in the striatum is more indicative of a predominantly dementing illness such as DLB [21]. Furthermore, LRP often involves the peripheral nervous system; including autonomic nuclei, ganglia and nerves subserving vasculature, intestines, heart, adrenal and salivary glands [18]. Of note, recent studies have discovered LBs in two patients with PD who had undergone transplantation of fetal mesencephalic dopaminergic neurones with long-term survival. Grafted cells, in these two patients, were not functionally impaired [22].

LRP has been described in both limbic (layer II) and neocortical structures (layers V and VI). Pathological change, in specific structures within these areas, has been studied meticulously in order to correlate clinical symptomatology with cortical LRP burden, and to differentiate between synucleinopathies. Of all the cortical areas studied, it appears that LRP burden in the parahippocampus is most indicative of dementia in this patient population, although in DLB cases, the pathology was more heterogeneous [23]. Similarly, in the entorhinal and anterior cingulate cortex (Brodmann area 24) LRP burden correlates well with cognitive deficits in patients with PD-D [14]. High LRP burden in the parahippocampus and amygdala correlate well with early visual hallucinations. Furthermore, LRP in the inferior temporal cortical structures is associated with earlier onset of hallucinations, and therefore with a greater likelihood of developing DLB [24].

The diverse pathological findings described above, which individually correlate with some clinical symptoms, have been consolidated in different ways in order to account for specific clinical syndromes. Since the findings in PD-D are quite heterogeneous, and even more so in DLB, pathological criteria for the diagnosis of these syndromes has been developed and validated. McKeith *et al.* have devised and revised criteria for the pathological diagnosis of DLB, taking into account the extent of LRP in specific brain regions, as well as ARP, and rating pathological burden in a semiquantitative fashion. In determining which clinical syndrome is most likely indicated by the pathological change being observed, the type of pathological change is as important as the distribution of such change. Therefore, the McKeith criteria assign a probability that the pathological change is consistent with the clinical syndrome of DLB, based not only on the LRP burden (which is directly related to the likelihood of the pathology representing DLB) and the ARP (which is inversely related to the likelihood of the pathology representing DLB [25]), but also on the areas involved. These criteria group cases into brainstem predominant, limbic or transitional, and diffuse neocortical, and the likelihood that the pathological changes represent the

DLB clinical syndrome is greater with more rostral and lesser with more caudal changes [26,27].

Progression of disease

The question of whether the aforementioned pathological changes and their distribution actually follow a distinct course of progression is central to understanding the patho-physiology of LBDs. Braak *et al.* meticulously studied a series of brains of patients with clinical PD, incidental LBs and LNs, and controls. Working under the assumption that there was a coherent progression of disease in these cases, they organized the samples in a sequential manner, and subsequently developed a staging system for LRP in this patient population. The staging system that emerged proposed a caudo-rostral progression of pathological change which began in the dorsal motor nucleus of the glossopharyngeal and vagus nerves, as well as the olfactory nucleus, and ascended to mesocortical and then neocortical structures. The first two stages are related to incidental LBD, the third and fourth stages with motor symptoms, and the later stages (five and six) to concurrent cognitive dysfunction [28]. Later studies by the same authors were able to correlate cognitive dysfunction with this staging system of LRP in patients with PD [29].

Multiple counter-examples to this staging system have since been proposed, whereby sparing of caudal regions with more rostral involvement has occurred, which implies that other pathological changes, aside from LBP, may be contributing [18]. Further evidence of this notion is that the existence of LRP—to the extent that meets pathological criteria for diagnosis of DLB—may occur in the absence of a clinical dementing syndrome [30]. More recent revisions of this staging system propose that the early sites of LRP are the olfactory bulb and enteric plexus of the stomach, and moreover propose that a neuro-trophic pathogen enters through the nasal or gastric mucosa and proceeds to the central nervous system via anterograde progression to temporal structures or through retrograde transport via peripheral ganglia, respectively [31].

A competing theory, which not only challenges Braak's proposed theory of disease progression but is also a unitary theory of pathophysiology for LBDs, identifies three distinct clinico-pathological subgroups. The first consists of a younger group of patients with a predominantly motor early phenotype which is consistent with caudo-rostral progression of pathological change. The second subgroup consists of patients that suffered a more aggressive course of disease, with an early onset of dementia and concomitant early neocortical involvement. The third subgroup identified represents patients with later onset of disease, and a subsequently shorter course, with a greater burden of pathological change that tended also to be more heterogeneous. This theory, and the data that support it, implies that a caudo-rostral progression of pathological change is only applicable to a subgroup of patients, and does not explain progression of disease in other subgroups, particularly those that follow a dementia-dominant clinical course [32].

Aetiologies underlying neurodegeneration

From the information presented above, we understand the specific pathology that is found in PD-D, where it occurs, how it correlates with clinical symptoms, how it can be correlated with clinical syndromes, and how it progresses; nevertheless the mechanisms that underlie these pathological changes remain unclear. Several theories have been developed to explain why the pathological changes that take place in LBDs actually occur. At the root of this discussion is the assumption that α-synuclein aggregation in LBs is the central neuropathological feature of these diseases, and this is supported by the finding that mutations in the α-synuclein gene lead to parkinsonism, the finding of aggregated α-synuclein with abnormal nitration, phosphorylation and ubiquitination, the development of neurodegeneration in transgenic animal models, and the aforementioned clinico-pathological correlation studies [21]. The finding that LBs are found in grafted neurones supports this assertion; however, the finding that LRP is present in patients without parkinsonism or cognitive dysfunction (incidental LBD) implies at least that LRP may not be the only mechanism underlying neurodegeneration in LBDs, which is certainly the case in more severe dementing syndromes such as DLB. Furthermore, some have theorized that there is a 'bystander' effect that occurs when multiple pathologies such as LRP and ARP coexist and may augment one another in these disease entities. Others suggest that the mere accumulation of abnormal proteins is not sufficient to account for the clinical symptoms, and instead, an assessment of the neurochemical changes that occur as a result of degeneration of neurones, particularly monoaminergic neurones, would more accurately represent the underlying pathophysiology. Certainly other changes, including vascular, and normal ageing changes, can and do contribute to degeneration of these neurones to differing degrees [18].

If we accept the assumption that α-synuclein pathology is indeed central to the pathophysiology of these diseases, it still remains unclear how exactly that occurs. The question of toxicity of α-synuclein has been posed, and remains largely unanswered; indeed, some have proposed that it may be the by-product of an effort by the cell to protect itself from neurodegeneration. Mechanisms of underlying degeneration include overproduction of α-synuclein, dysfunction of chaperones and other components of the ubiquitin–proteosome system, inflammation, oxitadive stress, excitotoxicity, mitochondrial dysfunction, growth factor deficiencies, prion-like mechanisms of cell injury, or a combination of these [33].

References

1 Parkinson J. An essay on the shaking palsy. Medical Classics, 1817; vol. 2(10): pp. 957–97.

2 Goldmann R, Gross AS, Hurtig HI. Cognitive impairment in Parkinson's disease and dementia with Lewy bodies: a spectrum of disease. Neurosignals 2008; 16: 24–34.

3 Cummings J. The dementias of Parkinson's disease: prevalence, characteristics, neurobiology, and comparison with dementia of Alzheimer type. Eur Neurol 1998; 28(Suppl 1): 15–23.

4 Aarsland D, Andersen K, Larsen JP, et al. Prevalence and characteristics of dementia in Parkinson disease: an 8-year prospective study. Arch Neurol 2003; 60: 387–92.

5 Emre M. Dementia in Parkinson's disease: cause and treatment. Curr Opin Neurol 2004; 17: 399–404.

6 Lewy F. Zür pathologischen Anatomie der Paralysis agitans. Dtsch Z Nervenheilk 1914; 1: 50–5.

7 Michael H, Polymeropoulos CL, Leroy E, et al. Mutation in the α-synuclein gene identified in families with Parkinson's disease. Science 1997; 276: 2045–7.

8 MG Spillantini, Schmidt ML, Lee VMY, Trojanowski JQ, Jakes R, Goedert M. α-Synuclein in Lewy bodies. Nature 1997; 388: 839–40.

9 Baba M, Nakajo S, Tu PH, et al. Aggregation of α-synuclein in Lewy bodies of sporadic Parkinson's disease and dementia with Lewy bodies. Am J Pathol 1998; 152: 879–84.

10 Shults CW. Lewy bodies. Proc Natl Acad Sci USA 2006; 103: 1661–8.

11 Galvin JE, Lee VM, Trojanowski JQ. Synucleinopathies: clinical and pathological implications. Arch Neurol 2001; 58: 185–90.

12 Hurtig HI, Trojanowski JQ, Galvin J, et al. Alpha-synuclein cortical Lewy bodies correlate with dementia in Parkinson's disease. Neurology 2000; 54: 1916–21.

13 Aarsland D, Perry R, Brown A, Larsen JP, Ballard AC. Neuropathology of dementia in Parkinson's disease: a prospective, community-based study. Ann Neurol 2005; 58: 773–6.

14 Kövari E, GG, François R, Herrmann PRH, Canuto A, Bouras C, Giannakopoulos P. Lewy body densities in the entorhinal and anterior cingulate cortex predict cognitive deficits in Parkinson's disease. Acta Neuropathol 2003; 106: 83–8.

15 Iqbal K, Grundke-Iqbal, I. Discoveries of tau, abnormally hyperphosphorylated tau and others of neurofibrillary degeneration: a personal historical perspective. J Alzh Dis 2006; 9: 219–42.

16 Bradley F, Boeve MH. Refining frontotemporal dementia with parkinsonism linked to chromosome 17. Arch Neurol 2008; 65: 460–64.

17 Tretiakoff C. Contribution a l'etude de l'anatomie pathologique du locus niger de Soemmering avec quelques dedutions relatives a la pathogenie des troubles du tonus musculaire et de la maladie de Parkinson, in. These de Paris; 1919.

18 Jellinger K. A critical reappraisal of current staging of Lewy-related pathology in human brain. Acta Neuropathol 2008; 116: 1–16.

19 Ma SY, Röyttä M, Rinne JO, Collan Y, Rinne UK. Correlation between neuromorphometry in the substantia nigra and clinical features in Parkinson's disease using disector counts. J Neurol Sci 1997; 151: 83–7.

20 Duda JE, Giasson BI, Mabon ME, Lee VMY, Trojanowski JQ. Novel antibodies to synuclein show abundant striatal pathology in Lewy body diseases. Ann Neurol 2002; 52: 205–10.

21 Lippa CF, Duda JE, Grossman M. DLB and PDD boundary issues: diagnosis, treatment, molecular pathology, and biomarkers. Neurology 2007; 68: 812–19.

22 Li JY, Englund E, Holton JL. Lewy bodies in grafted neurons in subjects with Parkinson's disease suggest host-to-graft disease propagation. Nature Med 2008; 14: 501–3.

23 Harding AJ, Halliday GM. Cortical Lewy body pathology in the diagnosis of dementia. Acta Neuropathol 2001; 102: 355–63.

24 Harding AJ, Broe GA, Halliday GM. Visual hallucinations in Lewy body disease relate to Lewy bodies in the temporal lobe. Brain 2002; 125: 391–403.

25 Merdes AR, Hansen LA, Jeste DV. Influence of Alzheimer pathology on clinical diagnostic accuracy in dementia with Lewy bodies. Neurology 2003; 60: 1586–90.

26 Fujishiro H, Ferman TJ, Boeve BF. Validation of the neuropathologic criteria of the Third Consortium for Dementia with Lewy Bodies for prospectively diagnosed cases. J Neuropathol Exp Neurol 2008; 67: 649–56.

27 McKeith IG, Dickson DW, Lowe J. Diagnosis and management of dementia with Lewy bodies. Neurology 2005; 65: 1863–72.

28 Braak H, Del Tredici K, Rüb U, de Vos RA, Jansen Steur EN, Braak E. Staging of brain pathology related to sporadic Parkinson's disease. Neurobiol Aging 2003; 24: 197–211.

29 Braak H, Rüb U, Jansen Steur EN, Del Tredici K, de Vos RAI. Cognitive status correlates with neuropathologic stage in Parkinson disease. Neurology 2005; 64: 1404–10.

30 Colosimo C, H.A., Kilford L, Lees AJ. Lewy body cortical involvement may not always predict dementia in Parkinson's disease. J Neurol Neurosurg Psychiatry 2003; 74: 852–6.

31 Hawkes CH, Del Tredicki K, Braak H. Parkinson's disease: a dual-hit hypothesis. Neuropathol Appl Neurobiol 2007; 33: 599–614.

32 Halliday G, Hely M, Reid W, Morris J. The progression of pathology in longitudinally followed patients with Parkinson's disease. Acta Neuropathol 2008; 115: 409–15.

33 Brundin P, Li J-Y, Holton JL, Lindvall O, Revesz T. Research in motion: the enigma of Parkinson's disease pathology spread. Nature Rev 2008; 9: 741–5.

Chapter 15

Cognitive impairment in non-demented patients with Parkinson's disease

Elise Caccappolo and Karen Marder

Introduction

Cognitive impairment is common in non-demented Parkinson's disease (PD) patients, including those with newly diagnosed disease [1–4]. A better understanding of the cognitive profile exhibited by this subset of patients could assist in defining the temporal pattern of cognitive impairment in non-demented patients and the prognostic significance of specific impairments, as well as identifying those patients at highest risk for developing dementia who might benefit from an intervention to delay or prevent cognitive decline.

Prevalence and incidence of cognitive impairment in PD

Prevalence estimates of cognitive impairment in non-demented PD patients vary widely, with 22–55% of PD patients fulfilling criteria for mild cognitive impairment (MCI) [5–6]. This group does not meet criteria for dementia, but exhibits cognitive performance that is worse than expected given age and education norms. The variability in prevalence estimates is secondary to methodological differences across studies such as the definition of cognitive dysfunction [7,8], neuropsychological test selection, patient population, and comparator group (e.g. normative data vs controls). For example, in a community-based study of 76 non-demented PD patients with longstanding disease, 45% of the sample were found to be non-impaired, while 55% exhibited cognitive impairment, defined as performance ≥2 standard deviations (SD) below a control group mean on one or more of three tests which assessed attention/executive abilities, visuospatial functioning, and immediate non-verbal memory [5]. Compared to the non-impaired PD patients, the cognitively impaired patients were older and had later age at disease onset which probably contributed to their poorer performance. More recently, a very large community-based study comparing 400 PD patients with a mean disease duration of 12 years to controls on a screening battery (Scales for Outcomes in Parkinson's disease – Cognition: SCOPA-COG) demonstrated that after taking age and education differences into account, 22% of the patients were cognitively impaired, defined as a score on the screening battery that fell ≥2 SD below the controls' score, with the most significant differences occurring on tests of executive functioning and memory [6].

Incidence studies of PD provide a more accurate estimate of cognitive impairment than prevalence studies, since the effects of motor impairment and medication effects are generally reduced. Also, survival rates are shorter in demented subjects so that cognitive dysfunction may be underestimated due to survival bias [9] and subjects in prevalence studies may have comorbid medical or psychiatric impairments that could contribute to cognitive decline, making incidence studies more helpful for investigating possible risk factors for cognitive dysfunction and dementia. Table 15.1 includes a list of clinic- and community-based incidence studies that illustrate the cognitive domains most frequently affected in early incident PD.

Two recent incidence studies provide similar rates of cognitive impairment in PD groups at the time of diagnosis [3,4]. In a population-based sample of 239 newly diagnosed PD patients, 36% of the group demonstrated cognitive impairment. Within this subgroup, 21% scored ≥1 SD below the mean on a pattern recognition memory test and were subsequently classified as having temporal lobe dysfunction, 13% scored below a cut-off score on a modified Tower of London test, which was associated with a frontostriatal type of deficit, and 15% were impaired on both measures, suggesting global impairment. Those patients who were cognitively intact (i.e. scoring >24 on the Mini-Mental State Examination (MMSE), within 1 SD of normative mean scores on the pattern recognition test, and above a cut-off score of 8/14 on the Tower of London test) were younger at the time of diagnosis [4]. In the second study, a comprehensive neuropsychological test battery was used to compare the performance of a community-based sample of 115 newly diagnosed PD patients with a mean disease duration of 19 months to that of 70 healthy controls. PD patients performed significantly worse across most tests, with 24% of the PD group classified as cognitively impaired. Impairment was defined as performance ≥2 SD below the normative sample mean score on at least three tests. The most substantial deficits were found on tests of executive function, memory, and complex attention/psychomotor speed (i.e. Digit Symbol subtest) [3].

Pattern of cognitive impairment in PD patients without dementia

Because the number of studies assessing the cognitive functioning of incident populations is relatively limited, the specific profile of cognitive impairment in non-demented PD remains not fully established. Available data consistently illustrate that deficits in executive functions are most prominent in early PD [3,13–15] and may include poor planning, sequencing, cognitive flexibility, and problem-solving ability as well as deficits in working memory and attention [4,11–12]. Visuospatial deficits including poor visual organization and visual construction, e.g. difficulty copying figures, matching figures or recognizing faces, have been identified in non-demented PD patients [16–18] and may occur early in the disease; for example, clock-drawing ability was impaired in 11% of Muslimović's newly diagnosed PD sample [3]. Aspects of memory are frequently impaired in non-demented patients and include encoding [19] and delayed recall [2,14] but recognition remains relatively well preserved, suggesting that storage of new information

Table 15.1 Studies of cognition in incident Parkinson's disease (PD)

Reference	PD group		Neuropsychological domains tested	Results (comparison of PD with control group or standardized scores)
	Mean age/PD duration	Clinical/community status		
Clinic-based				
Cooper et al. (1991) [10]	60 PD patients Age: 59.8 years Duration: 15.7 months 37 controls	– Patients in neurology outpatient clinics – Newly diagnosed, unmedicated	General intellect Memory Language Visuospatial Executive Motor control	PD patients showed significantly impaired performance on 10/15 cognitive tests Deficits found on tests of executive functioning: cognitive manipulation, working memory, set formation, and motor control
Owen et al. (1992) [11]	Subset of sample of 30 PD patients: 15 mild PD Duration: 18 months 44 controls	– Patients in general neurology clinic – No diagnosis of dementia – Unmedicated	Executive function Memory – Visual recall and recognition	PD patients significantly more impaired on attention task
Dujardin et al. (1999) [12]	17 PD patients Age: 63.2 (9.6) years Duration: 19.6 (13.4) months 17 controls	– Unmedicated – No significant depression or global cognitive impairment	Executive function – Stroop – Brown–Peterson paradigm	PD patients significantly more impaired on test of response inhibition (Stroop) than controls suggesting difficulty inhibiting a strong habitual response PD patients performed as well as controls on a dual-task measure requiring working memory (Brown–Peterson)
Muslimović et al. (2005) [3]	115 PD patients Age: 66.2 (10.1) years Duration: 18.8 (10.7) months 70 controls	– Participants in a longitudinal research project of functional status in PD – No global cognitive decline	Memory (verbal and visual) Executive Language Visuospatial Attention Psychomotor speed	24% of PD patients exhibited cognitive dysfunction (impaired performance on at least three neuropsychological tests) Deficits found on measures of: attention/executive function, psychomotor speed, visuospatial skills, memory, language

Table 15.1 (continued) Studies of cognition in incident Parkinson's disease (PD)

Reference	PD group Mean age/PD duration	Clinical/community status	Neuropsychological domains tested	Results (comparison of PD with control group or standardized scores)
Community-based				
Foltynie et al. (2004) [4]	159 PD patients Age: 70.6 years	– Newly diagnosed cohort using a community-based epidemiological approach – Cases identified over 3-month period	MMSE NART COWAT Semantic fluency Pattern recognition Memory Spatial recognition memory Tower of London BDI	8% scored <24 on mental status testing and were therefore considered demented. Of the remaining subjects, 36% demonstrated cognitive impairment. Within this subgroup, 21% were impaired on a pattern recognition memory test (memory), 13% were impaired on a modified Tower of London test (executive function), and 15% were impaired on both measures, suggesting global impairment
Aarsland et al. (2008) [2]	196 PD patients Age: 67.6 (9.2) years Duration: 2.3 (1.8) years 201 controls	– Community sample – Newly diagnosed, drug-naïve	CVLT-2 Silhouettes and cube subtests (VOSP) Category fluency Serial 7 subtest (MMSE) Stroop MADRS	PD patients were significantly impaired on all neuropsychological tests compared to controls, with largest effect sizes found for verbal memory and psychomotor speed 19% fulfilled criteria for MCI, of which: 62% naMCI-SD, 24% aMCI-SD, 11% aMCI-MD, 2.7% naMCI-MD

MMSE, Mini-Mental State Examination; NART, National Adult Reading Test; COWAT, Controlled Oral Word Association Test; BDI, Beck Depression Inventory; CVLT, California Verbal Learning Test; VOSP, Visual Object and Space Perception test; MADRS, Montgomery–Åsberg Depression Rating Scale; a/naMCI, amnestic/non-amnestic mild cognitive impairment; -SD, single domain; -MD, multiple domain.

occurs, but is not easily accessed [13,20]. Procedural memory is also impaired [21]. Language dysfunction is rarely reported in the non-demented PD population, with the exception of deficits in phonemic, semantic, and alternating fluency (e.g. shifting between types of categories or types of phonemic criteria), which have been found not only to exist [14,22–24], but to decline over time [24] and with disease severity as measured by Hoehn and Yahr stage [25] as well as to predict a later diagnosis of dementia [26–28]. Confrontation naming is generally intact in patients without dementia [29,30], but mild difficulty has also been documented [3].

Most of the deficits described in early PD may be explained at least in part by executive function deficits [31]. For example, visuospatial deficits may be due to executive dysfunction such as poor sequential organization, planning, abstraction and self-monitoring ability [16,18,32] or to deficits in visual attention [33]. In early PD, memory deficits typically reflect ineffective strategies in encoding and retrieval secondary to frontal dysfunction, such as poor executive control of attentional systems [34,35]. The finding that retrieval improves when patients are provided with cues, which assist by narrowing the search process, supports the role of frontal processes in memory impairment. Verbal fluency deficits may be attributed to executive dysfunction, such as an inability to generate efficient search strategies given that fluency tasks require self-initiated retrieval [14,24,36,37].

PD patients who exhibit early MCI are at a higher risk of developing dementia [26,38]. If the cognitive deficits found in incidence studies represent one end of a continuum of cognitive impairment, with dementia as an endpoint for a subset of patients, then the pattern of cognitive dysfunction associated with Parkinson's disease dementia can be assumed to reflect the same pattern of deficits, albeit more severe, as that exhibited by PD patients early in the disease process [39,40]. However, conversion to dementia is confounded by numerous risk factors including age at time of assessment [41,42] and PD subtype, i.e. patients with postural instability and gait disorder (PIGD) are at higher risk of converting to dementia than those with tremor (43) as well as the fact that the underlying pathology in patients with dementia may be heterogeneous including coexisting Alzheimer's disease (AD)-related pathology, diffuse cortical Lewy bodies and vascular changes, all of which may increase the severity or alter the pattern of cognitive impairment [44–46]. The question of whether DLB and PD-D represent different pathologies, or two clinico-pathological entities on the same disease spectrum, continues to be examined given their similar neuropsychological and clinical presentations [47].

The development of PD-D may lead not only to a worsening in the severity of those cognitive deficits found in non-demented PD patients, but to further impairments in domains other than executive functioning as additional brain regions become affected, including cortical regions [48]. Memory and learning performance in particular worsens, and in some studies, confrontation naming difficulties, considered to be sensitive to semantic memory [49], become apparent, as does visuospatial ability, which may be due to changes in visual perception [50,51]. A cortical cholinergic deficiency that is superimposed on the existing dopaminergic deficit is implicated in the progression of impairment, but some of these changes are also likely to be due to the comorbidities that frequently exist in many cases of PD.

Diagnosing cognitive impairment in PD patients

In general, neuropsychological tests vary in sensitivity and specificity as well as in available normative data, which, when combined with differences in premorbid functioning of individuals secondary to cultural and educational differences, results in considerable variability. Cognitive assessment of patients with PD may also be confounded by the motor difficulties and psychiatric symptoms experienced by many PD patients [52]. Cognitive impairment in PD is often broadly screened by means of the MMSE [53] with a score <24 generally accepted as indicating impairment [54]. However, the MMSE does not include measures of executive functioning, which, as discussed, is most often affected in early PD, but instead focuses on the domains of language and orientation, which may be preserved even in PD-D [55]. In addition, a ceiling effect is frequently found [52]. The MMSE has also been criticized for its lack of sensitivity even when a higher cut-off score of ≤26 is used [56,57]. The MMSE is most effective when differentiating PD patients with moderate or severe deficits from controls [58] as opposed to differentiating controls and mildly impaired patients [59]. A very recent study administered memory, executive function, and attention tests to 106 PD patients who obtained normal age and education-adjusted MMSE scores (mean score: 29.1) and found that 29% of the sample scored at least 1.5 SD below published normative means on at least two tests (for memory and executive abilities) or a single measure (for attention) [59].

Other screening batteries have been used in studies of PD-related cognitive functioning (Tables 15.2 and 15.3). For example, the cognitive section of the Cambridge Examination for Mental Disorders (CAMCOG) [71] includes all of the items from the MMSE so as to allow for the calculation of an MMSE total score (subsequently, the two measures correlate strongly, i.e. $r = 0.87$), but assesses additional cognitive areas such as perception (recognition of famous faces and objects from unusual angles) and abstract thinking (identifying similarities between objects) as well as functional status. When using a cut-off score of 80 (out of a maximum score of 107), the CAMCOG showed higher specificity for identifying dementia, defined by Diagnostic and Statistical Manual (DSM)-IV criteria, in PD patients than the MMSE [52] (CAMCOG-R) [61]. However, the CAMCOG's utility for identifying cognitive impairment in non-demented PD patients has yet to be formally assessed. Screening batteries designed to assess mild cognitive dysfunction, such as the Montreal Cognitive Assessment (MoCA) [63], can assist with identifying a more precise cognitive profile for non-demented PD patients. A comparison of the MMSE and MoCA scores for 88 PD patients revealed that the MoCA classified 32% of subjects scoring below a cut-off of 26/30 on the MMSE as having MCI, while the MMSE classified only 11% [69]. A more recent study compared the MoCA scores of 38 PD patients to their composite scores on a relatively brief neuropsychological battery (Hopkins Verbal Learning Test – Revised, Letter–Number Sequencing subtest from the WAIS-III, Stroop Color Word Test and fluency testing) and reported a correlation coefficient of 0.72 [70]. Although the sample size was small and the test battery was limited, this result suggests good convergent validity.

Table 15.2 Screening batteries used in Parkinson's disease (PD) studies

Battery	Tests/subscales	Comments
CAMCOG Cognitive section of the Cambridge Cognitive Examination (Roth *et al.*, 1986) [60]	Memory (short- and long-term, recall, recognition) Orientation Language Attention Praxis (construction) Perception Calculation Executive function	◆ Compared to MMSE, covers a broader range of cognitive functions, detects milder degrees of cognitive impairment, and avoids ceiling effects ◆ Contains 67 items grouped into 8 subscales ◆ Takes 25 min to administer ◆ Total possible score = 107, scores <80 used as cut-off for dementia ◆ Annual decline of 1.6 points in normals ◆ No age-and education-stratified norms available
CAMCOG-R Cognitive section of the Cambridge Cognitive Examination – Revised (Roth *et al.*, 1999) [61]	CAMCOG subscales + mental flexibility in verbal and visuospatial domains (ideational fluency and matrix reasoning)	◆ Includes two additional tests of executive function which do not contribute to overall score but are separately summed for a maximum score of 28 ◆ No cut-off score for dementia has been suggested
SCOPA-COG Scales for Outcomes in Parkinson's disease – Cognition (Marinus *et al.*, 2003) [62]	Immediate and delayed word recall Visual recall (block pointing in sequence) Digit span Counting backwards Reciting months backward Fist–palm–edge Set-shifting with dice Animal fluency Mental reconstruction of figures	◆ Developed for research purposes to compare PD groups ◆ Examines a narrow range of cognitive deficits specific to PD: memory, attention, executive and visuospatial functioning ◆ Consists of 10 items with maximum score of 43 ◆ Takes 10–15 min to administer
MoCA Montreal Cognitive Assessment (Nasreddine *et al.*, 2005) [63]	Memory Visuospatial functioning Executive functioning Attention Concentration Working memory Language Orientation	◆ Designed for clinicians to assess MCI ◆ Compared to MMSE, uses more demanding tests to assess executive functions, higher level language abilities, memory and complex visual reasoning ◆ Contains 8 subscales ◆ Takes 10 min to administer ◆ Total possible score: 30; score <26 used as cut-off for MCI ◆ No data on change scores, no norms available
PANDA Parkinson Neuropsychometric Dementia Assessment instrument(Kalbe *et al.*, 2008) [64]	Word-pair learning tasks – immediate and delayed recall Alternating verbal fluency Visuospatial task Working memory and attention Mood (depression)	◆ Designed for clinicians to assess cognitive functioning in PD ◆ Assesses functions typically affected in PD as well as depression ◆ Contains 5 subscales ◆ Takes 8–10 min to administer ◆ Total possible score: 30; score >18: normal; 15–17: mild cognitive dysfunction; <15: severe cognitive impairment/dementia ◆ Allows for score transformation so that scores are independent of age and education

Table 15.2 (continued) Screening batteries used in Parkinson's disease (PD) studies

Battery	Tests/subscales	Comments
PD-CRS Parkinson's Disease – Cognitive Rating Scale (Pagonabarraga *et al.*, 2008) [65]	Attention Working memory Stroop test Verbal fluencies Verbal memory Clock drawing Confrontation naming	◆ Developed to assess both subcortical and cortical functions ◆ Has not been subjected to extensive clinimetric evaluations

MMSE, Mini-Mental State Examination; MCI, mild cognitive impairment.

Screening measures designed to specifically evaluate cognitive impairment in PD can assist with more precisely identifying cognitive deficits in non-demented patients. The SCOPA-COG [62] was developed as a research tool to assess early cognitive changes independent of motor deficits in PD patients by selectively evaluating cognitive functions typically affected in PD including attention, memory, executive function and visuospatial ability. It demonstrated higher sensitivity in detecting differences between PD patients with mild disease severity (defined as Hoehn and Yahr Scale scores of 1 or 2) and normals than the MMSE [62]. In a separate study, 50 PD patients (58%) with normal MMSE scores were impaired on the SCOPA-COG, where impairment was defined as an overall score that was at least 2 SD below that of a control group; 14% of this cognitively impaired subgroup had a disease duration of less than 5 years [6]. The Parkinson Neuropsychometric Dementia Assessment Instrument (PANDA) [64] was, like the SCOPA-COG, designed to assess cognitive functions most typically affected in PD, with subscales that evaluate recall of a word-list, alternating verbal fluency, spatial imagery, and working memory/ attention. The PANDA also screens for depressive symptoms, which is appropriate given findings of lower cognitive performance in depressed (as opposed to non-depressed), non-demented PD patients [71] and the identification of depression as a risk factor for dementia in PD [37,41]. The PANDA demonstrated higher sensitivity for dementia as defined by DSM-IV criteria than the MMSE and higher sensitivity for mild cognitive disorder as defined by the International Classification of Diseases (ICD-10) [1,64]. In a cross-sectional study of 289 PD patients, cognitive impairment, defined as a PANDA score ≤14, was diagnosed in 44% of the sample, while only 17.5% of the sample obtained scores ≤24 on the MMSE [1]. Finally, the Parkinson's Disease – Cognitive Rating Scale (PD-CRS) [65] was developed to assess both predominantly subcortical (attention, working memory, verbal fluency, verbal memory, clock drawing) and nominally cortical (naming, copy of a clock) cognitive functions in PD. A goal of the scale's development was to provide a means of predicting dementia in PD. Patients classified as having MCI (scores of 0.5 on the Clinical Dementia Rating Scale) were differentiated from those with dementia by different scores on all of the subcortical items, as well as on naming and copying a clock (Tables 15.2 and 15.3). For each of these screening measures, poor performance has been associated with older age, longer disease duration, severity of extrapyramidal symptoms, and PIGD type.

Table 15.3 Studies using screening tools with Parkinson's disease (PD) populations

Study	Subjects	Study aim	Tests administered	Results
Hobson, Meara (1999) [52]	Community sample of 126 non-demented PD patients Mean age: 74 (8.3) years Mean duration: 7.7 (6.8) years	Compared the sensitivity and specificity of CAMCOG and MMSE for the detection of dementia in PD	CAMCOG MMSE GDS	CAMCOG had sensitivity of 95% vs 98% on MMSE CAMCOG had specificity of 94% vs 77% on MMSE 44% met DSM-IV criteria for dementia while 47% met CAMCOG criteria for dementia – compared with DSM-IV criteria, the CAMCOG misclassified 4 subjects as having and 3 as not having dementia
Hobson, Meara (2004) [66]	Community sample of 86 non-demented PD patients Mean age: 74 (8.6) years Mean duration: 6.7 (5.8) years 102 similarly aged normals	Compared PD patients to controls at follow-up	CAMCOG	At 4-year follow-up, 35% of the PD cohort had developed dementia according to DSM-IV criteria, compared to 7% of the controls
Athey et al. (2005) [67]	Community population of 94 PD patients who scored 25–30 on MMSE Mean age: 75 years Mean duration: 6.1 years	Compared the sensitivity and specificity of CAMCOG-R and MMSE for the detection of cognitive impairment in PD	CAMCOG-R	11% of subjects scored <80, suggesting dementia not picked up by MMSE Poorer performance on CAMCOG-R with age and more advanced disease stage, but not increasing disease duration
Athey, Walker (2006) [68]	Same cohort as in 2005 study: 85 PD patients Mean age: 75 years Mean duration: 5.7 years No control group	Examined cognitive decline over 13 months	CAMCOG-R	Significant decline in performance was seen across every domain, and was most marked in domains of orientation, expression, praxis and perception An overall decline of 3.9 points was demonstrated in those subjects with MMSE >24 during the 13-month period

Table 15.3 (continued) Studies using screening tools with Parkinson's disease (PD) population

Study	Subjects	Study aim	Tests administered	Results
Verbaan et al. (2007) [6]	Clinic-based sample of 400 PD Mean age: 60 (11.4) Mean duration: 10.5 (6.4) years 150 controls matched on age, sex and education	Evaluated cognitive functioning in a large cohort of PD patients	SCOPA-COG MMSE BDI	Controls performed significantly better than patients on the SCOPA-COG, each subdomain, and the MMSE 58% of patients with abnormal SCOPA-COG scores had normal MMSE scores PD patients scored lowest (as compared to controls) on executive functioning and memory tests MCI was not addressed, but 14% of patients with impaired cognition (≤ −2 SD of data of controls) had a disease duration <5 years
Zadikoff et al. (2007) [69]	88 PD patients with at least 5 years disease duration Mean age: 65 years Mean duration: 9.5 years	Compared the sensitivity and specificity of MoCA and MMSE to identify MCI in PD	MoCA MMSE	36% of patients who scored >25 on the MMSE scored <26 on the MoCA Range and SD of scores was larger with MoCA (7–30, 4.26) than with the MMSE (16–30, 2.55) More pronounced ceiling effect on MMSE (27 subjects scored 30) than on MoCA (4 subjects scored 30)
Gill et al. (2008) [70]	38 PD patients Mean age: 71 (10.5) years Mean duration: 6.6 (5.4) years	Compared MoCA to neuropsychological test battery	MoCA neuropsychological test MMSE Hopkins Verbal Learning Test – Revised Letter–Number Sequencing (WAIS-III) Stroop Test Phonemic fluency Category fluency	Range of scores was larger with MoCA (6–28) than with the MMSE (16 – 30) Ceiling effect was found on MMSE (4 subjects scored 30) but not on MoCA (0 subjects scored 30) 11 MCI subjects (scored <1.5 SD below norms on one neuropsychological test in either memory or executive functioning domain) had lower average MoCA score (23.3 ± 2.1) than MMSE score (27.4 ± 1.9)

Study	Sample	Comparison	Instruments	Results
Kalbe et al. (2008) [64]	124 PD patients subdivided into 3 groups: ◆ PD-D diagnosed according to DSM-IV criteria (n = 38) ◆ PD-MCD diagnosed according to ICD-10 (n = 40) ◆ No cognitive impairment (n = 46) 108 healthy controls	Compared PANDA to MMSE	PANDA Formal neuropsychological test batteries at three Parkinson clinics MMSE BDI	PANDA had specificity of 91% and sensitivity of 90% for PD-D Sensitivity of 77% for PD-D and PD-MCD
Riedel et al. (2008) [1]	289 PD patients (subset of 873 patients within epidemiological study) Mean age: 70 (8.6) years Mean duration: 6.7 (5.5) years	Compared PANDA to other diagnostic tools	PANDA MMSE Clock-drawing test MADRS	28.6% of patients met DSM-IV criteria for dementia PANDA revealed cognitive impairment (score ≤14) in 43.6%, clock-drawing test in 41.8%, MMSE (cut-off ≤24) in 50%

CAMCOG, Cognitive section of the Cambridge Cognitive Examination; MMSE, Mini-Mental State Examination; DSM, Diagnostic and Statistical Manual; GDS, Geriatric Depression Scale; SCOPA-COG, Scales for Outcomes in Parkinson's disease – Cognition; BDI, Beck Depression Inventory; MoCA, Montreal Cognitive Assessment; MCI, mild cognitive impairment; WAIS, Wechsler Adult Intelligence Scale; PANDA, Parkinson Neuropsychometric Dementia Assessment instrument; PD-D, Parkinson's disease with dementia; MCD, mild cognitive dysfunction; MADRS, Montgomery–Åsberg Depression Rating Scale.

Defining mild cognitive impairment in PD

As a concept, MCI, or more generally, cognitive functioning that reflects a decline from normal levels but does not meet criteria for dementia, may represent an intermediate stage of cognitive functioning that falls between normal ageing and early dementia [72,73]. Diagnostic criteria for this stage of functioning are, however, often vague, prompting investigators to operationalize strict criteria. For example, proposed diagnostic criteria for mild neurocognitive disorder are included in the Diagnostic and Statistical Manual – Text Revision (DSM-IV-TR) and require impairment in two areas of cognitive functioning such as memory, executive functioning, concentration, speed of thinking, and language as corroborated by neuropsychological testing; in addition, the cognitive dysfunction is expected to be associated with, at most, mild impairment in social or occupational functioning. Criteria required by the ICD-10 for a diagnosis of mild cognitive disorder (MCD) also requires cognitive impairment documented with formal neuropsychological testing. However, neither of these definitions provide cut-off scores for determining impairment (e.g. 1 or 1.5 SD below the mean) nor do they make recommendations regarding the neuropsychological tests to be used. Also, there are no universally accepted criteria for the degree of functional change that is considered appropriate for MCI. Functional assessment is frequently confounded by the presence of physical symptoms, particularly in PD patients where it is often unclear whether difficulties with activities of daily living (ADL) are due to motor or cognitive changes, and rating scales used to assess ADLs and instrumental ADLs in demented patients may lack the sensitivity and specificity needed for a mildly impaired population [74].

Applying the construct of MCI to PD

The lack of standardized diagnostic criteria for mild cognitive dysfunction in PD and other diseases has been addressed by applying established criteria typically used in AD populations [75]. In the setting of memory impairment, the construct of MCI has been conceived as representing the prodromal period of early AD [76], given that a high proportion of subjects with amnestic MCI progress to AD. Longitudinal investigations suggest conversion rates of 6–15% per year, with up to 70–80% of amnestic MCI patients progressing to probable AD within 10 years [56,77]. With PD patients, an MCI diagnosis may be valuable in terms of identifying subjects at high risk of conversion to dementia, which could prove helpful for clinical trials of neuroprotective agents. The identification of clinical subtypes of MCI, i.e. amnestic vs non-amnestic and single vs multiple domains within each of these categories, has fostered the application of MCI as a construct in other dementing disorders such as DLB, frontotemporal and vascular dementia [75].

Petersen's (2004) criteria for amnestic MCI requires the presence of a memory complaint and objective memory impairment for age, with all other domains within normal limits [72]. In general, memory performance that falls ≥1.5 SD below age- and education-matched normals is presumed to represent impairment. His criteria for multiple domain MCI and single domain non-memory MCI do not require memory impairment but do involve impaired performance in other cognitive domains, with intact or minimally impaired functioning. Specific information, however, about the assessment of functional status and the degree of change that is considered acceptable is unavailable. Similarly, individuals with cognitive performance that falls within normal limits for age but which represents a presumed decline from estimated levels of premorbid functioning often present diagnostic challenges, as do those with poor cognitive functioning that may be secondary to low education.

Two recent studies categorized PD patients using Petersen's criteria [2,10] and reported almost identical MCI rates of ~20%. Of these MCI patients, more subjects presented with single domain impairment than multiple domain dysfunction, with non-amnestic dysfunction representing the most common type of MCI. These similar findings are surprising given that the samples differed in size and demographics; i.e. Caviness *et al.* assessed 86 patients who were older (mean age of group: 76.4) and had longer disease durations (mean duration of group: 10.4 years) than the 196 non-demented, drug-naive subjects in Aarsland *et al.*'s community sample, which included control subjects (mean age: 67.6; duration: 2.3 years). Differences also existed in the methods used to classify MCI, as Caviness *et al.* retrospectively applied a diagnosis of MCI if subjects demonstrated performance at least 1.5 SD below the expected age-corrected mean score (based on normative values) on at least one of five designated cognitive domains, as shown by impaired performance on tests assumed to load on the domain. Based on this method, 21% of patients had MCI. Aarsland *et al.* created composite Z-scores for cognitive domains based on means and SD of the control group, and MCI was diagnosed if a composite score of ≥-1.5 SD was demonstrated on one or more domains, but only three possible domains were created based on factor analysis.

Subjects with multiple domain MCI may progress at high rates not only to AD but also to vascular dementia, while patients with single non-memory domain MCI progress to a variety of dementias, including frontotemporal dementia, Lewy body dementia, vascular dementia, primary progressive aphasia, AD or PD [75]. In a prospective study of 134 non-demented PD patients, 43% fulfilled criteria for a subtype of MCI adapted from Petersen *et al.*'s (2001) [73] criteria including amnestic MCI, multiple domain MCI or single non-memory domain MCI. Of this MCI subgroup, 62% developed dementia at a 4-year follow-up, defined as scores below the lowest quartile on the MMSE or below the 19th percentile on the Dementia Rating Scale; in addition, 20% of the initially cognitively intact patients were demented at follow-up [12]. In contrast to Petersen's findings in terms of the incidence rates of AD in amnestic MCI patients, single non-memory MCI, and multiple domain 'slightly impaired' MCI (i.e. impaired performance on at least two tests, without required memory impairment) patients were associated with the development of dementia, while amnestic MCI patients were not predictive of dementia in the setting of PD [12]. These contradictory findings may be attributable to the brief neuropsychological battery used to assess cognitive functioning. Of note, DLB patients were excluded from these analyses.

Neuroimaging studies of MCI in PD

Information about the potential pathophysiology of cognitive impairment in early PD has been provided by MRI studies. Memory impairment in non-demented PD patients was correlated with hippocampal atrophy [78], likewise cognitive impairment coincided with hippocampal volume loss in PD [79]. Few studies have examined imaging results for PD patients with MCI as defined with specific criteria. Recently, grey matter changes were studied with structural magnetic resonance imaging and voxel-based morphometry in eight PD patients with mean disease duration of 10 years who were diagnosed with MCI according to Petersen *et al.*'s (2001) criteria. Compared with cognitively intact PD patients (with mean disease duration of 14 years), the PD patients with MCI had reduced cortical grey matter density in the left middle frontal gyrus, precentral gyrus as well as in the left superior temporal lobe and right inferior temporal lobe patients [80].

Metabolic imaging has been used to identify patterns of regional metabolism in non-demented PD patients, including a pattern of increased pallido-thalamic and pontine activity in PD patients that corresponds with reductions in cortical motor regions [81,82]. Using F-fluorodeoxyglucose (FDG) positron emission tomography analyses on 15 non-demented PD patients, Huang *et al.* [83] identified a separate metabolic pattern characterized by reductions in medial frontal and parietal association areas and relative elevations in the cerebellar vermis and dentate nuclei that was specific to cognitive performance; when compared with neuropsychological test scores, this pattern correlated with memory and executive function performance. In a subsequent study, differences in regional metabolism were analysed for a group of 51 PD patients categorized by MCI subtype [84]. MCI was diagnosed if performance on one or more cognitive domains (executive, language, visuospatial, memory) fell ≥ 1.5 SD below normative values and MCI classifications of no impairment, single domain and multiple domain MCI were based on the severity of cognitive impairment. When compared to patients who were cognitively normal and healthy controls, multiple domain MCI patients exhibited metabolic reductions in the inferior parietal lobe and middle frontal gyrus, but patients with single domain MCI did not differ from controls or normal PD patients. However, hypermetabolism was found in the pons/cerebellum region for all three MCI groups, which may indicate a compensatory response to dopaminergic deficiency in the striatum.

Future directions

An increased focus on the cognitive impairment in non-demented PD patients has supplemented established information about the pathology of PD as well as suggesting potential predictors of PD-D, which could assist in the earliest application of available pharmacological and non-pharmacological therapies. Future efforts would be well directed toward better defining the temporal pattern of cognitive impairment in non-demented PD patients so as to more explicitly delineate the prognostic significance of specific patterns of impairment. To achieve this goal, a more precise definition of MCI is needed so that it could be used, much as Petersen's criteria are used in AD research, as an outcome in clinical trials or as a starting point for an enriched design in dementia trials. The identification of genetic mutations associated with PD, particularly in early onset PD, could help by identifying individuals at high risk for the development of PD. Assessing the cognitive functioning of carriers of specific mutations may help to determine whether specific cognitive impairments are manifest before motor signs.

Conclusions

Cognitive impairment is often found in non-demented PD patients when appropriate neuropsychological tests are administered. Such deficits are present even at the time of diagnosis in about 25–35% of the patients, and in cross-sectional studies prevalence rates of up to 55% have been reported. The profile of cognitive deficits varies but generally involves executive and attentional dysfunction in early stages, impairment in memory and visuospatial functions are also found, particularly as the disease progresses. Patients with MCI have a higher risk of conversion to dementia and future efforts may focus on intervention to delay or prevent further cognitive decline.

References

1 Riedel O, Klotsche J, Spottke A, *et al.* Cognitive impairment in 873 patients with idiopathic Parkinson's disease. J Neurol 2008; 255: 255–264.

2 Aarsland D, Bronnick K, Larsen JP, Tysnes OB, Alves G. Cognitive impairment in incident, untreated Parkinson disease: The Norwegian ParkWest Study. Neurology 2009; 72: 1121–26.

3 Muslimović D, Post B, Schmand B. Cognitive profile of patients with newly diagnosed Parkinson disease. Neurology 2005; 65, 1239–45.

4 Foltynie T, Brayne CEG, Robbins, TW, Barker RA. The cognitive ability of an incident cohort of Parkinson's patients in the UK. The CamPaiGN study. Brain 2004; 127: 550–560.

5 Janvin C, Aarsland D, Larsen JP, *et al.* Neuropsychological profile of patients with Parkinson's disease without dementia. Dement Geriatr Cogn Disord 2003; 15: 126–31.

6 Verbaan D, Marinus J, Visser M, *et al.* Cognitive impairment in Parkinson's disease. J Neurol Neurosurg Psychiatry 2007; 78: 1182–7.

7 Brown R, Marsden C. Internal versus external cues and the control of attention. Brain 1984; 111: 323–45.

8 Pillon B, Dubois B, Ploska A, Agid Y. Severity and specificity of cognitive impairment in Alzheimer's, Huntington's, and Parkinson's diseases and progressive supranuclear palsy. Neurology 1991; 41: 634–43.

9 Marder K, Leung D, Tang M, *et al.* Are demented patients with Parkinson's disease accurately reflected in prevalence surveys? A survival analysis. Neurology 1991; 41, 1240–3.

10 Caviness JN, Driver-Dunckley E, Connor DJ, *et al.* Defining mild cognitive impairment in Parkinson's disease. Mov Disord 2007; 22, 1272–7.

11 Janvin C, Aarsland D, Larsen J. Cognitive predictors of dementia in Parkinson's disease: a community-based, 4-year longitudinal study. J Geriatr Psychiatry Neurol 2005; 18: 149–54.

12 Janvin CC, Larsen JP, Aarsland D, Hugdahl K. Subtypes of mild cognitive impairment in Parkinson's disease: progression to dementia. Mov Disord 2006; 22, 1272–7.

13 Owen AM, James M, Leigh PN, *et al.* Fronto-striatal cognitive deficits at different stages of Parkinson's disease. Brain 1992; 115: 1727–51.

14 Cooper JA, Sagar HJ, Jordan N, *et al.* Cognitive impairment in early, untreated Parkinson's disease and its relationship to motor disability. Brain 1991; 114: 2095–2122.

15 Dujardin K, Degreef JF, Rogelet P, Defebvre L, Destee A. Impairment of the supervisory attentional system in early untreated patients with Parkinson's disease. J Neurol 1999; 246: 783–8.

16 Bondi MW, Kaszniak AW, Bayles KA Vance KT. Contributions of frontal system dysfunction to memory and perceptual abilities in Parkinson's disease. Neuropsychology 1993; 7: 89–102.

17 Levin BE, Llabre MM, Reisman S, *et al.* Visuospatial impairment in Parkinson's disease. Neurology 1991; 41: 365–9.

18 Stella F, Gobbi L, Gobbi S, Oliani M, Tanaka K, Pieruccini-Farla F. Early impairment of cognitive functions in Parkinson's disease. Arch Neuropsychiatry 2007; 65, 406–410.

19 Weintraub D, Moberg PJ, Culbertson WC, Duda JE, Stern MB. Evidence for impaired encoding and retrieval memory profiles in Parkinson's disease. Cogn Behav Neurol 2004; 17: 195–200.

20 Pillon B, Deweer B, Agid Y, Dubois B. Explicit memory in Alzheimer's, Huntington's and Parkinson's diseases. Arch Neurol 1993; 50: 374–9.

21 Saint-Cyr JA, Taylor AE, Lang. Procedural learning and neostriatal dysfunction in man. Brain 1988; 111: 941–59.

22 Flowers KA, Robertson C, Sheridan MR. Some characteristics of word fluency in Parkinson's disease. J Neurolinguistics 1996; 9: 33–46.

23 Pagonbarraga J, Kulisevsky J, Llebaria G, Garcia-Sanchez C, Pascual-Sedano B, Gironell A. Parkinson's disease-cognitive rating scale: a new cognitive scale specific for Parkinson's disease. Mov Disord 2008; 23: 998–1005.

24 Azuma T, Cruz RG, Bayles KA, Tomoeda CK, Montgomery EB. A longitudinal study of neuropsychological change in individuals with Parkinson's disease. Int J Geriatr Psychiatry 2003; 18: 1115–20.

25 Riepe MW, Kassubek J, Tracik J, Ebersach G. Screening for cognitive impairment in Parkinson's disease – which marker relates to disease severity? J Neural Transm 2006; 113: 1463–8.

26 Jacobs D, Marder K, Cote L, Sano M, Stern Y, Mayeux R. Neuropsychological characteristics of preclinical dementia in Parkinson's disease. Neurology 1995; 45: 1691–6.

27 Levy G, Jacobs D, Tang M, et al. Memory and executive function impairment predict dementia in Parkinson's disease. Mov Disord 2002; 17: 1221–6.

28 Williams-Gray CH, Foltynie T, Lewis SJ, Barker RA (). Cognitive deficits and psychosis in Parkinson's disease: a review of pathophysiology and therapeutic options. CNS Drugs 2006; 20: 477–505.

29 Levin BE, Llabre MM, Weiner WJ. Cognitive impairments associated with early Parkinson's disease. Neurology 1989; 39: 557–61.

30 Lewis FM, Lapointe LL, Murdoch BE. Language impairment in Parkinson's disease. Aphasiology 1998; 12: 193–206.

31 Crucian GP, Barrett AM, Schwartz RL, et al. Cognitive and vestibulo-proprioceptive components of spatial ability in Parkinson's disease. Neuropsychologia 2000; 38: 757–67.

32 Stern Y, Hermann A, Mayeux R, Rosen J. Prism adaptation in Parkinson's disease. J Neurol Neurosurg Psychiatry 1988; 51: 1584–1587.

33 Filoteo JV, Williams BJ, Rilling LM, Roberts, JW. Performance of Parkinson's disease patients on the Visual Search and Attention Test: impairment in single-feature but not dual-feature visual search. Arch Clin Neuropsychol 1997; 12: 621–34.

34 Pillon B, Boller F, Levy R, Dubois B. Cognitive deficits and dementia in Parkinson's disease. In: Boller F, Cappa S (eds). Handbook of neuropsychology. 2nd edn. Amsterdam: Elsevier, 2001; pp. 311–371.

35 Dubois B, Malapani C, Verin M, Rogelet P, Deweer B, Pillon B. Cognitive functions and the basal ganglia: the model of Parkinson disease. Rev Neurol (Paris) 1994; 150: 763–70.

36 Huber SJ, Shuttleworth EC, Paulson GW. Dementia in Parkinson's disease. Arch Neurol 1986; 43: 987–90.

37 Stern Y, Marder K, Tang M, Mayeux R. Antecedent clinical features associated with dementia in Parkinson's disease. Neurology 1993; 43: 1690.

38 Zgaljardic DJ, Borod JC, Foldi NS, et al. An examination of executive dysfunction associated with frontostriatal circuitry in Parkinson's disease. J Clin Exp Neuropsychol 2006; 28: 1127–44.

39 Zakzanis KK Freedman M. A neuropsychological comparison of demented and nondemented patients with Parkinson's disease. Appl Neuropsychol 1999; 6: 129–46.

40 Emre M. Dementia associated with Parkinson's disease. Lancet Neurology 2003; 2: 229–37.

41 Marder K, Tang MX, Cote L, Stern Y, Mayeux R. The frequency and associated risk factors for dementia in patients with Parkinson's disease. Arch Neurol 1995; 52: 695–701.

42 Levy G. The relationship of Parkinson disease with aging. Arch Neurol 2007; 64: 1242–6.

43 Levy G, Tang M, Cote L, et al. Motor impairment in PD relationship to incident dementia and age. Neurology 2000; 55: 539–44.

44 McKeith I, Burn D. Spectrum of Parkinson's disease, Parkinson's dementia, and Lewy-body dementia. Neurol Clin 2000; 18: 865–83.

45 Troster AI, Woods SP. Neuropsychological aspects of Parkinson's disease and parkinsonian syndromes. In Pahwa R, Lyons KE, Koller WC (eds). Handbook of Parkinson's disease, 3rd edn. New York: Marcel Dekker, 2003; pp. 127–157.

46 Braak, H, Rüb U, Jansen Steur ENH, Del Tredici K, de Vos RAI. Cognitive status correlates with neuropathologic stage in Parkinson disease. Neurology 2005; 64: 1404–10.

47 Kaufer DL, Tröster AI. Neuropsychology of dementia with Lewy bodies. In: Miller BL, Goldenberg G (eds). Handbook of clinical neurology: neuropsychology and behavior, Part I, 3rd edn. Amsterdam: Elsevier, 2008.

48 Braak H, Del Tredici K, Rub U, Jansen EN, Braak E. Staging of brain pathology related to sporadic Parkinson's disease. Neurobiol Aging, 2003; 24: 197–211.

49 Hart S. Language and dementia: a review. Psychol Med 1988; 18: 99–112.

50 Stern Y, Tang M, Jacobs D. Prospective comparative study of the evolution of probable Alzheimer's disease and Parkinson's disease dementia. J Int Neuropsychol Soc 1998; 4: 279–84.

51 Mosimann UP, Mather G, Wesnes KA, O'Brien JT, Burn DJ, McKeith IG. Visual perception in Parkinson disease dementia and dementia with Lewy bodies. Neurology 2004; 63: 2091–6.

52 Hobson P, Meara J. The detection of dementia and cognitive impairment in a community population of elderly people with Parkinson's disease by use of the CAMCOG neuropsychological test. Age Ageing 1999; 28: 39–43.

53 Folstein MF, Folstein SE, McHugh PR. Mini-Mental State: a practical method for grading the cognitive state of patients for the clinician. J Psychiatr Res 1975; 12: 189–98.

54 Tombaugh TN, McIntyre NJ. The Mini-Mental State Examination: a comprehensive review. J Am Geriatr 1992; 40: 922–35.

55 Jefferson AL, Cosentino SA, Ball S, et al. Errors produced on the Mini-Mental State Examination and Neuropsychological Test performance in Alzheimer's disease, ischemic vascular dementia, and Parkinson's disease. J Neuropsychiatry Clin Neuroscience 2002; 14: 311–20.

56 Tierney MC, Szalai JP, Dunn E, Geslani D, McDowell I. Prediction of probable Alzheimer disease in patients with symptoms suggestive of memory impairment: value of the Mini-Mental State Examination. Arch Fam Med 2000; 9: 527–32.

57 Monsch AU, Foldi NS, Ermini-Funfschilling DE, et al. Improving the diagnostic accuracy of the mini mental status examination. Acta Nerol Scand 1995; 92: 145–50.

58 Galasko D, Klauber MR, Hofstetter CR, Salmon DP, Lasker B, Thal LJ. The Mini-Mental State Examination in the early diagnosis of Alzheimer's disease. Arch Neurol 1990; 47: 49–52.

59 Mamikonyan E, Moberg P, Siderow A, et al. Mild cognitive impairment is common in Parkinson's disease patients with normal Mini-Mental State Examination (MMSE) scores. Parkinsonism Relat Disord 2009; 15: 226–31.

60 Roth M, Tym E, Mountjoy CQ, et al. CAMDEX: a standardized instrument for the diagnosis of mental disorder in the elderly with special reference to the early detection of dementia. Br J Psychiatry 1986; 149: 698–709.

61 Roth M, Huppert FA, Tym E, Mountjoy CQ. The Cambridge examination for Mental Disorders of the Elderly – Revised. Cambridge, MA: MIT Press, 1999.

62 Marinus J, Visser M, Verwey NA, et al. Assessment of cognition in Parkinson's disease. Neurology 2003; 61: 1222–8.

63 Nasreddine ZS, Phillips NA, Bedirian V, et al. The Montreal Cognitive Assessment, MoCA: a brief screening tool for mild cognitive impairment. J Am Geriatr Soc 2005; 53: 695–99.

64 Kalbe E, Calabrese P, Kohn N, et al. Screening for cognitive deficits in Parkinson's disease with the Parkinson neuropsychometric dementia assessment (PANDA) instrument. Parkinsonism Relat Disord 2008; 14: 93–101.

65 Pagonabarraga J, Kulisevsky J, Llebaria G, Garcia-Sanchez C, Pascual-Sedano B, Gironell A. Parkinson's Disease – Cognitive Rating Scale: a new cognitive scale specific for Parkinson's disease. Mov Disord 2008; 23: 998–1005.

66 Hobson P, Meara J. The detection of dementia and cognitive impairment in a community population of elderly people with Parkinson's disease by use of the CAMCOG neuropsychological test. Age Ageing 2004; 28: 39–43.

67 Athey RJ, Porter RW, Walker RW. Cognitive assessment of a representative community population with Parkinson's disease (PD) using the Cambridge Cognitive Assessment – Revised (CAMCOG-R). Age Ageing 2005; 34: 268–73.

68 Athey RJ, Walker. Demonstration of cognitive decline in Parkinson's disease using the Cambridge Cognitive Assessment (Revised) (CAMCOG-R). Int J Geriatr Psychiatry 2006; 21: 977–82.

69 Zadikoff C, Fox SH, Tang-Wai DF, et al. A comparison of the Mini Mental State Exam to the Montreal Cognitive Assessment in identifying cognitive deficits in Parkinson's disease. Mov Disord 2007; 23: 297–9.

70 Gill DJ, Freshman A, Blender JA, Ravina B. The Montreal Cognitive Assessment as a screening tool for cognitive impairment in Parkinson's disease. Mov Disord 2008; 23: 1043–6.

71 Huppert FA, Brayne C, Giill C, et al. CAMCOG-A concise neuropsychological test to assist dementia diagnosis: sociodemographic determinants in an elderly population sample. Br J Clin Psychol 1995; 34: 529–541.

72 Starkstein S, Petracca G, Chemerinski E, Merello M. Prevalence and correlates of parkinsonism in patients with primary depression. Neurology 2001; 57: 553–5.

73 Flicker C, Ferris SH, Reisberg B. Mild cognitive impairment in the elderly: predictors of dementia. Neurology 1991; 41: 1006–9.

74 Petersen RC, Smith G, Kokmen E, Ivnik RJ, Tangalos EG. Memory function in normal aging. Neurology 1992; 42: 396–401.

75 Albert SM, Michaels K, Padilla M, et al. Functional significance of mild cognitive impairment in elderly patients without a dementia diagnosis. Am J Geriatr Psychiatry 1999; 7: 213–220.

76 Petersen RC. Mild cognitive impairment as a diagnostic entity. J Intern Med 2004; 256: 183–94.

77 Petersen RC, Stevens JS, Ganguli MD, et al. Practice parameter: early detection of dementia: mild cognitive impairment (an evidence-based review). Report of the Quality Standards Subcommittee of the American Academy of Neurology. Neurology 2001; 56: 1133–42.

78 Petersen RC, Smith GE, Waring SC, Ivnik RJ, Tangalos EG, Kokmen E. Mild cognitive impairment: clinical characterization and outcome. Arch Neurol 1999; 56: 303–8.

79 Riekkinen P Jr, Kejonen Klaakso MP, Soininen H, Partanen K, Riekkinen M. Hippocampal atrophy is related to impaired memory, but not frontal function in non-demented Parkinson's disease patients. Neuroreport 1998; 9: 1507–11.

80 Camicioli R, Moore MM, Kinney A, Corbridge E, Glassberg K, Kaye JA. Parkinson's disease is associated with hippocampal atrophy. Mov Disord 2003; 18: 784–90.

81 Beyer MK, Janvin CC, Larsen JP, Aarsland D. A magnetic resonance imaging study of patients with Parkinson's disease with mild cognitive impairment and dementia using voxel-based morphometry. J Neurol Neurosurg Psychiatry 2007; 78: 254–59.

82 Eidelberg D, Moeller JR, Dhawan V, *et al.* The metabolic topography of parkinsonism. J Cereb Blood Flow Metab 1994; 14: 783–801.

83 Eidelberg D, Moeller JR, Kazumata K, *et al.* Metabolic correlates of pallidal neuronal activity in Parkinson's disease. Brain 1997; 120: 1315–24.

84 Huang C, Mattis P, Tang C, Perrine K, Carbon M, Eidelberg D. Metabolic brain networks associated with cognitive function in Parkinson's disease. NeuroImage 2007; 34: 714–23.

85 Huang C, Mattis P, Perrine K, Brown N, Dhawan V, Eidelberg D. Metabolic abnormalities associated with mild cognitive impairment in Parkinson disease. Neurology 2008; 70: 1470–77.

Chapter 16

Spectrum of Lewy body dementias: relationship of Parkinson's disease dementia to dementia with Lewy bodies

Clive Ballard and Dag Aarsland

Introduction

Dementia with Lewy bodies (DLB) and Parkinson's disease (PD) with dementia (PD-D) are characterized by parkinsonism and a dementia syndrome typically dominated by attentional, visuospatial and executive dysfunction and relatively well-preserved memory. Additional key symptoms are visual hallucinations, cognitive fluctuations, and sleep disturbances such as excessive daytime sleepiness and rapid-eye-movement (REM) sleep behavioural disorder (a parasomnia manifested by vivid, often frightening dreams associated with simple or complex behaviour during REM sleep) [1].

The distinction between DLB and PD-D as operationally defined within the standardized clinical criteria for DLB depends entirely upon the duration of parkinsonism prior to dementia. An arbitrary cut-off of 1 year had been chosen in the original consensus criteria for the clinical diagnosis of DLB [2]. Thus, PD-D would be diagnosed if dementia occurred more than 1 year after the onset of parkinsonism, whereas dementia prior to, or within, 1 year after onset of parkinsonism, was classified as DLB. The third report of the DLB Consortium [1] revised the operationalized diagnostic criteria for DLB. The report highlighted the unresolved issues in the relationship between DLB and PD-D by, on one hand, emphasizing the overall clinical and pathological similarities of the conditions, but at the same time maintaining the arbitrary 1-year rule for distinguishing the two syndromes for research studies. The importance of further research to resolve 'boundary issues' was also highlighted. Several key conceptual questions still remain unresolved, for example are these conditions distinct or part of the same spectrum? If they are distinct conditions, is the arbitrary 1-year rule a meaningful distinction between clinical entities with different clinical presentations? Addressing these issues is critical to take forward our understanding of this spectrum of conditions; establishing biological markers, determining prognostic indicators and, most importantly, in designing appropriate intervention studies and developing treatment paradigms across the dementias associated with Lewy bodies.

Studies directly comparing DLB and PD-D patients probably represent the best approach for resolving 'boundary issues', but methodological limitations have precluded clear conclusions in many of the comparative studies. For example, critical issues have included the selection of participants (i.e. whether community-based or hospital-based), whether participants were matched for severity of dementia, sample size, sensitivity and other psychometric properties of the tests used to characterize the patients, and diagnostic criteria and methods of diagnosis (e.g. diagnosis based on autopsy, prospective clinical assessment or retrospective chart review). In addition, many studies comparing neuropathology or neurochemistry in PD and DLB have not specified whether PD patients had dementia or not, and, if so, separately described the PD-D patients.

The aim of the current chapter is to summarize similarities and differences between DLB and PD-D from the best available information.

Comparative neuropathological, neurochemical and biomarker studies

Neuropathology

DLB and PD-D cannot be differentiated by neuropathology alone, in particular since usually only patients with end-stage disease come to autopsy. Both syndromes are associated with less cortical atrophy than is typical in Alzheimer's disease (AD). Medial temporal lobe structures are abnormal in both DLB and PD-D, although the severity of hippocampal atrophy is less marked than that seen in AD. Both DLB and PD-D have similar, significant atrophy and pathology in the amygdala [3].

Limbic and cortical Lewy bodies (LB) are the main substrate of the dementia syndrome in DLB and PD-D [4–6]. Several studies have suggested that in many cortical regions, the amount of Lewy body pathology does not differentiate DLB from PD-D or PD [5,6]. By contrast, data from the Newcastle brain bank (Table 16.1) indicate more pronounced cortical Lewy body pathology in DLB compared to PD-D in a range of cortical areas,

Table 16.1 Lewy body pathology: comparison between dementia with Lewy bodies (DLB) and Parkinson's disease with dementia (PD-D)

	DLB (n = 29)	PD-D (n = 11)	Evaluations
Age (years)	79.9 ± 4.8	74.2 ± 4.3	T = 3.3, P = 0.002
Female	17	5	χ^2 = 0.6, P = 0.46
MMSE closest to death	9.6 ± 9.1	12.2 ± 9.4	T = 0.7, P = 0.47
Duration of dementia	2.6 ± 1.8	2.1 ± 1.3	T = 0.9, P = 0.35
Duration of parkinsonism	1.2 ± 1.4	9.9 ± 6.9	T = 6.5, P < 0.0001
Frontal Lewy body density	1.2 ± 1.5	0.4 ± 0.3	T = 2.5, P = 0.02*
Transentorhinal Lewy body density	3.8 ± 2.9	1.8 ± 1.0	T = 3.1, P = 0.004*
Anterior cingulate Lewy body density	2.5 ± 2.4	1.4 ± 1.1	T = 2.0, P = 0.049*

MMSE, Mini-Mental State Examination.

although the prolonged duration of PD prior to dementia in this cohort may explain the magnitude of disparity in cortical Lewy body pathology. Other work has suggested a more specific regional pattern of differences in Lewy body density, with higher densities in parahippocampal and inferior temporal cortices in DLB compared with PD-D [7]. In both DLB and PD-D, cortical Lewy body pathology impacts upon phenotype. For example, the density of temporal lobe Lewy bodies in DLB correlates with the early occurrence of the characteristic well-formed visual hallucinations, and increasing Lewy body densities in limbic and frontal cortices in PD-D correlate with the severity of dementia [8,9].

The density of amyloid plaques has generally been reported to be higher in DLB than in PD-D, with the density of Aβ-positive plaques in many DLB patients being equivalent to that found in AD. While the amounts of Aβ deposition and cortical Lewy bodies correlate with dementia severity in DLB, this does not seem to be the case in PD-D [5]. Neurofibrillary tangles are typically substantially less pronounced than in AD, but may nevertheless influence the clinical phenotype, particularly in DLB [10,11].

One study has reported a marked Lewy body neurodegeneration in the striatum in DLB, but not in PD. PD-D patients had striatal neurodegeneration intermediate between PD and DLB [12]. By contrast, an important preliminary report focusing on striatal pathology in 28 brains, including 7 PD, 7 PD-D and 14 DLB has indicated that striatal α-synuclein pathology is similar in PD-D and DLB. Amyloid plaques were also similar in severity in the striatum in the two conditions [13].

Since clinically the main difference between DLB and PD-D is the different timing of dementia and parkinsonism, each with different biological underpinnings, it is likely that any pathological differences between the two syndromes are most pronounced early in the disease course and reflect different regional onset and progression with similar end-stage. Methodological difficulties make this hypothesis difficult to test. According to one influential hypothesis, the progression of alpha-synuclein pathology in PD is characterized by a systematic progression, beginning in brainstem and moving rostrally in predefined stages, with neocortical involvement in stages 5 and 6 [14]. Whereas this pattern of progression fits with many PD patients, the pattern in DLB suggests that the neocortex is involved from the onset of disease, and that some cases are without brainstem pathology. Emerging data are, however, not consistent with a unitary concept of the pathogenesis of Lewy body pathology. Cases with subcortical but no brainstem pathology [15], and with very high diffuse Lewy body load that either occur at onset of clinical disease or rapidly infiltrate the brain, with accompanying rapidly progressive clinical symptoms and short survival [16], have been reported. Exploring the cellular causes of these different clinical and pathological subtypes, broadly corresponding to younger patients with a slowly progressing motor parkinsonism and elderly subjects with more rapidly progressive disease, needs high priority.

Overall, studies consistently indicate higher amyloid pathology in DLB than in PD-D, but the literature is highly variable with markedly discrepant findings related to cortical Lewy body pathology and striatal pathology. One study from our group, examining the relationship between Lewy body pathology and the number of years of Parkinson's disease prior to dementia as a spectrum, demonstrated that there was substantially less cortical Lewy body pathology in patients with longstanding PD prior to dementia than in DLB patients, but that the differences were less pronounced in patients with 1–5 years of PD before dementia developed [17]. This study would support the concept of a continuum of Lewy body disease rather than two distinct diseases, and the different duration of PD-D in different studies may explain some of the discrepancies in results.

Of note, one recent study identified differential expression of α-synuclein, parkin and synphilin isoforms in different Lewy body diseases, suggesting the possibility that different molecular mechanisms lead to similar neuropathological changes even if the core neuropathological changes are similar, and that there are subtle disease-specific differences between DLB and PD [18].

Cerebrospinal fluid (CSF)

Studies of CSF have consistently shown characteristic changes of amyloid-beta and tau peptides in AD, but the initial studies focusing on DLB and PD-D have shown conflicting results. One study has reported an increase of an oxidated variant of amyloid-beta-peptide 1–40 relative to the sum of amyloid-beta-peptides in DLB compared to PD, but suggested that other species of amyloid are similar [19]. In a recent study, significantly reduced amyloid-beta-peptide 1–42 was reported in DLB compared to PD-D, whereas total and phosporylated tau did not differ significantly [20].

α-Synuclein is the pathological hallmark of DLB and PD-D, and appears to be the pathological substrate most closely related to progressive cognitive decline in these individuals. α-Synuclein is therefore a potentially attractive biomarker, and although recent progress has been made on the measurement of α-synuclein in the CSF, currently there are no studies directly comparing DLB and PD-D. However, results from recent studies have found similar or higher levels of total α-synuclein in CSF of AD and DLB patients, thus questioning the relevance of this measure as a biomarker of Lewy body disease, suggesting that it could rather be a marker of neurodegeneration [21]. These studies have all reported on total α-synuclein, and thus, as is the case with tau and p-tau, other species, for example phosphorylated α-synuclein, may be more specific markers of DLB and PD. For example, a recent autopsy study demonstrated similar levels of total α-synuclein in DLB and AD, but higher levels of soluble oligomers of α-synuclein in DLB compared to AD [22].

The small number of studies and the absence of longitudinal studies directly comparing CSF markers in DLB and PD-D makes it difficult to develop firm conclusions. Longitudinal studies in this field will play an important role in furthering our understanding of the similarities and differences in the evolution of pathology in DLB and PD-D.

Neurochemistry

The majority of neurochemical studies of DLB and PD-D have explored the dopamine and acetylcholine systems in neuropathological and in some functional neuroimaging studies. The findings overall suggest a similar profile of changes in the two dementias, but with some specific differences that may relate to phenotype. Marked cholinergic deficits have been reported in both DLB and PD-D in autopsy and PET studies. Cortical cholinergic deficits secondary to cell loss of forebrain nuclei are pronounced in DLB and PD-D, to a greater extent than in AD [e.g. 23,24] and associated with decreased performance on tests of attentional and executive functioning, but not with memory tests [25]. In addition, cholinergic deficits have also been reported in selected thalamic nuclei in PD-D [26]. In the insular cortex the cholinergic deficits were more marked in PD-D than DLB [27]. In DLB, but probably not in PD-D, there is a correlation between visual hallucinations and cholinergic deficits in the temporal cortex [28]. In addition, there is evidence linking cholinergic changes, in particular nicotinic modulation of thalamocortical circuitry, with the disturbed consciousness in patients with DLB [29]. Neuroimaging studies using single photon emission computed tomography (SPECT) ligands have also reported cholinergic receptor changes in DLB and PD-D, with increased muscarinic [30] and reduced nicotinergic binding in both dementias.

Although nigrostriatal dopamine changes occur in both syndromes, the severity and distribution of changes differ, with more marked nigral cell loss in PD-D than DLB, although this may be related to differences in disease duration. Importantly, there appears to be a postsynaptic dopaminergic upregulation in PD, but not in DLB, which may translate to the increased risk for neuroleptic sensitivity reactions in this group [31]. However, the interpretation of this study is difficult as there was no distinction between PD patients with and without dementia, and neuroleptic sensitivity is also prevalent in patients with PD and PD-D [32]. Preliminary data from our group show significantly higher frontal $5-HT_{1A}$ receptor binding density in DLB compared with PD-D, suggesting a distinct neurochemical feature of the two dementias [33]. Direct comparisons between DLB and PD-D patients have not yet been undertaken for a number of key neurochemical systems such as noradrenaline and glutamate. In addition, the association between neurochemical changes and clinical symptoms has rarely been explored.

One major animal model for PD, based on the assumption that dysfunction of the ubiquitine–proteasome system is a key element in the pathophysiology of PD, was recently found to be a relevant model also for DLB [34].

Studying the relationship between the time from onset of PD to dementia, we found that those with early dementia (i.e. less than 10 years after onset of PD) had similar morphological and neurochemical changes as those with DLB, whereas PD patients with late-onset dementia had less morphological cortical pathology (Lewy bodies, amyloid plaques, neurofibrillary tangles), but more severe cholinergic deficit in temporal cortex [17].

Comparative studies of clinical features in PD-D and DLB

Cognitive deficits

The overall profile of cognitive deficits is similar in the two syndromes, with both PD-D and DLB patients exhibiting significantly more marked executive and attention deficit, fluctuating attention, and less severe memory deficits than those with AD [23]. Some studies have reported more pronounced executive dysfunction in DLB than in PD-D, in particular in patients with mild dementia [35,36]. In addition, more pronounced auditory attentional disturbances were identified in PD-D compared to DLB [37]. The finding of more pronounced differences between DLB and PD-D in early rather than later disease is consistent with the findings on electroencephalogram (EEG) reported recently [38]. In contrast, a recent study of prepulse inhibition, a paradigm which enables the study of basic attention processes independent of task understanding and deliberate participation, demonstrated more pronounced impairment in DLB than PD-D [39]. Although studies based on group means provide important information, comparison of group means may disguise heterogeneity within the groups. Indeed, recent evidence has demonstrated that in PD and in PD-D, subgroups with different cognitive profiles exist: the majority of patients have an executive-visuospatial-dominant profile, whereas others have a memory-dominant profile [40,41]. Similarly, some DLB patients, probably those with more abundant AD-type changes, may lack the characteristic pattern of neuropsychological deficits usually associated with Lewy body diseases.

Neuropsychiatric symptoms

The profile of neuropsychiatric symptoms is also similar in DLB and PD-D. Persistent visual hallucinations are the most frequent psychiatric symptoms and are characteristic of both dementias [11,42–45]. Although misidentification syndromes and delusions are also common and have a similar phenomenology in both DLB and PD-D patients [46], they may be more prevalent in DLB than in PD-D, possibly due to morphological and/or neurochemical differences reported above. Depression is also common in both dementias [43–45]. Psychotic symptoms and depression are more frequent in DLB and PD-D than among people with AD, and the characteristic neuropsychiatric profile in DLB is less pronounced in those with more severe AD-type lesions [10,11].

Parkinsonism

A proportion of DLB patients do not have parkinsonism, sometimes even over a prolonged dementia of 5 years or more [47]. In the most detailed comparative study of parkinsonism to date, Burn *et al.* found that DLB patients had less severe parkinsonism than people with PD-D, but a similar severity of motor deficits compared to PD patients without dementia [48]. The severity of parkinsonism, however, appears to progress similarly

Table 16.2 Psychotic symptoms in dementia with Lewy bodies (DLB), Parkinson's disease with dementia (PD-D) and Alzheimer's disease (AD)

	DLB (*n* = 98)	PD-D (*n* = 48)	AD (*n* = 40)
Visual hallucinations	71(72%)	24 (50%)	10 (25%)
Auditory hallucinations	37 (38%)	10 (21%)	4 (10%)
Delusions	56 (57%)	14 (29%)	12 (30%)

Data from Ballard *et al.* (1999) [42] and Aarsland *et al.* (2001) [43].

in both conditions [47]. There are some subtle but important differences in key parkinsonian signs and symptoms. Postural instability and gait difficulties, predominantly mediated by non-dopaminergic lesions, are more pronounced in DLB and PD-D than in PD patients without dementia, whereas the opposite is true for tremor [48]. In addition, parkinsonian features tend to be more symmetrical in PD-D [49]. In a prospective study, those who had postural instability and gait difficulties-dominant PD at baseline, or who developed this after having tremor-dominant PD initially, had a higher risk of dementia compared to those who maintained a tremor-type PD [50]. Importantly, parkinsonism is a key factor explaining the functional impairment in DLB [51] as well as PD-D.

Cognitive and functional decline

Only one study has directly compared the course of cognitive decline in PD-D and DLB. This study reported that DLB and PD-D patients had a similar rate of decline on cognition over 2 years [52]. There are some indications that the course of disease is more severe in PD-D and DLB than in AD, although few longitudinal comparative studies have been done. The cognitive decline in PD-D [44] and DLB [53] seems to be similar to that in AD, but, consistent with the complex clinical symptoms in DLB, functional decline and mortality [53] progress more rapidly in DLB than in AD.

Structural and functional imaging

MIBG

Cardiac scintigraphy with ^{123}I-metaiodobenzylguanidine (MIBG) enables the quantification of postganglionic cardiac sympathetic innervation, and several studies have demonstrated reduced cardiac compared to mediastinal uptake in DLB and PD, as opposed to AD [54]. Direct comparative studies of DLB and PD-D are needed.

MRI

Using structural magnetic resonance imaging (MRI), the typical finding in DLB is relative preservation of hippocampus and medial temporal lobe volumes in comparison with AD. Other cortical and subcortical changes have also been reported in DLB, including the substantia innominata, hypothalamus and dorsal midbrain [55]. Similar changes have been reported in PD-D. However, the two studies comparing MRI in PD-D and DLB have conflicted, one reporting no differences [56] whereas the other found more pronounced cortical atrophy in DLB than in PD-D [57].

SPECT

SPECT studies of cerebral cortical blood flow have demonstrated characteristic patterns in DLB and PD-D. Cerebral perfusion deficits are confined mainly to either parietal or occipital regions or both in DLB as compared with AD, whereas reductions in all cortical areas have been reported in PD-D [58]. Comparative studies have reported slightly different regional patterns of cerebral blood flow in DLB and PD-D: in one study, DLB patients had a more markedly reduced blood flow in the frontal lobe [59]. In another study, the pattern was similar, but DLB patients had a more pronounced overall reduction of cerebral blood flow than PD-D patients [60]. Longitudinal studies have reported progressive reduction of frontal lobe blood flow in PD [61], but no significant change in PD-D [62]. Few studies have explored the associations between regional functional changes and specific clinical features. A recent longitudinal study reported correlations between increase in perfusion in midline posterior cingulate and decrease in hallucination severity, and between fluctuations of consciousness and increased thalamic and decreased inferior occipital perfusion [63].

SPECT functional imaging studies of dopamine transporter loss, visualized with tracers such as ^{123}I-N-3-fluoropropyl-2-β-carbomethoxy-3-β-(4-iodophenyl)-nortropane (FP-CIT) SPECT, have identified characteristic patterns in DLB and PD-D compared to PD patients without dementia, people with AD and normal controls. Characteristic differences are evident in the nigrostriatal dopamine system, demonstrating striatal abnormalities in PD and DLB, compared to AD and healthy controls [64,65]. A slightly different pattern in DLB and PD has been suggested, with PD and PD-D patients showing more left–right asymmetry and a more posterior striatal degeneration compared to DLB [64,65]. A similar rate of decline of striatal binding in PD-D and DLB has been shown [66]. The differences in the pattern of asymmetry are consistent with what has been reported in clinical studies of parkinsonism with regard to its symmetry [49].

Pittsburgh Compound B (PIB) imaging

The development of ^{11}C-labelled amyloid ligand PIB as a biomarker of cortical beta-amyloid burden has enabled *in vivo* assessment of amyloid burden. Although with some variation, the overall picture is that DLB patients have PIB binding similar to or less pronounced than AD patients, whereas PD-D patients have similar [67] or lower [68] PIB binding than DLB patients, consistent with pathological findings. The validity of PIB binding as a marker of amyloid pathology also in DLB and PD-D was supported in a recent finding of reduced ab1-42 in those patients with pathological binding. The overall conclusion to date is that PD-D has less amyloid burden than DLB, DLB somewhat less than AD [68].

Electrophysiology

Characteristic EEG changes have been reported in patients with DLB, such as slowing of background acivity and frequency variability. Two recent studies included both PD-D and DLB patients. In one study of patients with early and mild dementia [38], patients with DLB and PD-D had more posterior slowing and frequency variation than AD and healthy control subjects. At baseline, the changes were more common and severe in DLB than in PD-D, although at the 2-year follow-up, the changes in PD-D had become more pronounced. Interestingly, two subgroups of PD-D with and without cognitive fluctuations were identified, with EEG changes similar to the DLB group in PD-D with fluctuations, but not in those without. In contrast, in a study assessing mismatch negativity (MMN)—a component of the auditory event-related potential (ERP) considered to represent a basic automatic change detection system—pronounced changes with reduced MMN latency and areas were found in PD-D, but not in DLB or AD [37].

Genetic studies

Exciting studies over the last 5 years have identified several key genes involved in the development of PD, including the α-synuclein (*SNCA*), *parkin*, *DJ-1*, *LRRK2* and *PINK1*. The potential importance of these genes and other key genetic risk factors has not yet been elucidated for DLB. A recent systematic review of the available literature in respect to familial occurrence of dementia with parkinsonism explored the genetic evidence pertaining to PD-D and DLB. A substantial coincidental familial occurrence of dementia and parkinsonism was evident in the 24 families described in the review [69]. In 12 families the presentation of dementia and parkinsonism fulfilled current criteria for DLB in some family members and PD-D in others, implying that the same mutation in different members of the same family caused different clinical phenotypes. Patients with familial co-occurrence of dementia and parkinsonism displayed either mutations in the synuclein gene or showed positive correlations with the APOE3/4 and E4/4 alleles. Consistent with these observations, a three-generational Belgian family with different phenotypes involving dementia and/or parkinsonism [70] was described, with significant linkage to 2q35-q36. Together, these reports support the hypothesis of a common genetic underpinning of DLB and PD-D.

Treatment response

Cholinesterase inhibitors

In the only placebo-controlled trial of a cholinesterase inhibitor in patients with DLB, 120 patients were treated with rivastigmine (mean dose 7 mg) or placebo for 20 weeks [71]. The primary outcome measure was 30% improvement in a four-item subscore derived from the Neuropsychiatric Inventory (NPI) (delusions, hallucinations, apathy, depression), which was attained by 63% of people treated with rivastigmine and 30% of people treated with placebo, a significant difference on the observed case analysis. On the total NPI, there was a 3-point advantage for the rivastigmine-treated patients. Significant improvements were seen in attentional performance on computerized tests, with a non-significant 1-point advantage for the rivastigmine-treated patients on the Mini-Mental State Examination (MMSE). The only published large randomized, placebo-controlled, parallel group trial of a cholinesterase inhibitor in PD-D, also with rivastigmine [72], demonstrated that rivastigmine conferred benefit in comparison to placebo over 24 weeks of treatment, in 541 patients with PD-D (allocated 2:1 rivastigmine:placebo). Over the treatment period, the rivastigmine-treated patients had a 2-point advantage on the NPI, a 1-point advantage on the MMSE, an almost 3-point advantage on the ADAS-COG and also superiority on more specialized assessment of attention and executive function, all differences being statistically significant. Although there are always limitations to the interpretation of effect size comparisons across trials, the magnitude of benefit with rivastigmine treatment appears very similar in DLB and PD-D. There are no blinded studies directly comparing cholinesterase inhibitors in DLB and PD-D patients, but open-label trials also suggest that effect sizes and side-effects are similar [73].

In both syndromes, sudden withdrawal of cholinesterase inhibitors may be detrimental, and this may be particularly pronounced in PD-D [74].

Antipsychotics

Given the high frequency of psychotic symptoms in both DLB and PD-D, antipsychotic agents are frequently considered for DLB and PD-D patients. The only randomized controlled trial of an atypical antipsychotic in patients with dementia and PD indicated that quetiapine did not confer any greater benefit than placebo in the treatment of psychosis [75]. Importantly, severe neuroleptic sensitivity reactions have been identified as a major clinical issue in DLB. One study reported that 50% of neuroleptic-treated patients with DLB experienced severe drug sensitivity, with symptoms that included marked extrapyramidal features, confusion, autonomic instability, falls and accelerated mortality [76]. An accumulating literature of case reports and case series, as well as subsequent larger and more systematic reports, shows that severe sensitivity reactions occur with a wide range of typical and atypical antipsychotics, including clozapine, in DLB [77,78]. There is also evidence of similar poor tolerability in PD-D, albeit from fewer studies. A comparative study of DLB, PD-D, PD and AD examined neurolpetic sensitivity in 94 patients (15 with DLB, 36 with PD-D, 26 with PD, 17 AD). Severe neuroleptic sensitivity only occurred in patients with Lewy body disease (DLB 53%, PD-D 39%, PD 27%), but did not occur in AD. Thus, in the context of the current chapter, the severe neuroleptic sensitivity syndrome was common in both DLB and PD-D [32].

Responsiveness to levodopa

Motor symptoms contribute to the disability experienced by DLB and PD-D patients and are associated with an increased risk of falls. Acute levodopa challenge in 14 DLB patients yielded some improvement in UPDRS III score, finger tapping and walking test, but less so than in PD or PD-D [79,80]. Of the DLB patients, 36% were classified as 'responders' on levodopa challenge, compared with 70% of the PD-D and 57% of the PD patients. Although the majority of DLB patients seemed to tolerate the drug, 15% withdrew due to confusion and gastrointestinal problems. In an extension of this study [80], acute levodopa challenge considerably improved motor function and subjective alertness in all patients without compromising either reaction times or accuracy, but increased fluctuations were noted in both groups with dementia. Neuropsychiatric scores improved in patients with PD both with and without dementia on levodopa at 3 months. Conversely, in a more recent study limited efficacy and increased risk for psychosis was observed in DLB during 3 months of levodopa treatment [81]. Overall it would therefore appear that DLB patients are less responsive to levodopa than people with PD-D, but the relative impact on neuropsychiatric symptoms and cognition remains unresolved.

Clinicopathological dimensions rather than categories: personal interpretation

Overall there are many similarities, but also subtle differences, between DLB and PD-D and the number of direct comparative studies remains too limited to make firm conclusions. For context, it is also important to remember that marked differences exist *within* the two syndromes: some DLB patients have a very characteristic clinical profile with visuospatial and executive dysfunction, VH and parkinsonism, whereas others have a clinical profile more similar to that seen in patients with AD. Similarly, some PD patients develop dementia early in course, whereas others remain non-demented or develop it late in course; some develop VH or severe psychosis whereas others do not show these symptoms despite large doses of dopaminergic drugs.

Although there are no major brain differences between PD-D and DLB, subtle neurochemical and pathological differences are likely to subserve the subtle clinical differences. A more pronounced executive dysfunction in DLB may relate to the loss of the hippocampal projection to the frontal lobe in DLB but not PD, and more severe Lewy body pathology in inferior temporal lobe may relate to the higher frequency of visual hallucinations in DLB. The differential pattern of parkinsonian features in PD and DLB is in accordance with the differential striatal changes, with changes in PD-D patients being intermediate between those found in DLB and PD patients. Similarly, within the two syndromes, the severity of AD changes is associated with a less classical DLB phenotype. In PD-D, those who develop dementia early have more pronounced cortical morphological changes. More studies are needed to address the relationship between these syndromes, by understanding the relationship between the underlying pathological and neurochemical substrates, the clinical profile and course of PD-D and DLB. In addition, comparative studies so far conducted have been based purely upon the duration of PD prior to dementia, and no studies have yet used the new operationalized diagnostic criteria for PD-D [82] to undertake direct comparisons with DLB.

The available data strongly support a 'continuum' model, and indicate that any arbitrary clinical distinction between DLB and PD-D does not reflect the pattern of cortical neuropathological and neurochemical changes. As the majority of previous research has focused on the distinction between DLB and PD-D, future studies should combine DLB and PD-D patients and aim at disentangling empirically based subgroups within the continuum of LB dementia. This will enable further work to focus on the pathological and neurochemical processes underpinning the clinical phenotypes across the full spectrum, with the potential of understanding prognosis and to develop and evaluate new targeted treatment approaches.

Conclusions

DLB and PD-D are characterized by similar clinical presentations with parkinsonism, visual hallucinations, other psychotic symptoms, fluctuating cognition, REM sleep behavioural disorder, marked sensitivity to neuroleptic drugs and comparable treatment response to cholinesterase inhibitors. Although there are more similarities than differences, the absence of clinically significant parkinsonism in some DLB patients, the greater asymmetry of parkinsonism in PD-D, and the reduced levodopa responsiveness in DLB are noteworthy differences.

An arbitrary, but generally accepted, distinction has been made in current International Consensus diagnostic criteria between patients presenting with parkinsonism prior to the onset of dementia (PD-D), and developing parkinsonism and dementia concurrently (DLB). The clinical syndromes are very similar, yet it is a priority to understand the relationship between the duration of PD prior to dementia and the distribution of the major pathological and neurochemical disease substrates in order to produce an evidence-based diagnostic conceptualization. The few studies directly comparing PD-D and DLB using the current diagnostic definitions suggested that DLB patients have significantly higher cortical Lewy body density, greater amyloid pathology and more pronounced atrophy than those with PD-D, and that widespread neurofibrillary tangles are rare in both disorders. Within the PD-D group there seems to be less cortical AD pathology and less cortical Lewy body pathology in patients who had PD for 10 years or more before the onset of dementia. Even fewer reports have directly compared neurochemical changes in DLB and PD-D, suggesting severe cholinergic deficits in both conditions, but potential differences in cortical serotonergic function. The balance of evidence strongly indicates that DLB and PD-D are part of a continuum rather than distinct disorders.

References

1 McKeith IG, Dickson DW, Lowe J, *et al.* Diagnosis and management of dementia with Lewy bodies: third report of the DLB Consortium. Neurology 2005; 65: 1863–72.

2 McKeith IG, *et al.* Consensus guidelines for the clinical and pathologic diagnosis of dementia with Lewy bodies (DLB): Report of the Consortium on DLB International Workshop. Neurology 1996; 47: 1113–1124.

3 Cordato NJ, Halliday GM, Harding AJ, *et al.* Regional brain atrophy in progressive supranuclear palsy and Lewy body disease. Ann Neurol 2000; 47: 718–28.

4 Aarsland D, Perry R, Brown A, *et al.* Neuropathology of dementia in Parkinson's disease: a prospective, community-based study. Ann Neurol 2005; 58: 773–6.

5 Harding AJ, Halliday GM. Cortical Lewy body pathology in the diagnosis of dementia. Acta Neuropathol (Berl) 2001; 102: 355–63.

6 Tsuboi Y, Dickson DW. Dementia with Lewy bodies and Parkinson's disease with dementia: are they different?. Parkinsonism Relat Disord 2005; 11: 47–51.

7 Harding AJ, Broe GA, Halliday GM. Visual hallucinations in Lewy body disease relate to Lewy bodies in the temporal lobe. Brain 2002; 125: 391–403.

8 Samuel W, Galasko D, Masliah E, *et al.* Neocortical lewy body counts correlate with dementia in the Lewy body variant of Alzheimer's disease. J Neuropathol Exp Neurol 1996; 55: 44–52.

9 Kovari E, Gold G, Herrmann FR, *et al.* Lewy body densities in the entorhinal and anterior cingulate cortex predict cognitive deficits in Parkinson's disease. Acta Neuropathol (Berl) 2003; 106: 83–8.

10 Merdes AR, Hansen LA, Jeste DV, *et al.* Influence of Alzheimer pathology on clinical diagnostic accuracy in dementia with Lewy bodies. Neurology 2003; 60: 1586–90.

11 Ballard CG, Jacoby R, Del Ser T, *et al.* Neuropathological substrates of psychiatric symptoms in prospectively studied patients with autopsy-confirmed dementia with Lewy bodies. Am J Psychiatry 2004; 161: 843–9.

12 Duda JE, Giasson BI, Mabon ME, *et al.* Novel antibodies to synuclein show abundant striatal pathology in Lewy body diseases. Ann Neurol 2002; 52: 205–10.

13 Tsuboi Y, Uchikado H, Dickson DW. Neuropathology of Parkinson's disease dementia and dementia with Lewy bodies with reference to striatal pathology. Parkinsonism Relat Disord 2007; 13: 221–4.

14 Braak H, Del Tredici K, Rub U, *et al.* Staging of brain pathology related to sporadic Parkinson's disease. Neurobiol Aging 2003; 24: 197–211.

15 Parkkinen L, Pirttila T, Alafuzoff I. Applicability of current staging/categorization of alpha-synuclein pathology and their clinical relevance. Acta Neuropathol 2008; 115: 399–407.

16 Halliday G, Hely M, Reid W, *et al.* The progression of pathology in longitudinally followed patients with Parkinson's disease. Acta Neuropathol 2008; 115: 409–15.

17 Ballard C, Ziabreva I, Perry R, *et al.* Duration of Parkinsonism prior to dementia is associated with a distinct pattern of neuropathological and neurochemical substrates across the Lewy body dementia spectrum. Neurology 2006; 67: 1931–1934.

18 Beyer K, Domingo-Sabat M, Humbert J, *et al.* Differential expression of alpha-synuclein, parkin, and synphilin-1 isoforms in Lewy body disease. Neurogenetics 2008; 9: 163–72.

19 Bibl M, Mollenhauer B, Esselmann H, *et al.* CSF amyloid-beta-peptides in Alzheimer's disease, dementia with Lewy bodies and Parkinson's disease dementia. Brain 2006; 129: 1177–87.

20 Parnetti L, Tiraboschi P, Lanari A, *et al.* Cerebrospinal fluid biomarkers in Parkinson's disease with dementia and dementia with Lewy bodies. Biol Psychiatry 2008; 64: 850–5.

21 Ohrfelt A, Grognet P, Andreasen N, *et al.* Cerebrospinal fluid alpha-synuclein in neurodegenerative disorders-a marker of synapse loss?. Neurosci Lett 2009; 450: 332–5.

22 Paleologou KE, Kragh CL, MannDMA, *et al.* Detection of elevated levels of soluble α-synuclein oligomers in post-mortem brain extracts from patients with dementia with Lewy bodies. Brain [Epub: 20 January 2009].

23 Aarsland D, Ballard CG, Halliday G. Are Parkinson's disease with dementia and dementia with Lewy bodies the same entity?. J Geriatr Psychiatry Neurol 2004; 17: 137–45.

24 Bohnen NI, Kaufer DI, Ivanco LS, *et al.* Cortical cholinergic function is more severely affected in parkinsonian dementia than in Alzheimer disease: an in vivo positron emission tomographic study. Arch Neurol 2003; 60: 1745–8.

25 Bohnen NI, Kaufer DI, Hendrickson R, *et al.* Cognitive correlates of cortical cholinergic denervation in Parkinson's disease and parkinsonian dementia. J Neurol 2006; 253: 242–7.

26 Ziabreva I, Ballard CG, Aarsland D, *et al.* Lewy body disease: thalamic cholinergic activity related to dementia and parkinsonism. Neurobiol Aging 2006; 27: 433–8.

27 Pimlott SL, Piggott M, Owens J, *et al.* Nicotinic acetylcholine receptor distribution in Alzheimer's disease, dementia with lewy bodies, Parkinson's disease, and vascular dementia: in vitro binding study using 5-[(125)i]-a-85380. Neuropsychopharmacology 2004; 29: 108-16.

28 Ballard C, Piggott M, Johnson M, *et al.* Delusions associated with elevated muscarinic binding in dementia with Lewy bodies. Ann Neurol 2000; 48: 868–76.

29 Pimlott SL, Piggott M, Ballard C, *et al.* Thalamic nicotinic receptors implicated in disturbed consciousness in dementia with Lewy bodies. Neurobiol Dis 2006; 21: 50-6.

30 Colloby SJ, Pakrasi S, Firbank MJ, *et al.* In vivo SPECT imaging of muscarinic acetylcholine receptors using (R,R) 123I-QNB in dementia with Lewy bodies and Parkinson's disease dementia. Neuroimage 2006; 33: 423–9.

31 Piggott MA, *et al.* Nigrostriatal dopaminergic activities in dementia with Lewy bodies in relation to neuroleptic sensitivity: comparisons with Parkinson's disease. Biol Psychiatry 1998; 44: 765–74.

32 Aarsland D, Perry R, Larsen JP, *et al.* Neuroleptic sensitivity in Parkinson's disease and parkinsonian dementias. J Clin Psychiatry 2005; 66: 633–7.

33 Francis PT and Perry EK. Cholinergic andother neurotransmitter mechanisms in Parkinson's disease, Parkinson's disease dementia, and dementia with Lewy bodies. Mov Disord 2007; 22: 351–7.

34 MacInnes N, Iravani MM, Perry E, *et al.* Proteasomal abnormalities in cortical Lewy body disease and the impact of proteasomal inhibition within cortical and cholinergic systems. J Neural Transm 2008; 115: 869–78.

35 Downes JJ, Priestley NM, Doran M, *et al.* Intellectual, mnemonic, and frontal functions in dementia with Lewy bodies: a comparison with early and advanced Parkinson's disease. Behav Neurol 1998; 11: 173–83.

36 Aarsland D, Litvan I, Salmon D, *et al.* Performance on the dementia rating scale in Parkinson's disease with dementia and dementia with Lewy bodies: comparison with progressive supranuclear palsy and Alzheimer's disease. J Neurol Neurosurg Psychiatry 2003; 74: 1215–20.

37 Brønnick KS, Nordby H, Larsen JP, *et al.* Disturbance of automatic auditory change detection in dementia associated with Parkinson's disease: a mismatch negativity study. Neurobiol Aging [E-pub: doi 10.1016/j.neurobiolaging.2008.02.021].

38 Bonanni L, Thomas A, Tiraboschi P, *et al.* EEG comparisons in early Alzheimer's disease, dementia with Lewy bodies and Parkinson's disease with dementia patients with a 2-year follow-up. Brain 2008; 131: 690–705.

39 Perriol MP, Dujardin K, Derambure P, *et al.* Disturbance of sensory filtering in dementia with Lewy bodies: comparison with Parkinson's disease dementia and Alzheimer's disease. J Neurol Neurosurg Psychiatry 2005; 76: 106–8.

40 Foltynie T, Brayne CE, Robbins TW, *et al.* The cognitive ability of an incident cohort of Parkinson's patients in the UK. The CamPaIGN study. Brain 2004; 127: 550–60.

41 Janvin CC, Larsen JP, Aarsland D, *et al.* Subtypes of mild cognitive impairment in parkinson's disease: Progression to dementia. Mov Disord 2006; 21: 1343–9.

42 Ballard C, Holmes C, McKeith I, *et al.* Psychiatric morbidity in dementia with Lewy bodies: a prospective clinical and neuropathological comparative study with Alzheimer's disease. Am J Psychiatry 1999; 156: 1039–45.

43 Aarsland D, Ballard C, Larsen JP, *et al.* A comparative study of psychiatric symptoms in dementia with Lewy bodies and Parkinson's disease with and without dementia. Int J Geriatr Psychiatry 2001; 16: 528–36.

44 Aarsland D, Cummings JL. Psychiatric aspects of Parkinson's disease, Parkinson's disease with dementia, and dementia with lewy bodies. J Geriatr Psychiatry Neurol 2004; 17: 111.

45 Aarsland D, Bronnick K, Ehrt U, *et al.* Neuropsychiatric symptoms in patients with PD and dementia: frequency, profile and associated caregiver stress. J Neurol Neurosurg Psychiatry 2007; 78: 36–42.

46 Mosimann UP, Rowan EN, Partington CE, *et al.* Characteristics of visual hallucinations in Parkinson disease dementia and dementia with lewy bodies. Am J Geriatr Psychiatry 2006; 14: 153–6.

47 Ballard C, O'Brien J, Swann A, *et al.* One year follow-up of parkinsonism in dementia with Lewy bodies. Dementia Geriatr Cogn Disord 2000; 11: 219–22.

48 Burn DJ, Rowan EN, Minett T, *et al.* Extrapyramidal features in Parkinson's disease with and without dementia and dementia with Lewy bodies: a cross-sectional comparative study. Mov Disord 2003; 18: 884–9.

49 Gnanalingham KK, Byrne EJ, Thornton A, *et al.* Motor and cognitive function in Lewy body dementia: comparison with Alzheimer's and Parkinson's diseases. J Neurol Neurosurg Psychiatry 1997; 62: 243–52.

50 Alves G, Larsen JP, Emre M, *et al.* Changes in motor subtype and risk for incident dementia in Parkinson's disease. Mov Disord 2006; 21: 1123–30.

51 McKeith IG, Rowan E, Askew K, *et al*. More severe functional impairment in dementia with lewy bodies than Alzheimer disease is related to extrapyramidal motor dysfunction. Am J Geriatr Psychiatry 2006; 14: 582–8.

52 Burn DJ, Rowan EN, Allan LM, *et al*. Motor subtype and cognitive decline in Parkinson's disease, Parkinson's disease with dementia, and dementia with Lewy bodies. J Neurol Neurosurg Psychiatry 2006; 77: 585–9.

53 Hanyu H, Sato T, Hirao K, *et al*. Differences in clinical course between dementia with Lewy bodies and Alzheimer's disease. Eur J Neurol 2009; 16: 212–7.

54 Taki J, Yoshita M, Yamada M, *et al*. Significance of 123I-MIBG scintigraphy as a pathophysiological indicator in the assessment of Parkinson's disease and related disorders: it can be a specific marker for Lewy body disease. Ann Nucl Med 2004; 18: 453–61.

55 Whitwell JL, Weigand SD, Shiung MM, *et al*. Focal atrophy in dementia with Lewy bodies on MRI: a distinct pattern from Alzheimer's disease. Brain 2007; 130: 708–19.

56 Burton EJ, McKeith IG, Burn DJ, *et al*. Cerebral atrophy in Parkinson's disease with and without dementia: a comparison with Alzheimer's disease, dementia with Lewy bodies and controls. Brain 2004; 127: 791–800.

57 Beyer MK, Larsen JP, Aarsland D. Gray matter atrophy in Parkinson disease with dementia and dementia with Lewy bodies. Neurology 2007; 69: 747–54.

58 Colloby S, O'Brien J. Functional imaging in Parkinson's disease and dementia with Lewy bodies. J Geriatr Psychiatry Neurol 2004; 17: 158–63.

59 Kasama S, Tachibana H, Kawabata K, *et al*. Cerebral blood flow in Parkinson's disease, dementia with Lewy bodies, and Alzheimer's disease according to three-dimensional stereotactic surface projection imaging. Dement Geriatr Cogn Disord 2005; 19: 266–75.

60 Mito Y, Yoshida K, Yabe I, *et al*. Brain 3D-SSP SPECT analysis in dementia with Lewy bodies, Parkinson's disease with and without dementia, and Alzheimer's disease. Clin Neurol Neurosurg 2005; 107: 396–403.

61 Firbank MJ, Molloy S, McKeith IG, *et al*. Longitudinal change in 99mTcHMPAO cerebral perfusion SPECT in Parkinson's disease over one year. J Neurol Neurosurg Psychiatry 2005; 76: 1448–51.

62 Firbank MJ, Burn DJ, McKeith IG, *et al*. Longitudinal study of cerebral blood flow SPECT in Parkinson's disease with dementia, and dementia with Lewy bodies. Int J Geriatr Psychiatry 2005; 20: 776–82.

63 O'Brien J T, Firbank MJ, Mosimann UP, *et al*. Change in perfusion, hallucinations and fluctuations in consciousness in dementia with Lewy bodies. Psychiatry Res 2005; 139: 79–88.

64 O'Brien JT, Colloby S, Fenwick J, *et al*. Dopamine transporter loss visualized with FP-CIT SPECT in the differential diagnosis of dementia with Lewy bodies. Arch Neurol 2004; 61: 919–25.

65 Walker Z, Costa DC, Walker RW, *et al*. Striatal dopamine transporter in dementia with Lewy bodies and Parkinson disease: a comparison. Neurology 2004; 62: 1568–72.

66 Colloby SJ, Williams ED, Burn DJ, *et al*. Progression of dopaminergic degeneration in dementia with Lewy bodies and Parkinson's disease with and without dementia assessed using 123I-FP-CIT SPECT. Eur J Nucl Med Mol Imaging 2005; 32: 1176–85.

67 Maetzler W, Liepelt I, Reimold M, *et al*. Cortical PIB binding in Lewy body disease is associated with Alzheimer-like characteristics. Neurobiol Dis 2009; 34: 107–12.

68 Gomperts SN, Rentz DM, Moran E, *et al*. Imaging amyloid deposition in Lewy body diseases. Neurology 2008; 71: 903–10.

69 Kurz MW, Schlitter AM, Larsen JP, *et al*. Familial occurrence of dementia and parkinsonism: a systematic review. Dementia Geriatr Cogn Disord 2006; 22: 288–95.

70 Bogaerts V, Engelborghs S, Kumar-Singh S, *et al*. A novel locus for dementia with Lewy bodies: a clinically and genetically heterogeneous disorder. Brain 2007; 130: 2277–91.

71 McKeith I, Del Ser T, Spano P, *et al*. Efficacy of rivastigmine in dementia with Lewy bodies: a randomised, double-blind, placebo-controlled international study. Lancet 2000; 356: 2031–6.

72 Emre M, Aarsland D, Albanese A, *et al*. Rivastigmine for dementia associated with Parkinson's disease. N Engl J Med 2004; 351: 2509–18.

73 Thomas AJ, Burn DJ, Rowan EN, *et al*. A comparison of the efficacy of donepezil in Parkinson's disease with dementia and dementia with Lewy bodies. Int J Geriatr Psychiatry 2005; 20: 938–44.

74 Minett TS, Thomas A, Wilkinson LM, *et al*. What happens when donepezil is suddenly withdrawn? An open label trial in dementia with Lewy bodies and Parkinson's disease with dementia. Int J Geriatr Psychiatry 2003; 18: 988–93.

75 Kurlan R, Cummings J, Raman R, *et al*. Alzheimer's Disease Cooperative Study Group. Quetiapine for agitation or psychosis in patients with dementia and parkinsonism. Neurology 2007; 68: 1356–63.

76 McKeith I, Fairbairn A, Perry R, *et al*. Neuroleptic sensitivity in patients with senile dementia of Lewy body type. Br Med J 1992; 305: 673–8.

77 Ballard C, Grace J, McKeith I, *et al*. Neuroleptic sensitivity in dementia with Lewy bodies and Alzheimer's disease. Lancet 1998; 351: 1032–3.

78 Sadek J, Rockwood K. Coma with accidental single dose of an atypical neuroleptic in a patient with Lewy Body dementia. Am J Geriatr Psychiatry 2003; 11: 112–3.

79 Molloy S, McKeith IG, O'Brien JT, *et al*. The role of levodopa in the management of dementia with Lewy bodies. J Neurol Neurosurg Psychiatry 2005; 76: 1200–3.

80 Molloy SA, Rowan EN, O'Brien JT, *et al*. (2006). Effect of levodopa on cognitive function in Parkinson's disease with and without dementia and dementia with Lewy bodies. J Neurol Neurosurg Psychiatry 2006; 77: 1323–8.

81 Goldman JG, Goetz CG, Brandabur M, *et al*. Effects of dopaminergic medications on psychosis and motor function in dementia with Lewy bodies. Mov Disord 2008; 23: 2248–50.

82 Emre M, Aarsland D, Brown R, *et al*. Clinical diagnostic criteria for dementia associated with Parkinson's disease. Mov Disord 2007; 22: 1689–1707.

Chapter 17

Spectrum of disorders with parkinsonism and dementia

Jaime Kulisevsky and Javier Pagonabarraga

Introduction

Advances on the neuropathological basis of dementia in the past 5–10 years have expanded our knowledge on the different nosological entities that cause dementia associated with parkinsonism. While dementia has been clearly defined as a frequent and disabling condition associated with Parkinson's disease (PD) [1], and dementia with Lewy bodies is currently considered the second commonest cause of neurodegenerative dementia in older people [2], the actual prevalence and impact of cognitive deficits in other neurodegenerative diseases associated with dementia and parkinsonism have not been so clearly described.

In the 1970s, severe cognitive dysfunction leading to prototypical 'subcortical' dementia was described in patients with progressive supranuclear palsy (PSP) [3]. Patients with corticobasal degeneration (CBD) are known to suffer from profound language and visuospatial disturbances with major impact on global cognitive function [4]. Furthermore, some patients with PSP or CBD may present with cognitive decline [5], and CBD pathology has been described in patients with a clinical diagnosis of frontotemporal dementia [6]. Although dementia has been proposed to be an exclusion criterion for the diagnosis of multiple system atrophy (MSA), several recent studies have reported prominent cognitive deficits in patients with MSA as compared with control subjects [7,8].

Frontal–subcortical circuits link basal ganglia with regions of the frontal lobe and thalamus in functional systems that regulate motor function, cognition, emotions, and behaviour [9]. Hence, dysfunction of frontal–subcortical circuits may account for the frequent coexistence of cognitive and behavioural disturbances with parkinsonism in patients with basal ganglia disorders. Cognitive dysfunction in diseases with parkinsonism usually involves a pattern of deficits characterized by impairment in cognitive domains subserved by frontal or frontostriatal and parietal cognitive networks, namely attention and concentration, executive functions, verbal fluency, praxis, and visuospatial functioning [10,11]. A list of major neurodegenerative disorders associated with dementia and parkinsonism is presented in Table 17.1.

Table 17.1 Spectrum of major neurodegenerative disorders associated with dementia and Parkinsonism

---

- ◆ Tauopathies:
  - Progressive supranuclear palsy (PSP)
  - Corticobasal degeneration (CBD)
  - Frontotemporal lobar degeneration (FTLD)
    - Pick's disease
    - Frontotemporal dementia with parkinsonism (FTDP)
    - Multiple system tauopathy with presenile dementia (MSTD)
- ◆ α-Synucleinopathies:
  - Lewy body disease
    - Parkinson's disease
    - Dementia with Lewy bodies
  - Multiple system atrophy (MSA)
- ◆ Tardopathies [TAR-DNA binding protein-43 (TDP-43) proteinopathies]:
  - Frontotemporal lobar degeneration with ubiquitin-positive inclusions (FTLD-U)
  - Frontotemporal lobar degeneration with motor neuron disease (FTLD-MND)
- ◆ Amyloidopathies
  - Sporadic Alzheimer's disease
  - Familial Alzheimer's disease associated with mutations in the genes encoding amyloid precursor protein (*APP*), presenilin 1 (*PSEN1*), or presenilin 2 (*PSEN2*).
- ◆ Miscellaneous
  - Fragile X-associated tremor/ataxia syndrome (FXTAS)
  - Spinocerebellar ataxias (SCA type 2, 17, 21)
  - Fahr's syndrome (bilateral striopallidodentate calcification)
  - Huntington's disease

Tauopathies and cognitive dysfunction

Progressive supranuclear palsy (PSP)

PSP is an adult-onset neurodegenerative disorder characterized by atypical akinetic–rigid syndrome, usually non-responsive to levodopa, early postural instability and vertical supranuclear-gaze palsy. Recent epidemiological studies have shown that the disorder is more common than previously recognized, with an average annual incidence for ages 50–99 years around 5.3 cases per 100 000 population [12].

Although in their seminal paper Steele *et al.* [13] reported cognitive impairment in seven out of the nine patients they evaluated, and that the characteristic pattern of neuropsychological deficits observed in PSP gave rise to the term 'subcortical dementia' [3], traditionally more attention has been focused on the motor and oculomotor abnormalities present in PSP that may aid in the differentiation from PD, than to the cognitive and behavioural disturbances associated with PSP. Behavioural and cognitive changes occur in 50–90% of patients with PSP, often within the first year of the disease [14,15]. In cross-sectional studies, frequency of dementia in PSP is close to 55% [16].

Cognitive changes were initially reported by Albert et al. and characterized as a prototypical 'subcortical dementia' [3]. This pattern of deficits was differentiated from those in patients with 'cortical dementia', who usually present with aphasia, apraxia, or agnosia; it was suggested that the symptoms found in PSP were similar to those that had previously been described in patients with frontal lobe lesions [11,17]. The 'subcortical dementia' described by Albert *et al.* was characterized by a cluster of neuropsychological deficits including forgetfulness, slowing of thought process, emotional or personality changes (apathy, depression, irritability) and impaired ability to manipulate acquired knowledge [3]. The neuropsychological–mechanistic basis for all these deficits seems to be the prolonged time lag in carrying out mental functions, rather than primary dysfunction of the cortical systems responsible for individual cognitive domains. Hence, cognitive functions may be performed strikingly better if the patient is given sufficient time to respond. As PSP was thought to almost exclusively affect subcortical nuclei (including the pallidum, caudate nucleus, red nucleus, subthalamic nucleus, and substantia nigra), the authors proposed that cognitive impairment in PSP was due to bilateral frontal–subcortical dysfunction [3]. In fact, neuroimaging studies have shown that PSP affects both presynaptic and postsynaptic aspects of dopaminergic and cholinergic systems, which project to the prefrontal cortex, leading to early cognitive dysfunction [18–21].

PSP patients have dramatically slowed information processing speed, early and severe executive dysfunction with problems in allocating attentional resources, difficulty in planning, shifting conceptual sets and prominent recall deficits with moderate forgetfulness [22,23]. These cognitive defects can be also found in patients with PD and other akinetic–rigid syndromes, but patients with PSP show a greater impairment in attention, processing speed, set-shifting, and categorization abilities than those with PD or MSA [24,25]. Slowing of information processing speed and execution of responses is especially prominent in PSP. In order to assess whether this slowness is directly related to cognitive dysfunction or to the bradykinetic syndrome, Dubois *et al.* measured reaction times using tasks with different levels of cognitive complexity, but the same amount of motor demands [26]. They found that central processing time in PSP is significantly increased when performing complex situations, as compared to both PD and a control group, whereas in the PD group cognitive speed was similar to that of controls. These results have been further replicated in studies using event-related potentials showing dramatically increased response latencies in complex attentional tasks in PSP that have not been observed in other dementias or parkinsonian syndromes [27].

Executive functions are clearly altered in PSP, with impairment in most tests assessing frontal lobe functions [23]. In particular, PSP patients show impairment in tasks of working memory, reasoning, problem-solving, conceptualization, planning, and social functions [28,29]. Characteristically, PSP patients show perseverative errors during performance of executive tasks, as well as problems with response inhibition which are not common in other parkinsonian syndromes such as PD or MSA [28]. Similar to patients with focal prefrontal lesions, PSP patients show decreased ability to inhibit previously learned cognitive responses, whereas PD patients show more evident deficits in the maintenance of new cognitive programmes [30]. This cognitive dissociation has been linked to differential involvement of the medial prefrontal cortex (associated with impaired response inhibition) [31], and dysfunction of circuits connecting the striatum with the dorsolateral prefrontal cortex (associated with impairment in set maintenance) [32]. The inability to inhibit inappropriate responses has been claimed as a useful clinical marker that helps to discriminate PSP from PD [33]. The 'applause sign' – the inability to stop clapping hands after three times – was observed in 71% of PSP patients, but in none of the PD patients [33]. Perseverative behaviours – due to the inability to stop an automatic activity once it has been released – have been related to dysfunction of the medial aspects of the prefrontal cortex and the caudate nucleus [34].

Overall, there seems to be a more diffuse impairment of prefrontal-based cognitive functions in PSP as compared to PD. Recently, degeneration in the prefrontal cortex has been shown in PSP, beyond the well-established degeneration of subcortical nuclei [15]. Clinical heterogeneity and atypical presentations frequently result in misdiagnosis at the early stages of PSP [35]. Recently, Williams *et al.* identified two clinical phenotypes in pathologically proven PSP patients [36]. Patients with Richardson's syndrome (RS) (54% of all cases) developed the classical symptoms associated with PSP, with early onset of postural instability and falls, supranuclear vertical gaze palsy and a more severe cognitive dysfunction. By contrast, patients with PSP–parkinsonism (PSP-P) phenotype (32% of all cases) were characterized by asymmetric onset, tremor, moderate initial therapeutic response to levodopa, and were frequently misdiagnosed as PD. More recently, a third clinical phenotype has been described [15]. In a prospective study of 152 patients with a clinical diagnosis of PSP given after 5 years of disease duration, 20% had predominant cognitive dysfunction and behavioural changes at disease onset associated with mild instability and absent or mild oculomotor disturbances. The most common initial mis-diagnosis in this group was dementia, frontotemporal dementia in particular (35%). Volumetric magnetic resonance imaging (MRI) studies have shown that PSP patients have greater loss of grey matter volume in both the medial and lateral aspects of the pre-frontal cortex compared with MSA and PD, which correlates with the degree of executive dysfunction but not with motor dysfunction [37]. In PSP patients with predominant cog-nitive versus parkinsonian symptoms, a specific and higher atrophy in the prefrontal lobe has been found bilaterally, involving both grey and white matter [38], which supports the hypothesis that cognitive impairment in PSP is a direct consequence of the degeneration of prefrontal cortex along with degeneration of subcortical nuclei.

Behavioural changes are also a frequent and characteristic feature in PSP [39]. In a descriptive study of neuropsychiatric symptoms in PSP, almost all patients suffered from moderate-to-severe apathy (91%), and 36% exhibited disinhibition. Depression (18%), anxiety (18%), and irritability (9%) were infrequent, and hallucinations or delusions were not reported [40]. Apathy was significantly associated with executive dysfunction, suggesting that both cognitive dysfunction and apathy in PSP are mediated by a common pathology, i.e. degeneration of prefrontal areas or dysfunction in the frontal–subcortical circuits [40,41]. The importance of apathy in PSP is further demonstrated by the fact that PSP can be discriminated from PD and AD by more severe apathy and less frequent depression [42,43]. Frequent association of apathy with disinhibition provides further evidence as to the role of dysfunction in the orbitofrontal and medial–frontal circuits with regard to behavioural disturbances in PSP [42]. This role has been supported in recent volumetric MRI studies showing frontal atrophy to correlate with behavioural changes in PSP [44]. Although hallucinations have been infrequently reported, they can be present in 9–16% of patients diagnosed with PSP [45,46].

All these findings demonstrate that PSP is a disorder with heterogeneous clinical presentation covering a broad spectrum of symptoms that may manifest either as a predominat motor disease resembling PD, an atypical parkinsonism with predominant instability, oculomotor disturbances and cognitive impairment, or as a predominant dementing disease with prominent and early behavioural disturbances resembling FTD.

Corticobasal degeneration (CBD)

CBD is a progressive neurodegenerative disorder that typically presents with asymmetrical parkinsonism and cognitive dysfunction. In the initial clinical descriptions of CBD, symptoms of cortical dysfunction were confined to ideomotor and limb-kinetic apraxia, and in some cases alien hand, whereas clinically relevant cognitive and behavioural disturbances were reported to appear only in more in advanced stages of the disease [47,48].

The presence of cognitive impairment in CBD is now widely recognized. In the last two decades detailed neuropsychological assessment of autopsy-proven cases showed not only that cognitive deficits are common in CBD, but also that they may be present from the early stages of the disease and may help in differential diagnosis [5]. In clinico-pathological studies, a specific pattern of cognitive impairment was evident at the time of presentation, whereas characteristic motor abnormalities were present in fewer than half of the patients [49]. Reviewing the natural history of 14 patients with autopsy-proven CBD, Wenning *et al.* observed that 64% of them presented with ideomotor apraxia and 36% with features of 'cortical-type' dementia at the first visit. As the disease progressed, development of lateralized and focal cognitive symptoms (i.e. aphasia in 36%) and a progressive frontal syndrome led to the diagnosis of dementia in 6 out of 14 patients (43%); 58% of patients suffered from apathy, irritability, or disinhibited behaviour [50]. Subsequent larger clinical series confirmed the importance of cognitive deficits in CBD showing that 25% (36 out of 147) of CBD patients presenting with predominant motor symptoms developed dementia during the course of the disease [51]. Further clinico-pathological studies broadened the clinical spectrum of CBD, demonstrating that it can present with various clinical syndromes. Beyond the classical corticobasal syndrome (unilateral and asymmetric parkinsonism, dystonia, ideomotor apraxia, and myoclonus), CBD may also present with progressive non-fluent aphasia, speech apraxia, PSP-like syndrome (vertical supranuclear gaze palsy, early postural instability), or a posterior cortical atrophy syndrome [52]. Conversely, the classical corticobasal clinical syndrome may be an atypical presentation of other neurodegenerative diseases such as AD [53], PSP, or Creutzfeldt–Jakob disease [54].

Typical symptoms of frontotemporal dementia have also been described in CBD at disease onset, in the absence of classical corticobasal features [55,56]. In autopsy studies a pathological diagnosis of CBD was not uncommon (30% of tau-positive cases) in patients with a clinical diagnosis of frontotemporal dementia [6].

The neuropsychological pattern and severity of cognitive dysfunction in CBD is highly variable between patients. The most characteristic symptoms are asymmetric limb apraxia (usually ideomotor and limb-kinetic, with deficits in posture imitation, symbolic gesture execution, and object utilization), constructional and visuospatial difficulties, executive dysfunction, acalculia, and progressive non-fluent aphasia [4,57] (Table 17.2).

The most frequent cognitive symptom in CBD is apraxia, being present in up to 70% of patients [59]. Limb apraxia in CBD is asymmetric and most often ideomotor in nature. Ideomotor apraxia impairs the ability of using tools or mimicking their use, but preserves the recognition of the pattern and temporal sequence of actions when performed by others [60]. Limb-kinetic apraxia (usually coexisting with ideomotor apraxia) has been reported less often in CBD; it can be differentiated from ideomotor apraxia by its more distal, unilateral nature, impairing only the performance of fine finger movements and hand postures, and affecting all kind of movements, regardless of their instrumental purpose (impairment of transitive and intransitive movements) [61]. Ideational apraxia, the impairment in the conceptualization and planning of a sequence of complex motor behaviour, is infrequent in CBD, and develops in advanced stages of the disease [60]. Visual–perceptive difficulties, the difficulty in perceiving the spatial relationships of visual stimuli, are responsible for the constructional apraxia observed in CBD, especially in patients with predominant right hemisphere frontoparietal degeneration [62]. Patients with constructional apraxia are unable to assemble into action motor behaviours that require the integration of spatial relationships [63]. In CBD, it is mainly seen as a progressive impairment in drawing and writing, which is frequent in early disease or may even be the presenting feature [64].

Aphasia and speech difficulties are common in CBD and serve as good clinical markers in differentiation from PD, PSP, and MSA [65,66]. Language disturbances in CBD resemble those in FTD patients with a non-fluent progressive aphasia phenotype [65]. Clinicopathological studies confirmed the presence of speech and language disturbances in CBD [5], although detailed neuropsychological investigations are needed to disclose

Table 17.2 Pattern of cognitive and behavioural disturbances in corticobasal degeneration

- ◆ Cognitive dysfunction [4]:
  - Limb apraxia (ideomotor, limb-kinetic, ideational)
  - Constructional apraxia
  - Visuospatial difficulties (line orientation, figure rotation, motion perception)
  - Executive dysfunction (medial and lateral prefrontal cortex deficits)
  - Acalculia
  - Progressive non-fluent aphasia
  - Speech apraxia
- ◆ Behavioural disturbances [58]:
  - 75% depression
  - 40% apathy
  - 20% irritability
  - 20% agitation
  - <10% disinhibition

their actual prevalence and severity in the early stages. Neuropsychological studies assessing language in CBD have shown that most patients (65%) develop progressive aphasia during the course of the illness [67]. In particular, language at baseline is more impaired in CBD patients with primarily cognitive presentation, although the evolution to aphasia is similar in both primarily motor and cognitive forms as the disease progresses [68]. Aphasia has been shown to be present in 44% of autopsy-proven CBD cases [4].

Impairment on tests of frontal lobe function is one of the most consistent findings in CBD [69]. Measures of working memory, set-shifting, set acquisition, resistance to interference, conceptualization, mental flexibility, and social judgement [70] have been shown to be early and severely affected [57]. As mentioned above for PSP, these deficits highlight the extensive degeneration of lateral and medial prefrontal cortex and frontal–subcortical circuits in tauopathies.

Visuospatial skills are usually impaired, with poor performance on tests of line orientation, mental rotation of figures and perception of motion. These deficits reflect predominantly dysfunction of the dorsal visual pathways involving the parieto-occipital cortex rather than dysfunction of the ventral visual stream, which is more involved in the perception of shapes, colours, and object identification [24,69].

Findings of memory impairment in CBD are inconsistent, some studies reporting episodic memory deficits whereas others finding no alterations in memory. Episodic memory as opposed to semantic memory is better preserved in CBD compared to AD, suggesting that dysfunction of semantic networks in the anterior and lateral aspects of the temporal cortex, rather than hippocampal/medial temporal degeneration, may account for the memory deficits seen in CBD [71].

Frontotemporal dementia with parkinsonism

In 1996, an international consensus conference was held in order to define the cognitive, behavioural, and motor disturbances of families with frontotemporal dementia with parkinsonism linked to chromosome 17 (FTDP-17) [72]. The group discussed 25 families with similar symptoms of familial adult-onset behavioural disturbances, frontal lobe type dementia and parkinsonism. Thirteen kindreds were identified with sufficient evidence for linkage of this phenotype to chromosome 17 [72]. These families shared common – although heterogeneous – clinical features, with symptoms starting typically in the fifth decade, patients developing behavioural (disinhibition, loss of personal awareness, apathy, mental rigidity, defective judgement, stereotyped behaviours and hyper-orality with hyperphagia) and cognitive (speech disturbances with non-fluent aphasia, echolalia and palilalia, mutism, executive dysfunction, relative preservation of memory, orientation, and visuospatial functions) disturbances typical of frontotemporal lobar degeneration. Either early or during the course of the disease, patients usually exhibited parkinsonian symptoms with early postural instability, absence of resting tremor, poor response to levodopa and, occasionally, supranuclear ophthalmoplegia or apraxia of eyelid opening [72–75]. It was decided to classify these patients under the term FTDP-17, and the need to identify the gene or genes responsible for this disorder was emphasized [72].

In the past 5 years, advances in immunohistochemistry and molecular genetics have expanded our knowledge on different disorders that can manifest FTDP-17 phenotype.

In many kindreds with FTDP-17, mutations in the gene encoding the microtubule-associated protein tau (MAPT) on chromosome 17 have been found, with patients showing tau-positive inclusions on neuropathology [76]. In several other kindreds ubiquitin-positive inclusions were described, but no associated tau pathology or mutations in the *MAPT* gene were observed. In 2006, this group of patients was better defined by the identification of mutations in the gene encoding progranulin (*PGRN*), which is only 1.7 Mb centromeric to MAPT on chromosome 17. Symptomatology of patients with *MAPT* and *PGRN* mutations is almost identical to that previously described as FTDP-17, although some clinical features may help to differentiate patients with *MAPT* or *PGRN* mutations [77]. In *FTDP* with *MAPT* mutations, the phenotypes of mild cognitive impairment, probable Alzheimer disease, semantic dementia, or corticobasal syndrome have rarely been described, few cases have been diagnosed with amyotrophic lateral sclerosis, and no cases with symptoms of posterior cortical atrophy or suggestive of dementia with Lewy bodies have been reported. In FTDP with PRGN mutations the syndromic diagnoses have been more variable, patients presenting with predominant memory impairment, limb apraxia, parkinsonism or visuospatial dysfunction. The development of a corticobasal syndrome has been frequent in the cases reported thus far [78].

In summary, the nosological entity previously called FTDP-17 is now known to include patients with different mutations and different neuropathological features. Waiting for the discovery of new mutations to come, current terminology for patients developing symptoms of FTDP should indicate whether those patients are carrying or likely to carry mutations in the *MAPT* or *PRGN* genes.

α-Synucleinopathies and cognitive dysfunction

Parkinson's disease dementia and dementia with Lewy bodies, prototypical synucleinopathies associated with dementia and parkinsonism, are the main topic of this book and covered extensively in other chapters. The other relatively common form of synucleinopathies – MSA – will be discussed here.

Multiple system atrophy

MSA is an adult-onset, sporadic, progressive neurodegenerative disorder that presents clinically with autonomic symptoms and motor impairment. The profile of motor impairment varies across patients and includes a variable combination of poorly levodopa-responsive parkinsonism, cerebellar ataxia and corticospinal tract dysfunction. Eighty per cent of MSA patients present with predominant parkinsonism (MSA-P) caused by striatonigral degeneration, and the remaining 20% with cerebellar ataxia (MSA-C) associated with olivo-ponto-cerebellar atrophy [79]. Neuropathologically, MSA is defined as an α-synucleinopathy, characterized by degeneration of striatonigral and olivopontocerebellar structures. The cellular loss is accompanied by profuse aggregates of distinctive cytoplasmic inclusions within oligodendroglial cells (GCIs), formed by filamentous α-synuclein and a number of other proteins [80].

As for CBD, original descriptions of patients with MSA put the emphasis on the movement disorder characteristic of the disease. To date, a few studies have focused on associated cognitive and behavioural disturbances. Although in the initial diagnostic criteria dementia was proposed to be an exclusion criterion for the diagnosis of MSA [79], several subsequent studies have reported prominent cognitive defects in patients with MSA when compared with control subjects [7,8].

The first study to prospectively assess cognitive function in MSA with comprehensive neuropsychological testing was published in 1992 by Robbins *et al.* [81]. The authors used tests sensitive to frontal lobe dysfunction, memory and learning deficits, and compared performance with a control group. Neuropsychological deficits were found, which were compatible with a prominent frontal-lobe-like syndrome, with significant deficits in all three frontal tests and verbal fluency, in the absence of consistent impairment in language, visual perception, memory or learning. Neuropsychological performance, however, was heterogeneous, with a group of patients showing high degree of intellectual functions despite severe physical disability, some with deficits restricted to tests sensitive for frontal lobe dysfunction and others exhibiting a broader range of impairment, with clear deficits on executive tasks, memory, and language [81]. Recently, a case of MSA presenting with prominent semantic language deficits has been reported [82]. Previous studies have consistently reported a selective impairment of executive functions in MSA. However, memory and visuospatial deficits similar to the pattern of cognitive impairment seen in PD have also been observed [83]. In several cross-sectional studies, MSA and PD patients displayed a similar profile of cognitive dysfunction, performing poorly in the visuospatial organization, construction and visuomotor ability tests [84,85]. Patients with MSA are impaired on tests of verbal fluency, working memory, attentional set-shifting, set acquisition, planning, free recall in verbal memory tests, and response inhibition [86,87]. In one study, executive deficits in MSA were found to be of similar severity to that in PD, but less severe than that seen in PSP [14]. In another cross-sectional study, however, executive dysfunction in MSA was more severe and diffuse than in PD [86]. In the only longitudinal study yet reported, PD and MSA patients showed a similar overall cognitive performance and a similar pattern of cognitive impairment at baseline, except for a higher impairment of verbal fluency in MSA. However, after a mean follow-up of 21 months, patients with MSA deteriorated significantly more than those with PD [24].

The only study that focused on cognitive defects in MSA-C (mean disease duration of 4.6 years) showed evidence of mild cognitive impairment, with impaired verbal memory and executive function; none of the patients fulfilled criteria for dementia [8]. A recent comparative study of cognitive defects in MSA-P (mean disease duration 3.2 years) and MSA-C (mean disease duration 2.6 years), showed MSA-P patients to present with more severe and widespread cognitive dysfunction, with impairments in verbal fluency, executive function, visuospatial and constructional tests [7]. Patients with MSA-C showed milder impairment, only in visuospatial and constructional functions. Neuropsychological impairment in MSA-P was correlated with decreased perfusion in the prefrontal cortex and posterior parietal lobes (^{99m}Tc-ethylcysteine dimmer single photon emission computed tomography), whereas cognitive impairment in MSA-C correlated with cerebellar hypoperfusion [7]. In keeping with these findings, a recent study identified three groups of patients with MSA with a differential degree of cognitive impairment and a different pattern of deficits in glucose metabolism as assessed by fluorodeoxiglucose positron emission tomography [88]. Patients in group I had a significantly shorter disease duration, frequent memory impairment, executive dysfunction and hypometabolism in the frontal cortex. Patients in groups II and III displayed multiple domain cognitive deficits, had more severe motor impairment and showed hypometabolism not only in the frontal but also in the parietotemporal cortex and bilateral caudate nucleus. All these findings demonstrate the frequent and progressive nature of cognitive deficits in MSA, and that cognitive impairment is related to cortical hypometabolism beginning in the frontal and spreading to the parietotemporal cortex [88]. Several recent neuroimaging studies have demonstrated that cortical atrophy in MSA is more severe than previously had been considered. MSA is associated with volume loss in widespread cortical regions, particularly involving the lateral prefrontal cortex, but also the orbitofrontal cortex, posterior parietal cortex, hippocampus, insula, caudate nucleus, putamen, primary sensorimotor cortex, corpus callosum, and supplementary motor area [89–91].

In the diagnostic criteria for MSA the presence of dementia is considered as a non-supporting feature. This imposes a selection bias in research studies which include patients with a clinical diagnosis, and the accuracy of data regarding cognitive impairment and dementia in studies using retrospective clinical information of autopsy-proven cases of MSA is limited. Furthermore, it is worth noting that most published studies comparing cognition in PD, PSP and MSA did not include PD or PSP patients with dementia – this selection bias may limit the generalization of their results.

Even though it has been shown that the degree of cognitive impairment is of similar severity in PD and MSA, and that the degree of cortical atrophy seems to be even greater in MSA, there are no published studies on the actual prevalence of dementia in MSA. A shorter disease duration, and the fact that dementia does not appear as a major complaint in patients with otherwise severe and very disabling motor symptoms, may account for the lack of data on dementia in MSA [89]. A recent paper attemping to characterize the prevalence and nature of cognitive impairments in MSA recruited 58 MSA patients over a period of 10 years, 10 of whom were diagnosed with dementia. Cognitive decline preceded onset of motor symptoms in three. While there were no demographic differences (age at onset, gender, duration of disease, or severity of cerebellar dysfunction) between patients with and without dementia, they found that the ratios of ^{123}I-metaidobenzylguanidine (MIBG) cardiac scintigraphy were significantly decreased in demented patients. White matter lesions were evident in these patients, and frontal atrophy was prominent in patients whose cognitive decline was preceded by onset of motor symptoms [92].

Overall, data presented here clearly demonstrate that cognitive impairment is common in MSA and is of similar severity to age- and education-matched patients with PD.

Symptomatic forms of dementia associated with parkinsonism

In addition to the array of primary neurodegenerative disorders associated with a combination of dementia and parkinsonism, a number of disorders affecting the brain can lead to a similar clinical presentation. Such disorders include a wide range of disparate aetiologies including cerebrovascular disease (in particular subcortical vascular encephalopathy and multiple lacunar infarcts), normal pressure hydrocephalus, prion diseases, other infections and drug intoxications. These disorders are mentioned in Chapter 18 and will not be elaborated further here. It should suffice to say that in most cases the disease history including the onset, the course and the temporal sequence of symptoms, the presence of other neurological and systemic findings, appropriate laboratory and imaging studies would reveal the correct diagnosis.

Conclusions

Disorders affecting basal ganglia share a distinctive pattern of cognitive deficits. A predominantly frontostriatal pattern of cognitive impairment, consisting of a frontal lobe-like syndrome without genuine cortical deficits such as amnesia, apraxia, aphasia, or agnosia is the common pattern. Recent pathological data, however, have demonstrated widespread, moderate-to-severe cortical damage in patients with PSP, CBD, and MSA. The greater cognitive impairment of patients with PSP in prefrontal-based cognitive functions is probably related to the substantial frontal deafferentation along with direct involvement of premotor and prefrontal areas. Likewise, progressive and significant cortical dysfunction in prefrontal and posterior parietal areas explains the predominantly dysexecutive and visuospatial nature of deficits found in patients with MSA. Recent advances in immunocytochemistry and molecular genetics have helped to refine the nosological entity of FTDP-17. Mutations in the *MAPT* or *PGRN* genes may account for the clinical and pathological heterogeneities previously described in such patients. Hence the term 'frontotemporal dementia with parkinsonism' seems more appropriate than FTDP-17.

References

1 Goetz CG, Emre M, Dubois B. Parkinson's disease dementia: definitions, guidelines, and research perspectives in diagnosis. Ann Neurol 2008; 64(Suppl 2): S81-92.

2 McKeith I, Mintzer J, Aarsland D, et al. Dementia with Lewy bodies. Lancet Neurol 2004; 3: 19–28.

3 Albert ML, Feldman RG, Willis AL. The 'subcortical dementia' of progressive supranuclear palsy. J Neurol Neurosurg Psychiatry 1974; 37: 121–30.

4 Graham NL, Bak TH, Hodges JR. Corticobasal degeneration as a cognitive disorder. Mov Disord 2003; 18: 1224–32.

5 Bergeron C, Davis A, Lang AE. Corticobasal ganglionic degeneration and progressive supranuclear palsy presenting with cognitive decline. Brain Pathol 1998; 8: 355–65.

6 Hodges JR, Davies RR, Xuereb JH, et al. Clinicopathological correlates in frontotemporal dementia. Ann Neurol 2004; 56: 399–406.

7 Kawai Y, Suenaga M, Takeda A, et al. Cognitive impairments in multiple system atrophy: MSA-C vs MSA-P. Neurology 2008; 70: 1390–6.

8 Burk K, Daum I, Rub U. Cognitive function in multiple system atrophy of the cerebellar type. Mov Disord 2006; 21: 772–6.

9 Cummings JL. Frontal–subcortical circuits and human behavior. Arch Neurol 1993; 50: 873–80.

10 Salmon DP, Filoteo JV. Neuropsychology of cortical versus subcortical dementia syndromes. Semin Neurol 2007; 27: 7–21.

11 Cummings JL, Benson DF. Subcortical dementia. Review of an emerging concept. Arch Neurol 1984; 41: 874–9.

12 Schrag A, Ben-Shlomo Y, Quinn NP. Prevalence of progressive supranuclear palsy and multiple system atrophy: a cross-sectional study. Lancet 1999; 354: 1771–5.

13 Steele JC, Richardson JC, Olszewski J. Progressive supranuclear palsy. A heterogeneous degeneration involving the brain stem, basal ganglia and cerebellum with vertical gaze and pseudobulbar palsy, nuchal dystonia and dementia. Arch Neurol 1964; 10: 333–59.

14 Bak TH, Crawford LM, Hearn VC, Mathuranath PS, Hodges JR. Subcortical dementia revisited: similarities and differences in cognitive function between progressive supranuclear palsy (PSP), corticobasal degeneration (CBD) and multiple system atrophy (MSA). Neurocase 2005; 11: 268–73.

15 Kaat LD, Boon AJ, Kamphorst W, Ravid R, Duivenvoorden HJ, van Swieten JC. Frontal presentation in progressive supranuclear palsy. Neurology 2007; 69: 723–9.

16 Menza MA, Cocchiola J, Golbe LI. Psychiatric symptoms in progressive supranuclear palsy. Psychosomatics 1995; 36: 550–4.

17 Nauta WJ. The problem of the frontal lobe: a reinterpretation. J Psychiatr Res 1971; 8: 167–87.

18 Pirker W, Asenbaum S, Bencsits G, et al. [123I]beta-CIT SPECT in multiple system atrophy, progressive supranuclear palsy, and corticobasal degeneration. Mov Disord 2000; 15: 1158–67.

19 Kim YJ, Ichise M, Ballinger JR, et al. Combination of dopamine transporter and D2 receptor SPECT in the diagnostic evaluation of PD, MSA, and PSP. Mov Disord 2002; 17: 303–12.

20 Shinotoh H, Namba H, Yamaguchi M, et al. Positron emission tomographic measurement of acetylcholinesterase activity reveals differential loss of ascending cholinergic systems in Parkinson's disease and progressive supranuclear palsy. Ann Neurol 1999; 46: 62–9.

21 Asahina M, Suhara T, Shinotoh H, Inoue O, Suzuki K, Hattori T. Brain muscarinic receptors in progressive supranuclear palsy and Parkinson's disease: a positron emission tomographic study. J Neurol Neurosurg Psychiatry 1998; 65: 155–63.

22 Litvan I, Grafman J, Gomez C, Chase TN. Memory impairment in patients with progressive supranuclear palsy. Arch Neurol 1989; 46: 765–67.

23 Grafman J, Litvan I, Stark M. Neuropsychological features of progressive supranuclear palsy. Brain Cogn 1995; 28: 311–20.

24 Soliveri P, Monza D, Paridi D, et al. Neuropsychological follow up in patients with Parkinson's disease, striatonigral degeneration-type multisystem atrophy, and progressive supranuclear palsy. J Neurol Neurosurg Psychiatry 2000; 69: 313–18.

25 Borroni B, Turla M, Bertasi V, Agosti C, Gilberti N, Padovani A. Cognitive and behavioral assessment in the early stages of neurodegenerative extrapyramidal syndromes. Arch Gerontol Geriatr 2008; 47: 53–61.

26 Dubois B, Pillon B, Legault F, Agid Y, Lhermitte F. Slowing of cognitive processing in progressive supranuclear palsy. A comparison with Parkinson's disease. Arch Neurol 1988; 45: 1194–9.

27 Johnson R, Jr., Litvan I, Grafman J. Progressive supranuclear palsy: altered sensory processing leads to degraded cognition. Neurology 1991; 41: 1257–62.

28 Grafman J, Litvan I, Gomez C, Chase TN. Frontal lobe function in progressive supranuclear palsy. Arch Neurol 1990; 47: 553–8.

29 Robbins TW, James M, Owen AM, et al. Cognitive deficits in progressive supranuclear palsy, Parkinson's disease, and multiple system atrophy in tests sensitive to frontal lobe dysfunction. J Neurol Neurosurg Psychiatry 1994; 57: 79–88.

30 Partiot A, Verin M, Pillon B, Teixeira-Ferreira C, Agid Y, Dubois B. Delayed response tasks in basal ganglia lesions in man: further evidence for a striato-frontal cooperation in behavioural adaptation. Neuropsychologia 1996; 34: 709–21.

31 Dillon DG, Pizzagalli DA. Inhibition of action, thought, and emotion: a selective neurobiological review. Appl Prev Psychol 2007; 12: 99–114.

32 Monchi O, Petrides M, Mejia-Constain B, Strafella AP. Cortical activity in Parkinson's disease during executive processing depends on striatal involvement. Brain 2007; 130: 233–44.

33 Dubois B, Slachevsky A, Pillon B, Beato R, Villalponda JM, Litvan I. "Applause sign" helps to discriminate PSP from FTD and PD. Neurology 2005; 64: 2132–3.

34 Nigg JT. On inhibition/disinhibition in developmental psychopathology: views from cognitive and personality psychology and a working inhibition taxonomy. Psychol Bull 2000; 126: 220–46.

35 Osaki Y, Ben-Shlomo Y, Lees AJ, et al. Accuracy of clinical diagnosis of progressive supranuclear palsy. Mov Disord 2004; 19: 181–9.

36 Williams DR, de Silva R, Paviour DC, et al. Characteristics of two distinct clinical phenotypes in pathologically proven progressive supranuclear palsy: Richardson's syndrome and PSP-parkinsonism. Brain 2005; 128: 1247–58.

37 Paviour DC, Price SL, Jahanshahi M, Lees AJ, Fox NC. Longitudinal MRI in progressive supranuclear palsy and multiple system atrophy: rates and regions of atrophy. Brain 2006; 129: 1040–9.

38 Josephs KA, Whitwell JL, Dickson DW, et al. Voxel-based morphometry in autopsy proven PSP and CBD. Neurobiol Aging 2008; 29: 280–9.

39 Kulisevsky J, Litvan I, Berthier ML, Pascual-Sedano B, Paulsen JS, Cummings JL. Neuropsychiatric assessment of Gilles de la Tourette patients: comparative study with other hyperkinetic and hypokinetic movement disorders. Mov Disord 2001; 16: 1098–1104.

40 Litvan I, Mega MS, Cummings JL, Fairbanks L. Neuropsychiatric aspects of progressive supranuclear palsy. Neurology 1996; 47: 1184–9.

41 Cordato NJ, Halliday GM, Caine D, Morris JG. Comparison of motor, cognitive, and behavioral features in progressive supranuclear palsy and Parkinson's disease. Mov Disord 2006; 21: 632–8.

42 Levy ML, Cummings JL, Fairbanks LA, et al. Apathy is not depression. J Neuropsychiatry Clin Neurosci 1998; 10: 314–19.

43 Aarsland D, Litvan I, Larsen JP. Neuropsychiatric symptoms of patients with progressive supranuclear palsy and Parkinson's disease. J Neuropsychiatry Clin Neurosci 2001; 13: 42–9.

44 Cordato NJ, Pantelis C, Halliday GM, et al. Frontal atrophy correlates with behavioural changes in progressive supranuclear palsy. Brain 2002; 125: 789–800.

45 Williams DR, Lees AJ. Visual hallucinations in the diagnosis of idiopathic Parkinson's disease: a retrospective autopsy study. Lancet Neurol 2005; 4: 605–10.

46 Diederich NJ, Leurgans S, Fan W, Chmura TA, Goetz CG. Visual hallucinations and symptoms of REM sleep behavior disorder in Parkinsonian tauopathies. Int J Geriatr Psychiatry 2008; 23: 598–603.

47 Riley DE, Lang AE, Lewis A, et al. Cortical–basal ganglionic degeneration. Neurology 1990; 40: 1203–12.

48 Rinne JO, Lee MS, Thompson PD, Marsden CD. Corticobasal degeneration. A clinical study of 36 cases. Brain 1994; 117(Pt 5): 1183–96.

49 Murray R, Neumann M, Forman MS, et al. Cognitive and motor assessment in autopsy-proven corticobasal degeneration. Neurology 2007; 68: 1274–83.

50 Wenning GK, Litvan I, Jankovic J, et al. Natural history and survival of 14 patients with corticobasal degeneration confirmed at postmortem examination. J Neurol Neurosurg Psychiatry 1998; 64: 184–9.

51 Kompoliti K, Goetz CG, Boeve BF, et al. Clinical presentation and pharmacological therapy in corticobasal degeneration. Arch Neurol 1998; 55: 957–961.

52 Wadia PM, Lang AE. The many faces of corticobasal degeneration. Parkinsonism Relat Disord 2007; 13(Suppl 3): S336–40.

53 Alladi S, Xuereb J, Bak T, et al. Focal cortical presentations of Alzheimer's disease. Brain 2007; 130: 2636–45.

54 Moreaud O, Monavon A, Brutti-Mairesse MP, Grand S, Lebas JF. Creutzfeldt–Jakob disease mimicking corticobasal degeneration clinical and MRI data of a case. J Neurol 2005; 252: 1283–4.

55 Boeve BF, Josephs KA, Drubach DA. Current and future management of the corticobasal syndrome and corticobasal degeneration. Handb Clin Neurol 2008; 89: 533–48.

56 Boeve BF, Lang AE, Litvan I. Corticobasal degeneration and its relationship to progressive supranuclear palsy and frontotemporal dementia. Ann Neurol 2003; 54(Suppl 5): S15–19.

57 Pillon B, Blin J, Vidailhet M, et al. The neuropsychological pattern of corticobasal degeneration: comparison with progressive supranuclear palsy and Alzheimer's disease. Neurology 1995; 45: 1477–83.

58 Litvan I, Cummings JL, Mega M. Neuropsychiatric features of corticobasal degeneration. J Neurol Neurosurg Psychiatry 1998; 65: 717–21.

59 Soliveri P, Piacentini S, Girotti F. Limb apraxia in corticobasal degeneration and progressive supranuclear palsy. Neurology 2005; 64: 448–53.

60 Leiguarda R, Lees AJ, Merello M, Starkstein S, Marsden CD. The nature of apraxia in corticobasal degeneration. J Neurol Neurosurg Psychiatry 1994; 57: 455–9.

61 Leiguarda RC, Merello M, Nouzeilles MI, Balej J, Rivero A, Nogues M. Limb-kinetic apraxia in corticobasal degeneration: clinical and kinematic features. Mov Disord 2003; 18: 49–59.

62 Sawle GV, Brooks DJ, Marsden CD, Frackowiak RS. Corticobasal degeneration. A unique pattern of regional cortical oxygen hypometabolism and striatal fluorodopa uptake demonstrated by positron emission tomography. Brain 1991; 114(Pt 1B): 541–56.

63 Zadikoff C, Lang AE. Apraxia in movement disorders. Brain 2005; 128: 1480–97.

64 Mimura M, White RF, Albert ML. Corticobasal degeneration: neuropsychological and clinical correlates. J Neuropsychiatry Clin Neurosci 1997; 9: 94–8.

65 Graham NL, Bak T, Patterson K, Hodges JR. Language function and dysfunction in corticobasal degeneration. Neurology 2003; 61: 493–9.

66 Frattali CM, Grafman J, Patronas N, Makhlouf F, Litvan I. Language disturbances in corticobasal degeneration. Neurology 2000; 54: 990–2.

67 Kertesz A, Martinez-Lage P, Davidson W, Munoz DG. The corticobasal degeneration syndrome overlaps progressive aphasia and frontotemporal dementia. Neurology 2000; 55: 1368–75.

68 McMonagle P, Blair M, Kertesz A. Corticobasal degeneration and progressive aphasia. Neurology 2006; 67: 1444–51.

69 Soliveri P, Monza D, Paridi D, et al. Cognitive and magnetic resonance imaging aspects of corticobasal degeneration and progressive supranuclear palsy. Neurology 1999; 53: 502–7.

70 Dubois B, Slachevsky A, Litvan I, Pillon B. The FAB: a Frontal Assessment Battery at bedside. Neurology 2000; 55: 1621–6.

71 Massman PJ, Kreiter KT, Jankovic J, Doody RS. Neuropsychological functioning in cortical-basal ganglionic degeneration: differentiation from Alzheimer's disease. Neurology 1996; 46: 720–6.

72 Foster NL, Wilhelmsen K, Sima AA, Jones MZ, D'Amato CJ, Gilman S. Frontotemporal dementia and parkinsonism linked to chromosome 17: a consensus conference. Conference Participants. Ann Neurol 1997; 41: 706–15.

73 Lynch T, Sano M, Marder KS, et al. Clinical characteristics of a family with chromosome 17-linked disinhibition–dementia–parkinsonism–amyotrophy complex. Neurology 1994; 44: 1878–84.

74 van Swieten JC, Stevens M, Rosso SM, et al. Phenotypic variation in hereditary frontotemporal dementia with tau mutations. Ann Neurol 1999; 46: 617–26.

75 van Swieten JC, Rosso SM, van Herpen E, Kamphorst W, Ravid R, Heutink P. Phenotypic variation in frontotemporal dementia and parkinsonism linked to chromosome 17. Dement Geriatr Cogn Disord 2004; 17: 261–4.

76 Hutton M, Lendon CL, Rizzu P, et al. Association of missense and 5'-splice-site mutations in tau with the inherited dementia FTDP-17. Nature 1998; 393: 702–5.

77 Baker M, Mackenzie IR, Pickering-Brown SM, et al. Mutations in progranulin cause tau-negative frontotemporal dementia linked to chromosome 17. Nature 2006; 442: 916–19.

78 Boeve BF, Hutton M. Refining frontotemporal dementia with parkinsonism linked to chromosome 17: introducing FTDP-17 (MAPT) and FTDP-17 (PGRN). Arch Neurol 2008; 65: 460–4.

79 Gilman S, Wenning GK, Low PA, et al. Second consensus statement on the diagnosis of multiple system atrophy. Neurology 2008; 71: 670–6.

80 Wenning GK, Stefanova N, Jellinger KA, Poewe W, Schlossmacher MG. Multiple system atrophy: a primary oligodendrogliopathy. Ann Neurol 2008; 64: 239–46.

81 Robbins TW, James M, Lange KW, Owen AM, Quinn NP, Marsden CD. Cognitive performance in multiple system atrophy. Brain 1992; 115(Pt 1): 271–91.

82 Apostolova LG, Klement I, Bronstein Y, Vinters HV, Cummings JL. Multiple system atrophy presenting with language impairment. Neurology 2006; 67: 726–7.

83 Pillon B, Dubois B, Agid Y. Testing cognition may contribute to the diagnosis of movement disorders. Neurology 1996; 46: 329–34.

84 Testa D, Fetoni V, Soliveri P, Musicco M, Palazzini E, Girotti F. Cognitive and motor performance in multiple system atrophy and Parkinson's disease compared. Neuropsychologia 1993; 31: 207–10.

85 Pillon B, Gouider-Khouja N, Deweer B, et al. Neuropsychological pattern of striatonigral degeneration: comparison with Parkinson's disease and progressive supranuclear palsy. J Neurol Neurosurg Psychiatry 1995; 58: 174–9.

86 Monza D, Soliveri P, Radice D, et al. Cognitive dysfunction and impaired organization of complex motility in degenerative parkinsonian syndromes. Arch Neurol 1998; 55: 372–8.

87 Paviour DC, Winterburn D, Simmonds S, et al. Can the frontal assessment battery (FAB) differentiate bradykinetic rigid syndromes? Relation of the FAB to formal neuropsychological testing. Neurocase 2005; 11: 274–82.

88 Lyoo CH, Jeong Y, Ryu YH, et al. Effects of disease duration on the clinical features and brain glucose metabolism in patients with mixed type multiple system atrophy. Brain 2008; 131: 438–46.

89 Watanabe H, Saito Y, Terao S, et al. Progression and prognosis in multiple system atrophy: an analysis of 230 Japanese patients. Brain 2002; 125: 1070–83.

90 Konagaya M, Konagaya Y, Sakai M, Matsuoka Y, Hashizume Y. Progressive cerebral atrophy in multiple system atrophy. J Neurol Sci 2002; 195: 123–7.

91 Brenneis C, Seppi K, Schocke MF, et al. Voxel-based morphometry detects cortical atrophy in the Parkinson variant of multiple system atrophy. Mov Disord 2003; 18: 1132–8.

92 Kitayama M, Wada-Isoe K, Irizawa Y, Nakashima K. Assessment of dementia in patients with multiple system atrophy. Eur J Neurol 2009 Feb 19 [Epub ahead of print]

Chapter 18

Diagnosis of dementia in Parkinson's disease

Murat Emre

Introduction

In essence, diagnosis of dementia in a patient with Parkinson's disease (PD) is no different from diagnosing dementia in any given patient. The diagnostic approach can be conceptualized as a two-step process: diagnosis of dementia and differential diagnosis with regard to its aetiology. The first step involves excluding other conditions which can mimic dementia, as well as the evaluation of whether mental impairment is severe enough to affect normal functioning by itself in order to fulfil the current definition of dementia. The second step includes the assessment of the aetiology, i.e. whether dementia is due to PD by excluding other potential causes. Although rather straightforward in a patient with a typical history and symptoms of PD, this step involves considering other conditions which can present with dementia and Parkinsonism, particularly in patients for whom the history is not reliable or when atypical features are present.

As compared to other patients with suspected dementia, diagnosis of dementia in patients with PD can be more difficult. There are several confounding factors related to the disease itself, its treatment and comorbid conditions which are more frequent in this patient population. These include adverse effects of medication, acute or prolonged confusion due to systemic abnormalities or diseases and presence of depression, all of which can mimic symptoms of dementia. At times, severe motor impairment renders it difficult to judge whether impairment in function, a prerequisite to diagnose dementia, is due to mental or motor dysfunction. Conditions that can mimic dementia in patients with PD are listed in Table 18.1 and the general approach to diagnosis is summarized below.

Diagnosis of dementia

Diagnosing dementia in patients with PD is principally a clinical undertaking, with little help from auxillary methods. The diagnostic process involves several components including a careful history from patients and their family members with emphasis on typical features of PD-D [1], assessment of cognitive functions, behavioural symptoms and activities of daily living (ADL). In typical cases auxillary examinations are of least help – they usually serve the purpose of excluding alternative etiologies in suspected patients.

Table 18.1 Conditions which may mimic dementia in patients with Parkinson's disease (PD)

◆ Worried patients or their families
◆ Mild cognitive impairment of PD
◆ Depression
◆ Acute or prolonged confusion (delirium)
◆ Adverse effects of drugs

Taking the history

Along with cognitive testing, a detailed history is the most powerful tool for the diagnosis of dementia. Of particular interest are the mode of onset of mental dysfunction, the profile and the time course of cognitive and behavioural symptoms, the presence of typical features for PD-D, presence/absence of depressive symptoms or symptoms and signs of acute confusion. Typically, cognitive impairment due to PD has an insidious onset and slow progression. Current treatment and recent changes in medication should be reviewed, in particular administration of drugs known to cause mental dysfunction such as anticholinergics, along with recently initiated treatments and changes in doses.

PD patients who are in the course of developing dementia frequently present with typical early symptoms. It is useful to specifically ask for the presence of such features when taking the history from patients and their family members. Changes in sleep–wake cycle are frequent, including excessive daytime sleepiness, disturbance of night sleep and brief confusion or transient hallucinations on awakening. Rapid-eye-movement (REM) sleep behaviour disorder (RBD; dream-enacting behaviour such as speaking, screaming, or movements in sleep) may be seen also in patients without dementia; it is, however, more common in demented patients and may precede development of dementia by many years. Prior to overt psychosis, 'phantom boarder' phenomenon or 'feeling of presence' may develop where the patients believe that somebody is standing behind them or there is somebody else in the house, although they do not see this person. Development of hallucinations or psychosis shortly after initiating dopaminergic medication may be another early sign of incipient dementia. The presence of visual hallucinations, usually well-formed, coloured objects, insects, animals or humans should also be specifically asked for. Patients and their families may not volunteer this information because of fear that the patients are going 'mad', but may admit it when asked. Other early signs include loss of interest, apathy, social withdrawal, forgetfulness, inattentiveness and difficulties with concentration when reading a book, watching a movie or following a conversation. Early signs of functional impairment include difficulties in handling personal or family finances, navigating or finding directions especially in unfamiliar, but sometimes also in familiar, environments.

Assessment of cognitive functions

Cognitive functions can be examined either by using formal, validated scales or by administering several tests for each cognitive domain. For each purpose one can use either simple scales or a limited number of easy-to-administer bedside tests for screening purposes, or more elaborate scales and more complex neuropsychologcial tests for a detailed and quantitative evaluation. A two-level approach, simpler screening scales and tests for practising physicians, or a more detailed assessment for complex cases or for research purposes, was also proposed in the recent recommendations for the diagnosis of PD-D published by a Task Force of the Movement Disorder Society [2].

Composite cognitive scales

Simple, easy-to-administer and less time-consuming scales include those which are not specific for PD, as well as those developed specifically for screening patients with PD (Table 18.2). General purpose scales, such as the most widely known Mini-Mental State Examination (MMSE), can be used for brief screening. The Montreal Cognitive Assessment (MoCA) is probably more sensitive to detect cognitive deficits in PD, as it includes a more detailed assessment of executive functions [3]. Addenbrooke's Cognitive Examination scale takes longer to complete compared with the other screening batteries [4]. However, it offers the advantages that a more complete and extensive cognitive evaluation can be achieved, and an MMSE score can be extracted from this scale.

Screening batteries specifically developed for PD include the Parkinson Neuropsy-chometric Dementia Assessment (PANDA) [5], and the Mini-Mental Parkinson [6]. These scales specifially include tests assessing common deficits seen in patients with PD. Another screening instrument which focuses on impairment in frontal–executive functions, one of the core deficits in PD-D, and also including assessment of some behavioural symptoms, is the Frontal Assessment Battery (FAB) [7].

More elaborate scales are reserved for a more detailed and quantitative assessment, and these are usually administered in the context of research studies or in early stage patients with high education who can show a normal performance on simple screening scales. These also include two categories: those not specific for PD, and those specifically developed to assess

Table 18.2 Composite scales which can be used to evaluate cognitive functions in Parkinson's disease (PD)

A. Screening scales
- ◆ General purpose scales
  - Mini Mental State Examination (MMSE)
  - Montreal Cognitive Assessment (MoCA)
  - Addenbrooke's Cognitive Assessment
  - Frontal Assessment Battery (FAB)
- ◆ PD-specific scales
  - Mini-Mental Parkinson
  - Parkinson Neuropsychometric Dementia Assessment (PANDA)

B. More quantitative scales
- ◆ General purpose scales
  - Alzheimer Disease Assessment Scale – cognitive section (ADAS-COG)
  - Mattis Dementia Rating Scale (DRS)
- ◆ PD-specific scales
  - Scales for Outcomes in Parkinson's disease – Cognition (SCOPA-COG)
  - Parkinson Disease – Cognitive Rating Scale (PD-CRS)

typical deficits in PD. Among the established and validated scales in the former group are the most widely used composite cognitive scale, the Alzheimer Disease Assessment Scale – cognitive section (ADAS-COG) [8], and the Mattis Dementia Rating Scale (DRS) [9], which is more sensitive for PD as it includes an extensive executive functions component. Scales for Outcomes in Parkinson's disease – Cognition (SCOPA-COG) [10] and Parkinson Disease – Cognitive Rating Scale (PD-CRS) [11] were both specifically developed to assess cognitive functions in patients with PD, and can also be used for follow-up purposes to assess change over time.

When using composite scales and trying to interpret their scores, it is important that one should not consider only the total score, but also the profile of deficits. For example a score of 27 on MMSE is nominally a normal score. This score, however, may be abnormal in a well-educated patient when the errors include difficulties copying the intersecting pentagons, failing to remember one out of three words, and one mistake on subtracting serial 7s. These show typical deficits in attention, visuospatial function, and free recall and may indicate an abnormal performance in this particular patient despite a nominally normal MMSE score.

Neuropsychological tests

A full neuropsychological evaluation, with several tests for each cognitive domain, including attention, memory, language, praxis, visuospatial and executive functions, tailored for the age, education and the general mental status of the patient, is the most appropriate way to assess cognitive functions. This is, however, time-consuming and needs special expertise to choose the tests, perform them, and interpret their results. For the practising neurologist, easy-to-administer bedside tests may be sufficient to rapidly assess the cognitive status of the patient. In accordance with the profile of cognitive impairment in PD-D, several simple tests for the most-affected cognitive domains can be administered (Table 18.3). These include serial 7s (subtracting 7s from 100 backwards) or months/days

Table 18.3 Neuropsychological tests to evaluate individual cognitive domains

A. Bedside tests
- ◆ Attention: serial 7s, months or days backwards
- ◆ Memory: learning a 3–5-word list, or a 5-item address, with delayed free recall, recall after cueing and recognition
- ◆ Executive functions: verbal (lexical and category) fluency, clock-drawing test
- ◆ Visual–spatial functions: copying intersecting pentagons or a 3-dimensional cube; imitating hand figures such as butterfly figure or intercalating fingers
- ◆ Language: spontaneous speech (word-finding difficulties, pauses), naming common and rarer objects, understanding complex sentences

B. More comprehensive tests
- ◆ Attention: forward and backward digit span, continuous performance tests
- ◆ Memory: Rey Auditory Learning, California Verbal Learning, Buschke Selective Reminding Tests
- ◆ Executive functions: Wisconsin Card Sorting, Stroop, Tower of London tests, Trails A–B
- ◆ Visual–spatial functions: Rey–Osterreich Complex Figure, Picture Completion, Recognizing Embedded Figures, Line Orientation and Benton Facial Recognition tests
- ◆ Language: Boston Naming Test

recited backwards to assess attention; verbal fluency (both lexical and semantic) and clock-drawing test for executive functions; copying a three-dimensional cube or intersecting pentagons, mimicking complex hand figures (such as intercalating fingers) to assess visuospatial functions; and simple memory tests such as learning a three-to-five word list or a five-item address, assessing both free recall and recognition (after cueing and after providing alternatives) following sufficient learning trials. The most yielding are probably verbal fluency and clock-drawing tests, which are described below.

Lexical fluency task consists of naming as many words as possible which start with a certain letter within one minute. The letters used in the English language are F, A and S, personal and geographical names are not allowed. The semantic fluency test requires naming as many objects as possible within a minute, which belong to a certain semantic category, such as animals or vegetables. Both tests are sensitive measures of executive functions, specifically of internally cued search strategies. The cut-off scores vary depending on age, culture, and education; usually 12–14 words for each letter or items in each category are regarded as normal. The clock-drawing test taps executive functions such as planning as well as visuospatial functions. The patient is given an empty circle of about 5 cm in diameter on a blank sheet, with the centre and the top marked, and asked to place all the numbers of a clock in the appropriate location and then to draw the arms of the clock to indicate 11:10. The following are evaluated: whether the patient starts with an adequate planning by placing 12, 3, 6 and 9 first; whether all the numbers are located in the right place; whether the whole circle is used; and whether 11:10 is correctly indicated.

Examples of more eloborate neuropsychological tests are listed in Table 18.3. These include forward and backward digit span, and continous performance tests for attention; Wisconsin Card Sorting, Tower of London, or Stroop tests for assessing planning, mental set-building and set-shifting, trails A–B test for psychomotor speed and set-shifting for the assessment of various components of executive functions; California Verbal Learning, Rey's 15 words and 15 shapes or Bushke's Selective Reminding test for memory; copying Rey–Osterreich complex figure, picture completion test, recognizing embedded figures, line orientation and face recognition tests to assess visuospatial functions; and Boston Naming test for confrontational naming. The extent of testing and type of tests should be tailored according to the age, intellectual capacity and general condition of the patient.

Assessment of behavioural symptoms

At bedside or in the office setting, the most efficient and practical way to assess behavioural symptoms is through a semistructured interview with the patient and a well-informed family member. As patients and caregivers may not voluntarily report psychotic symptoms, these should be specifically asked for, in particular the existence of typical symptoms such as infidelity, phantom boarder or 'feeling of presence' delusions and visual hallucinations, typically of insects, animals or people. A tactful way of asking may be: 'Patients with this disease may sometimes have dreams when they are awake, does this happen to you?' Likewise loss of interest and motivation, apathy, social withdrawal, depressive symptoms such as sadness and anhedonia, excessive daytime sleepiness, transient confusion and disorientation on awakening and symptoms of RBD must be explored.

The most widely used formal scale to assess behavioural and neuropsychiatric symptoms is the Neuropsychiatric Inventory [12]. There are 10- and 12-item versions, and also the possibility to capture caregiver burden. The scale is easy to use with screening questions for each symptom answered by an informed caregiver. When the occurrence of a particular symptom is confirmed the severity is measured semiquantitatively by assessing the frequency of its occurrence and the grade of discomfort caused by it.

Assessment of functional impairment

This is probably the most difficult part of the assessment, yet the most critical one to ascertain the diagnosis of dementia as per current definitions. It is generally less difficult to decide if a patient has functional impairment. The more difficult part is to judge whether and how much of the functional impairment is due to motor vs mental dysfunction. This can be especially difficult in patients who have severe motor impairment, in particular axial involvement such as postural imbalance and speech disorder, symptoms which are more frequent in demented PD patients. Elderly patients may have stopped taking care of themselves for many years, simply because it is more convenient to rely on their caregivers for ADL. In such cases it may be difficult to judge whether they have any functional impairment as they do not attempt to do much by themselves.

Given all these limitations the most direct and useful way to assess functional impairment is to ask the family members what the patient was able to do before cognitive symptoms become apparent, that s/he is not able to do anymore. Instrumental (such as handling financies and money, shopping, traveling alone) and basic ADL (such as choosing clothes, dressing, bathing, personal hygiene), as well as occupational and social activities should be probed by asking lead-questions. Once newly developed functional impairment is acknowledged, one should attempt to qualify if the impairment is more due to mental or motor dysfunction. Questions for various daily activities should be asked, based on the age, sex, social and occupational status of the patient. It was proposed that the ability of a patient to organize and remember his/her own medication schedule can be used to assess functional impairment, as all PD patients receive medication [2].

Although there is none specifically developed for PD, ADL scales such as Alzheimer Disease Consortium Study – Acitivities of Daily Living (ADCS-ADL) scale [13] or Disability Assessment in Dementia (DAD) [14] scale can be used to quantitatively assess functional impairment.

Auxillary methods

These include laboratory examinations and neuroimaging, and occasionally electrophysiological investigations such as electoencephalography may be needed. Laboratory examinations may help to differentiate acute confusion (delirium) from dementia, and also to exclude or reveal other causes of dementia such as metabolic, endocrine or toxic disorders. One should not forget that PD patients with mental dysfunction are usually elderly people – they are also prone to other causes of dementia which can affect the elderly population at large. Therefore, a basic laboratory screening should be performed in PD patients who develop mental dysfunction, including haematological, biochemical, and urine tests. The array of laboratory examinations can be limited or expanded based on the clinical presentation. In typical cases with an insidious onset and slow progression, laboratory examinations may not be necessary.

In a patient with established, longstanding PD who then develops symptoms of dementia with a clinical presentation typical for PD-D, a renewed structural imaging may not be necessary. There is no single pattern of atrophy in computed tomography or magnetic resonance imaging (MRI) scan that would help to diagnose dementia in individual patients; nevertheless imaging may help to exclude alternative diagnosis. Findings in structural and functional imaging are described in detail in Chapter 10, whereas those relevant for diagnosis are summarized below.

In structural imaging with MRI there is a 4-fold increased rate of whole-brain atrophy and also more cortical atrophy in PD-D compared with non-demented PD and controls [15]. In general, medial temporal lobe atrophy including the hippocampus and parahippocampal gyrus is more severe in AD patients, with more severe atrophy of the thalamus and parieto-occipital lobes in patients with PD-D [16].

Functional imaging will rarely be required for routine diagnosis. In rCBF single photon emission computed tomography (SPECT), PD-D patients often demonstrate frontal hypoperfusion or bilateral temporoparietal deficits [17]. Perfusion deficits in precuneus and inferior lateral parietal regions, areas associated with visual processing, have also been described in PD-D, compared with AD where perfusion deficits are found in a more anterior and inferior location [18]. Reduced metabolism in temporoparietal regions of patients with PD-D compared with PD is also observed in ^{18}F-fluorodeoxyglucose–positron emission tomography (^{18}F-FDG-PET) studies [19], both PD-D and DLB patients demonstrating similar patterns of decreased metabolism in bilateral inferior and medial frontal lobes, and right parietal lobe [20].

FP-CIT SPECT demonsrates the integrity of nigrostriatal dopaminergic terminals and can help to differentiate Lewy body-related dementias from AD with extrapyramidal features, e.g. due to neuroleptic use. Significant reductions were found in ^{123}I-FP-CIT binding in the caudate, anterior and posterior putamens in subjects with DLB and PD-D compared to those with AD and controls, the greatest loss in all three areas being seen in patients with PD-D [21].

Another imaging method which can differentiate Lewy body-related dementias from other disorders such as AD is MIBG-SPECT. ^{123}I-Metaiodobenzylguanidine (^{123}I-MIBG) is an analogue of noradrenaline, and its imaging with SPECT can be used to quantify postganglionic sympathetic cardiac innervation. The heart:mediastinum (H:M) ratio is lower in PD and in other related diseases such as multiple system atrophy and DLB, but normal in patients with AD [22,23].

Finally, another method, still in its infancy with regard to routine diagnosis, is imaging of specific protein depositions in the brain. Imaging of α-synuclein is not yet achieved in humans, but amyloid burden can be quantified using substances binding to beta-amyloid. In PET studies with the Pittsburgh Compound B (PIB), mean cortical levels of amyloid were increased two-fold in AD [24], and by 60% in DLB [25]. In PD-D mean cortical amyloid load was not significantly elevated, although 20% of individuals showed an AD pattern of increased PIB uptake [26]. Once established with reliable cut-off values, quantitative assessment of amyloid vs α-synuclein burden may help in differential diagnosis.

Diagnostic criteria for PD-D

Until recently, there have been no specific criteria for the diagnosis of PD-D. In clinical practice diagnosis was made empirically, diagnosis in research studies was mainly based on the Diagnostic and Statistical Manual (DSM)-IV criteria, which groups 'dementia due to PD' along with 'other causes of dementia' without providing specifics. This gap was recognized by the Movement Disorder Society, and a Task Force of international experts was instituted to develop specific clinical diagnostic criteria for PD-D [27].

According to these criteria, the first step in the diagnostic process is the diagnosis of Parkinson's disease in accordance with the UK Brain Bank criteria for the diagnosis of PD. The second step involves identification of a dementia syndrome diagnosed on the basis of history, clinical and mental examination, with insidious onset, slow progression and typical clinical features (Table 18.4). The later steps involve screening for other conditions, in the presence of which diagnosis of dementia would be uncertain or impossible. Diagnostic certainty relies on the presence of typical or atypical cognitive and behavioural features as well as the presence or absence of other conditions. Based on these features, diagnostic criteria are described for 'probable'and 'possible' PD-D (Table 18.5). A probable PD-D is diagnosed when dementia with typical features develops on the background of established PD and in the absence of any other conditions which may contribute to, or cause, dementia. A diagnosis of possible PD-D is justified when either there is one or more atypical clinical feature, or in the presence of one or more conditions which would make the diagnosis of PD-D uncertain.

Differential diagnosis

As mentioned above, diagnosis of dementia in patients with PD can be difficult because of several confounders, notably the presence of severe motor and speech impairment, as well as comorbidities such as depression, systemic disorders and adverse events of drugs. The onset, the course and the pattern of neuropsychological and behavioural symptoms, the presence or absence of systemic and laboratory findings are important factors to decide whether the patient is suffering from dementia associated with PD or from conditions which can mimic dementia. Once these are excluded and a dementia syndrome is diagnosed, other disorders with combined motor and mental dysfunction should be excluded before diagnosing PD-D.

The main prerequisite for the diagnosis of PD-D is that dementia develops in the background of established PD. Yet, this may not always be easy to ascertain, especially in those patients who develop dementia relatively soon after developing motor symptoms or

Table 18.4 Clinical features of dementia associated with Parkinson's disease (PD-D) (from Emre *et al.* [27])

I. **Core features**
1. Diagnosis of PD according to Queen Square Brain Bank criteria
2. A dementia syndrome with insidious onset and slow progression, developing within the context of established PD and diagnosed by history, clinical, and mental examination, defined as:
   - Impairment in more than one cognitive domain
   - Representing a decline from premorbid level
   - Deficits severe enough to impair daily life (social, occupational, or personal care), independent of the impairment ascribable to motor or autonomic symptoms

II. **Associated clinical features**
1. Cognitive features:
   - Attention: impaired. Impairment in spontaneous and focused attention, poor performance in attentional tasks; performance may fluctuate during the day and from day to day
   - Executive functions: impaired. Impairment in tasks requiring initiation, planning, concept formation, rule-finding, set-shifting or set maintenance; impaired mental speed (bradyphrenia)
   - Visuospatial functions: impaired. Impairment in tasks requiring visual–spatial orientation, perception, or construction
   - Memory: impaired. Impairment in free recall of recent events or in tasks requiring learning new material, memory usually improves with cueing, recognition is usually better than free recall
   - Language: core functions largely preserved. Word-finding difficulties and impaired comprehension of complex sentences may be present
2. Behavioural features:
   - Apathy: decreased spontaneity; loss of motivation, interest, and effortful behaviour
   - Changes in personality and mood including depressive features and anxiety
   - Hallucinations: mostly visual, usually complex, formed visions of people, animals or objects
   - Delusions: usually paranoid, such as infidelity, or phantom boarder (unwelcome guests living in the home) delusions
   - Excessive daytime sleepiness

III. **Features which do not exclude PD-D, but make the diagnosis uncertain**
   - Coexistence of any other abnormality which may by itself cause cognitive impairment, but judged not to be the cause of dementia, e.g. presence of relevant vascular disease in imaging
   - Time interval between the development of motor and cognitive symptoms not known

IV. **Features suggesting other conditions or diseases as cause of mental impairment, which, when present, make it impossible to reliably diagnose PD-D**
   - Cognitive and behavioural symptoms appearing solely in the context of other conditions such as:
     - Acute confusion due to
       (a) Systemic diseases or abnormalities
       (b) Drug intoxication
     - Major depression according to DSM-IV
   - Features compatible with 'probable vascular dementia' criteria according to NINDS-AIREN (dementia in the context of cerebrovascular disease as indicated by focal signs in neurological examination such as hemiparesis, sensory deficits, and evidence of relevant cerebrovascular disease by brain imaging *and* a relationship between the two as indicated by the presence of one or more of the following: onset of dementia within 3 months after a recognized stroke, abrupt deterioration in cognitive functions, and fluctuating, stepwise progression of cognitive deficits)

Table 18.5 Diagnostic criteria for probable and possible PD-D (from Emre *et al.* [27])

Probable PD-D

A. Core features: both must be present

B. Associated clinical features:
- ♦ Typical profile of cognitive deficits including impairment in at least two of the four core cognitive domains (impaired attention which may fluctuate, impaired executive functions, impairment in visuospatial functions, and impaired free recall memory which usually improves with cueing)
- ♦ The presence of at least one behavioural symptom (apathy, depressed or anxious mood, hallucinations, delusions, excessive daytime sleepiness) supports the diagnosis of 'probable' PD-D; however, lack of behavioural symptoms does not exclude the diagnosis

C. None of the group III features present

D. None of the group IV features present

Possible PD-D

A. Core features: both must be present

B. Associated clinical features:
- ♦ Atypical profile of cognitive impairment in one or more domains, such as prominent or receptive-type (fluent) aphasia, or pure storage-failure type amnesia (memory does not improve with cueing or in recognition tasks) with preserved attention
- ♦ Behavioural symptoms may or may not be present

OR:

C. One or more of the group III features present

D. None of the group IV features present

when this temporal relationship cannot be determined. In such patients, other disorders that present with parkinsonism and dementia should be considered in the differential diagnosis, including other neurodegenerative diseases and symptomatic forms. Applying the UK Brain Bank diagnostic criteria for PD as well as the diagnostic criteria for PD-D would easily exclude the alternative diagnosis in the majority of patients. There remains, however, a group of patients where a careful differential diagnosis becomes necessary. Other disorders which present with a combination of parkinsonism and cognitive dysfunction are listed in Table 18.6 and are briefly summarized below.

The main degenerative disorder which overlaps with PD-D is DLB. The clinical and pathological features of DLB and PD-D grossly overlap; clinically it is the time course of the symptoms and presenting features that differentiate these two disorders. The clinical and pathological overlap between these two conditions led to the suggestion that they represent two clinical entitites on the spectrum of Lewy body-related dementias, with different temporal and spatial sequences of events [28,29]. The original Consortium Criteria for DLB stipulated that mental dysfunction should precede motor symptoms by at least 1 year or that they should occur within 1 year of each other [30]. There is, however, no clinical or pathological basis to suggest a fixed time interval between the development of motor vs mental symptoms in differentiating PD-D from DLB. In fact, it is often difficult to determine retrospectively when cognitive or behavioural changes emerged in relation to motor symptoms. These aspects were acknowledged in the subsequent revision of the DLB criteria, and accordingly it was proposed that the '1-year rule' between the onset of

Table 18.6 Disorders which may present with parkinsonism and dementia

---

- ◆ Degenerative disorders
  - Dementia with Lewy bodies
  - Progressive supranuclear palsy
  - Corticobasal ganglionic degeneration
  - Frontotemporal dementia–parkinsonism complex
  - Multiple system atrophy
- ◆ Symptomatic forms
  - Cerebrovascular disease (subcortical vascular encephalopathy, lacunar state)
  - Normal-pressure hydrocephalus
  - Drug intoxications such as with neuroleptics, anticonvulsants

---

dementia and parkinsonism should be maintained in research studies in which distinction is made between DLB and PD-D [31]. In practice, however, it is suggested that the diagnosis of PD-D should be entertained when dementia develops following the diagnosis of idiopathic PD, whereas the diagnosis of DLB is warranted when the symptoms of dementia precede or coincide with the development of motor symptoms. The diagnostic difficulty mostly arises when the temporal relationship between the occurrence of motor vs mental dysfunction is unknown or uncertain. In cases where this temporal relationship cannot be determined, it may be easier to use a more generic term such as 'Lewy body disease'.

Other degenerative disorders that can present with a combination of parkinsonism and mental dysfunction include progressive supranuclear palsy, corticobasal ganglionic degeneration, frontotemporal dementia–parkinsonism complex and occasional cases of multiple system atrophy. Symptomatic forms of dementia associated with extrapyramidal features include cerebrovascular disease (in particular subcortical vascular encephalopathy and lacunar state), normal-pressure hydrocephalus and drug intoxications, such as with neuroleptics or anticonvulsants, e.g. valproate.

A detailed history including a review of current treatment, deliberate questioning for features known to be associated with PD-D and use of appropriate neuropsychological tests are the essential tools in differential diagnosis. Laboratory investigations and neuroimaging may reveal the presence of alternative aetiologies or may help to exclude them. The pattern of atrophy or the presence of vascular pathology in structural imaging, and the selective distribution of hypometabolism in functional imaging may be helpful. FP-CIT SPECT may help to differentiate patients with PD-D from AD patients with extrapyramidal symptoms. Auxillary investigations may be particularly helpful in the differential diagnosis of atypical or complex cases.

Conclusions

Diagnosis of dementia associated with PD is a two-step process. The first step involves exclusion of other causes of mental dysfunction and an evaluation of how severe daily functioning is impaired due to cognitive deficits. A detailed history, an adequate evaluation of cognitive functions, behavioural symptoms and ADL are the main diagnostic tools, whereas auxillary examinations are of less help in standard cases. Application of clinical diagnostic criteria for PD-D facilitates the diagnostic process. Although not necessary when dementia with typical features for PD-D develops in the context of established PD, differential diagnosis with regard to other causes of parkinsonism associated with dementia may be required in complex cases.

References

1 Emre M. Dementia associated with Parkinson's disease. Lancet Neurology 2003; 2: 229–37.

2 Dubois B, Burn D, Goetz C, *et al.* Diagnostic procedures for Parkinson's disease dementia: recommendations from the Movement Disorder Society task force. Mov Disord 2007; 22: 2314–24.

3 Nasreddine ZS, Phillips NA, Bedirian V, *et al.* The Montreal Cognitive Assessment, MoCA: a brief screening tool for mild cognitive impairment. J Am Geriatr Soc 2005; 53: 695–9.

4 Mioshi E, Dawson K, Mitchell J, Arnold R, Hodges J. The Addenbrooke's Cognitive Examination Revised (ACE-R): a brief cognitive test battery for dementia screening. Int J Geriatr Psychiatry 2006; 21: 1078–5.

5 Kalbe E, Calabrese P, Kohn N, *et al.* Screening for cognitive deficits in Parkinson's disease with the Parkinson neuropsychometric dementia assessment (PANDA) instrument. Parkinsonism Relat Disord 2008; 14: 93–101.

6 Mahieux F, Fénelon G, Flahault A, Manifacier MJ, Michelet D, Boller F. Neuropsychological prediction of dementia in Parkinson's disease. J Neurol Neurosurg Psychiatry 1998; 64: 178–83.

7 Dubois B, Slachevsky A, Litvan I, Pillon B. The FAB: a Frontal Assessment Battery at bedside. Neurology 2000; 55: 1621–6.

8 Rosen WG, Mohs RC, Davis KL. A new rating scale for Alzheimer's disease. Am J Psychiatry 1984; 141: 1356–64.

9 Mattis S. Dementia Rating Scale. Odessa, FL: Psychological Assessment Resources Inc., 1988.

10 Marinus J, Visser M, Verwey NA, *et al.* Assessment of cognition in Parkinson's disease. Neurology 2003; 61: 1222–8.

11 Pagonabarraga J, Kulisevsky J, Llebaria G, García-Sánchez C, Pascual-Sedano B, Gironell A. Parkinson's disease-cognitive rating scale: a new cognitive scale specific for Parkinson's disease. Mov Disord 2008; 23: 998–1005.

12 Cummings JL, Mega M, Gray K, Rosenberg-Thompson S, Carusi DA, Gornbein J. The Neuropsychiatric Inventory: comprehensive assessment of psychopathology in dementia. Neurology 1994; 44: 2308–14.

13 Galasko D, Bennett D, Sano M, *et al.* An inventory to assess activities of daily living for clinical trials in Alzheimer's disease. The Alzheimer's Disease Cooperative Study. Alzheimer Dis Assoc Disord 1997; 11(Suppl 2): S33–9.

14 Gélinas I, Gauthier L, McIntyre M, Gauthier S. Development of a functional measure for persons with Alzheimer's disease: the disability assessment for dementia. Am J Occup Ther 1999; 53: 471–81.

15 Burton EJ, McKeith IG, Burn DJ, O'Brien JT. Brain atrophy rates in Parkinson's disease with and without dementia using serial magnetic resonance imaging. Mov Disord 2005; 20: 1571–6.

16 Burton EJ, McKeith IG, Burn DJ, Williams ED, O'Brien JT. Cerebral atrophy in Parkinson's disease with and without dementia: a comparison with Alzheimer's disease, dementia with Lewy bodies amnd controls. Brain 2004; 127: 791–800.

17 Bissessur S, Tissingh G, Wolters EC, Scheltens P. rCBF SPECT in Parkinson's disease patients with mental dysfunction. J Neural Transm 1997; Suppl 50: 25–30.

18 Firbank MJ, Colloby SJ, Burn DJ, McKeith IG, O'Brien JT. Regional cerebral blood flow in Parkinson's disease with and without dementia. Neuroimage 2003; 20: 1309–19.

19 Peppard RF, Martin WR, Carr GD, *et al*. Cerebral glucose metabolism in Parkinson's disease with and without dementia. Arch Neurol 1992; 49: 1262–8.

20 Yong SW, Yoon JK, An YS, Lee PH. A comparison of cerebral glucose metabolism in Parkinson's disease, Parkinson's disease dementia and dementia with Lewy bodies. Eur J Neurol 2007; 14: 1357–62.

21 O'Brien JT, Colloby S, Fenwick J, *et al*. Dopamine transporter loss visualized with FP-CIT SPECT in the differential diagnosis of dementia with Lewy bodies. Arch Neurol 2004; 61: 919–25.

22 Yoshita M. Differentiation of idiopathic Parkinson's disease from striatonigral degeneration and progressive supranuclear palsy using iodine-123 meta-iodobenzylguanidine myocardial scintigraphy. J Neurol Sci 1998; 155: 60–7.

23 Yoshita M, Taki J, Yamada M. A clinical role for [(123)I]MIBG myocardial scintigraphy in the distinction between dementia of the Alzheimer's type and dementia with Lewy bodies. J Neurol Neurosurg Psychiatry 2001; 71: 583–8.

24 Edison P, Archer HA, Hinz R, *et al*. Amyloid, hypometabolism, and cognition in Alzheimer disease. An [11C]PIB and [18F]FDG PET study. Neurology 2007; 68: 501–8.

25 Rowe CC, Ng S, Ackermann U, *et al*. Imaging b-amyloid burden in aging and dementia. Neurology 2007; 68: 1718–25.

26 Edison P, Rowe CC, Rinne JO, *et al*. Amyloid load in Parkinson's disease dementia and Lewy body dementia measured with [11C]PIB-PET. J Neurol Neurosurg Psychiatry 2008, 24 Jul [Epub ahead of print].

27 Emre M, Aarsland D, Brown R, *et al*. Clinical diagnostic criteria for dementia associated with Parkinson's disease. Mov Disord 2007; 22: 1689–1707.

28 Lippa CF, Duda JE, Grossman M, *et al*. DLB and PDD boundary issues: diagnosis, teatment, molecular pathology and biomarkers. Neurology 2007; 68: 812–19.

29 Lippa CF, Emre M. Characterizing clinical phenotypes: the Lewys in their life or the life of their Lewys?. Neurology 2006; 67: 1910–11.

30 McKeith IG, Galasko D, Kosaka K, *et al*. Consensus guidelines for the clinical and pathologic diagnosis of dementia with Lewy bodies (DLB): report of the consortium on DLB international workshop. Neurology 1996; 47: 1113–24.

31 McKeith IG, Dickson DW, Lowe J, *et al*. Diagnosis and management of dementia with Lewy bodies: third report of the DLB Consortium. Neurology 2005; 65: 1863–72.

Chapter 19

Management of Parkinson's disease dementia and dementia with Lewy bodies

Ian McKeith and Murat Emre

Introduction

The management of the Lewy body dementias (PD-D and DLB) can be one of the most complex tasks facing neurologists, psychiatrists, geriatricians, primary care physicians or others caring for such patients [1]. On the one hand there lies the risk of provoking severe neuroleptic sensitivity reactions which can sometimes be fatal [2], on the other are the potentially gratifying beneficial effects of cholinesterase inhibitors (ChE-Is) [3]. Polypharmacy is the norm with multiple pharmacological treatment, targets including motor impairment, cognitive deficits, psychiatric symptoms and autonomic dysfunction. Non-pharmacological treatments similarly need to be directed towards a variety of symptom complexes. Depending on availability of resources it is apparent that the best delivery of care to a person with PD-D or DLB and his or her carers, will be devised and reviewed by a multidisciplinary team of experienced specialists and delivered, when possible, in the patient's home, minimizing the need for multiple hospital attendances. The general principles described below are applicable to most patients with a Lewy body-related dementia [4], the details of administration, dosing and response varying more on the individual person's symptom mix rather than any particular diagnostic label (PD-D or DLB) which they might carry [5].

Making and disclosing the diagnosis

Clinical diagnostic approach and criteria have been dealt with earlier in this volume. Suffice it to say that the new operationalized criteria [5,6] should assist clinicians to make more confident and reliable diagnoses than previously. Common problems which remain in diagnosing PD-D are deciding whether cognitive impairment is severe enough to warrant a dementia diagnosis [7] and the extent to which activities of daily living impairment is due to motor and autonomic impairment alone. The distinction between PD-D and DLB also causes difficulties for some, but for the purposes of clinical management this should not be regarded as particularly important – a diagnosis of Lewy body dementia or Lewy body disease with dementia should be adequate for most situations. The key is that the clinician is able to give a confident diagnostic label to the patient and family and follow this up with explanations to common questions, e.g. has the person with PD developed another disorder to explain the dementia, such as Alzheimer's disease (AD), or whether the onset of confusion and hallucinations are the side-effects of medication or a consequence of disease progression. For lay persons, who do not have a grounding in neuroanatomy and physiology, it can be difficult to understand how a single disorder can produce such widely variable symptoms as tremor, instability, constipation, hallucinations, sleep disturbance and cognitive impairment. Time spent at this early stage in explaining the diagnosis and mechanisms underlying symptoms, and checking out how well the patient and family understand what they have been told, is an essential part of forming the therapeutic alliance which will be required for the next stages of management. This is a particularly important step in developing non-pharmacological management strategies which need to address the manifestations of dementia in general plus the additional unique features of PD-D and DLB. The latter include fluctuating levels of cognitive and communicative ability which are particularly perplexing and stressful for carers [8]. Useful materials to aid in this process can be found on a variety of websites, produced by carer support organizations [9], specialist clinics [10], or by government bodies [11].

Making a problem list, managing antiparkinsonian medications and non-pharmacological approaches

Having negotiated a common framework and terminology for diagnosis and understanding, the next step is to produce a problem list, working systematically through the domains of motor, cognitive, neuropsychiatric, autonomic function and sleep. Having established this list, the next step is to ask the patient and carer to identify the symptoms that they find most disabling or distressing and which carry highest priority for treatment. There may be discrepant views about this which have to be resolved, e.g. a carer may complain that his/her sleep is being disrupted by the patient's nocturnal restlessness, whereas the patient is more preoccupied with motor slowness through the day. Patients with a long-established history of PD will usually be familiar with the concept of trading benefits of treatment in one domain against potential adverse events in another, e.g. dyskinesias, worsening of nightmares or emergence of hallucinations, as the cost of improved mobility with increased dopaminergic drug dose. What needs to be additionally stated is that some wearing- off of dopaminergic drug responsiveness may occur as a consequence of disease progression, at that same time as the emergence of side-effects starts to become disproportionate to dose elevation. In other words chasing maintenance of motor function by continuing to increase antiparkinsonian drugs may not only become less effective than in the earlier stages of PD, but the risk of precipitating or exacerbating cognitive and psychiatric symptoms in particular is increased. The therapeutic ratio of these agents begins therefore to fall and the potential for unwanted symptoms to persist becomes greater, even after the medication which clearly precipitated their onset is withdrawn. This phenomenon of confusional states and visual hallucinations following closely on the heels of changes in antiparkinsonian treatments is generally interpreted as the symptoms having been 'caused' by medications. The reality is, however, that dementia and related symptoms in PD typically occur because of diffuse spread of the disease process, cortical involvement in particular producing a vulnerable cerebral substrate. Substances which affect neurotransmitter systems can under such circumstances 'bring forward in time' symptoms which were destined to emerge eventually, independent of such treatment. There is unlikely ever to be a randomized controlled trial of this proposition, but there is substantial corroborating clinical experience and circumstantial evidence.

In addition to providing adequate information to the patient and the family about the disease, other non-pharmacological measures should be taken including sufficient mental and physical activation, avoidance of aggravating factors such as undue sensory stimuli and inappropriate environmental factors. Before initiating a pharmacological treatment, other conditions which can trigger or aggravate mental dysfunction should be excluded. These include systemic abnormalities and diseases, depression, adverse events of antiparkinson medication and treatment for concomitant diseases. Drugs which can cause mental dysfunction, such as anticholinergics, tricyclic antidepressants and benzodiazepines should be discontinued. Before reverting to medication the need for treatment, especially of behavioural symptoms, should be determined, based on symptom frequency, severity and burden. In principle, one drug should be introduced at a time with low doses and titrated up as needed. Non-specific treatment for behavioural symptoms should be tapered and discontinued, once sufficient symptom control is attained.

Specific treatments for cognitive impairment

Cholinesterase inhibitors

Evidence suggests that cholinergic deficit is a major biochemical substrate of cognitive dysfunction in PD-D and DLB [12]. Cholinesterase inhibitors (ChE-Is) inhibit the enzyme acetylcholinesterase, which breaks down acetylcholine in the synaptic cleft, terminating its postsynaptic effects. Through this inhibition the synaptic half-life of acetylcholine is prolonged and cholinergic transmission is enhanced. The first report with a ChE-I in PD-D was of a small, open-label study with tacrine, the first ChE-I which became available for clinical use [13], which suggested favourable effects on mental symptoms without worsening of motor functions. All available ChE-Is including donepezil, rivastigmine and galantamine have subsequently been tested in PD-D and DLB. Despite open-label designs and small sample sizes in most of these studies, a consistent pattern was seen with improvements in cognitive and behavioural symptoms [3]. Worsening of motor symptoms, usually a dose-related increase in tremor, was seen only in a few cases. These preliminary findings prompted the initiation of one large-scale, placebo-controlled randomized trial with rivastigmine in DLB, and two studies in PD-D, one with rivastigmine and the other with donepezil. The first [14] to be conducted assessed the effect of rivastigmine in DLB patients over a period of 20 weeks, followed by a 3-week withdrawal period. A total of 120 patients with a clinical diagnosis of probable DLB, and a Mini-Mental State Examination (MMSE) score between 10 and 23, were treated with up to 12 mg per day of rivastigmine (mean dose 7 mg/day) or placebo. A four-item subscore of the Neuropsychiatric Inventory

Table 19.1 Changes from baseline in the primary and secondary efficacy parameters in the EXPRESS study [14]

Scale	Rivastigmine	Placebo	P-value
Primary			
ADAS-COG	2.1	−0.7	<0.001
ADCS-CGIC	3.8	4.3	0.007
Secondary			
ADCS-ADL	−1.1	−3.6	0.02
NPI	2.0	0.0	0.02
CDR Power of attention	31.0	−142.7	0.009
MMSE	0.8	−0.2	0.03
Verbal fluency	1.7	−1.1	<0.001
Ten-point clock drawing test	0.5	−0.6	0.02

NPI, Neuropsychiatric Inventory; MMSE, Mini-Mental State Examination.

Positive values indicate improvements and negative values deteriorations.

(NPI), comprising delusions, hallucinations, apathy and depression, was used as the primary efficacy criterion [15]. Approximately twice as many patients on rivastigmine (63.4%) than on placebo (30.0%) showed at least a 30% improvement from baseline on their NPI-4 scores ($P = 0.001$), with psychotic features resolving almost completely in more than half of the treated patients. These symptoms re-emerged during a 3-week washout period. Statistically non-significant improvements were also seen at 20 weeks in MMSE score and Clinical Global Impression of Change (CGIC)-plus rating, in favour of the rivastigmine-treated group. Parkinsonian signs did not worsen on treatment, although emergent tremor was noted in four rivastigmine-treated patients. Predominant adverse effects were cholinergic in nature and the frequency of nausea (37%), vomiting (25%), anorexia (19%) and somnolence (9%) was significantly higher in the rivastigmine-treated patients. Most adverse events were rated as either mild or moderate, but seven of 59 patients receiving rivastigmine withdrew for this reason (not significantly different from the placebo group). Long-term follow-up of some of the study participants [16] found MMSE and NPI scores to be stable over the first 12 months of treatment, then to gradually worsen, although not significantly so, even 2 years after baseline. UPDRS motor scores tended to improve, probably because some antiparkinsonian treatment was initiated during this time.

In the EXPRESS study 541 patients with mild-to-moderate PD-D were assigned to rivastigmine or placebo over 24 weeks [17]. Rivastigmine was slowly titrated with monthly increments of 3 mg/day over the first 16 weeks up to 12 mg/day and then maintained at the highest tolerated dose for another 8 weeks; the mean dose at the end of the study was 8.6 mg/day. Primary efficacy parameters included the ADAS-COG for the assessment of cognitive functions and a CGIC scale for the assessment of overall changes from baseline. Both primary endpoints showed statistically significant improvements on rivastigmine treatment compared with placebo. Patients on rivastigmine showed a 2.1 improvement in ADAS-COG at week 24, whereas patients on placebo deteriorated by 0.7 points ($P < 0.001$). The mean score for the CGIC at week 24 was 3.8 in the rivastigmine and 4.3 in the placebo group (score 4 indicating no change, lower scores indicating improvement and higher scores indicating worsening from baseline). More patients on rivastigmine showed any degree of improvement (40.8% vs 29.7% on placebo) and more patients on placebo had any degree of deterioration (42.5% on placebo vs 33.7% on rivastigmine) ($P = 0.007$). Similarly, all secondary efficacy measures revealed statistically significant differences in favour of rivastigmine including neuropsychiatric symptoms (NPI), the clock-drawing test, verbal fluency, computer-based attention tests and MMSE score (Table 19.1). Activity of daily living scores showed a minimal worsening from baseline in patients on rivastigmine, whereas those on placebo did worsen significantly more. Adverse events were significantly more frequent with rivastigmine, mainly nausea (29.0% vs 11.2%) and vomiting (16.6.% vs 1.7%) on rivastigmine and placebo, respectively. Worsening of parkinsonian symptoms was more frequently reported on rivastigmine (27.3% vs 15.6 % on placebo), this was principally driven by worsening of tremor (10.2% vs 3.9%). UPDRS motor scores did not, however, reveal any significant differences between the groups.

In order to assess the long-term effects of rivastigmine, the EXPRESS study had a further 6-month extension during which all patients received active treatment [18]. The results demonstrated that the beneficial effects seen during the first 6 months were largely maintained, although treatment effects started to decline. Patients who initially received placebo and then switched to rivastigmine showed similar benefits to those who had been on rivastigmine for the whole duration of the study, but not in all parameters, suggesting potential benefits of starting treatment earlier. Importantly, there was no evidence of worsening motor function over the course of 1 year of treatment [19].

The second large randomized, double-blind, placebo-controlled study in PD-D used donepezil [20] in which 550 patients with mild-to-moderate PD-D were randomized into three groups to receive either placebo, donepezil 5 mg or donepezil 10 mg for 24 weeks. The primary efficacy parameters were ADAS-COG and a global measure of change from baseline (CIBIC-plus). At week 24, there was a 0.3-point improvement in ADAS-COG on placebo, 2.45-point improvement on 5 mg and 3.72-point improvement on 10 mg. These differences did not reach statistical significance in the primary analysis because of a country interaction, but did so when this was controlled for ($P < 0.001$). The CIBIC-plus showed statistically significant superiority for 10 mg, but not for 5 mg. Statistically significant differences in favor of donepezil were also found on some secondary measures including MMSE, Brief Test of Attention and Verbal Fluency Test, whereas there were no statistically significant differences from placebo on the activities of daily living scale Disability Assessment in Dementia and the behavioural scale NPI. UPDRS motor scores did not reveal any significant worsening of motor functions on donepezil.

Using CHE-Is in practice: predictors of outcome, side-effects and discontinuation

Visual hallucinations are known from postmortem studies to be associated with more severe cholinergic deficits in the Lewy body dementias [21], and patients with hallucinations might therefore be expected to benefit more from cholinergic enhancement. This was demonstrated to be the case in both the DLB [22] and the PD-D study with rivastigmine [23]. The presence of visual hallucinations in Lewy body disease is also associated with a greater degree of impairment in attentional performance and a faster rate of cognitive decline, the common factor probably being greater cholinergic deficit, presumably mediated in part by activity of the enzyme butyryl-cholinesterase [24] which may increase in functional importance as acetylcholinesterase levels diminish. Other clinical indicators suggestive of central cholinergic failure and therefore potentially predictive of a good ChE-I response include apathy and daytime drowsiness. In practice the majority of PD-D and DLB patients will have such symptoms, visual hallucinations, or both. Given the lack of any demonstrable alternatives, a trial of a ChE-I seems to be the preferred action for any PD-D or DLB patient with significant cognitive impairments.

The side-effect profile of ChE-Is in Lewy body dementias is broadly similar to that reported in the larger AD population, but there are additional effects to be considered which probably reflect the pre-existing impact of the disease on cholinergic autonomic activity. The drugs are generally well-tolerated at doses in the usual AD range with dropout rates reported from 10% to 31%. In addition to the well-recognized gastrointestinal side-effects, troublesome hypersalivation, rhinorrhoea and lacrimation occurred in about 15% of DLB and PD-D patients treated with donepezil, and postural hypotension, falls and syncope in up to 10%. The same open-label study found no difference in treatment responsiveness or side-effect profile when PD-D and DLB patients were compared [25]. Worsening parkinsonism occurred in 9% of patients on 10 mg of donepezil, but rarely was this clinically significant and it could usually be improved by dose reduction. Abrupt withdrawal of ChE-I is associated with rapid return of neuropsychiatric symptoms and cognitive decline in DLB and PD-D [26]. Although reinstatement of treatment may reverse such deterioration, it is recommended that patients with Lewy body-related dementias who are assessed as responding to ChE-I are maintained on treatment long term. Since attempts at switching from one ChE-I to another may be associated with clinically significant withdrawal effects [27], this treatment strategy should be considered carefully and patients who are switched should be closely monitored. A preliminary comparison of datasets from treatment studies in DLB using different ChE-Is suggests that there are no major differences between the available agents [28].

Rivastigmine has a marketing approval for treatment of patients with mild-to-moderate PD-D, both in the EU and the USA. Licensing approval has not been sought for any of the other CHE-Is in PD-D, nor for the use of any of them in DLB. Much prescribing is therefore 'off label', creating difficulties for those drafting good practice guidelines and dealing with reimbursement issues. Given the scale of the clinical problem and the lack of safe alternatives, this is an unsatisfactory situation and there is a good case for investment in more clinical trials, particularly those measuring longer-term outcomes, cost-effectiveness and practical aspects of drug administration.

NMDA antagonists and dopaminergic drugs

The N-methyl-D-aspartate (NMDA) antagonist memantine is approved for the treatment of moderate to severe AD. Conflicting results had been described in few case reports or case series in patients with DLB, reporting both worsening or improvement in equal measure [29,30]. In a small case series, good tolerability and possible benefits had been suggested in patients with PD-D [31]. Recently, three double-blind, randomized control-led studies comparing memantine with placebo have been reported. The first, a study of 22 weeks duration, included 25 patients with PD-D [32]. At the end of the study there were no significant differences between the two groups on any efficacy parameters, how-ever, 6 weeks after withdrawal more patients who had been treated with memantine deteriorated on a global scale ($p=0.04$), suggested that they had had some beneficial effects while being treated. The second study lasted 24 weeks and included 72 patients with either PD-D or DLB of mild to moderate severity [33]. The primary endpoint, the global change score CGIC was significantly in favour of memantine ($p=0.03$), the effect was stronger in the PD-D group. Except for the improved speed in an attentional task in the memantine group, there were no other significant differences in secondary outcome measures between the two groups.

A larger randomized, double blind, placebo controlled, 24 weeks trial in 199 patients with mild to moderate PD-D or DLB has just been completed. In the total population the CGIC analysis revealed that the mean CGIC score was lower (better) and there were more patients with an improvement or remaining stable under memantine treatment, and more patients on placebo deteriorated. The difference was not statistically significant in the total population and in the PD-D group. In the DLB group, however, it reached sta-tistical significance. Likewise in the DLB group, patients treated with memantine showed significant improvement in NPI total score at 24 weeks, compared to patients treated with placebo. There were no consistent effects of memantine on cognitive tests in either the PD-D or DLB groups [34].

The effects of dopaminergic treatment on mental functions have barely been studied in patients with PD-D, most formal studies having been performed in non-demented patients. The results have been equivocal, describing either no effects, or improvement in some and worsening in other functions. In one of the few studies which specifically included demented patients, subjects with PD, PD-D or DLB were tested for cogni-tive functions and behavioural symptoms after acute levodopa challenge and following 3 months of treatment. After acute challenge, patients reported improvement in subjective alertness, but fluctuations increased; reaction time and accuracy remained unchanged in those with PD-D. After 3 months of treatment neuropsychiatric scores improved both in PD and PD-D, mean global cognitive score was better, but attention and memory scores were worse in PD patients without dementia. Reaction time became slower in those with PD-D, but there were no patients with marked deterioration [35].

Drug treatment of psychiatric and behavioural symptoms

In common with other types of dementia, it is the psychiatric and behavioural symptoms which cause greatest distress to patients and carers, and which eventually lead to requests for treatment and institutional care [36]. In Lewy body dementias such symptoms are frequent and contribute to greater impairment in quality of life and costs of care than AD patients with equivalent cognitive impairments [37,38]. In addition to the cognitive effects of ChE-Is described above, the same agents have also been reported to improve a range of neuropsychiatric symptoms in PD-D and DLB, particularly apathy, visual hallucinations, anxiety, sleep disturbance and delusions [3]. It is probable that these behavioural effects are largely mediated via improvements in attention and cognitive processing. Since cognitive and neuropsychiatric symptoms often go hand in hand, the choice of a ChE-I as first-line drug treatment is often directed at both domains.

Agitation and related behaviours are less likely to improve with ChE-Is and may even be aggravated as the patient becomes more activated. The mainstay of treatment for agitation, aggression and psychotic symptoms in dementia has generally been with D2 receptor antagonists, but these drugs, particularly traditional neuroleptic agents, can provoke severe neuroleptic sensitivity reactions in up to 50% of DLB patients and 25% of PD-D with a 2–3-fold increased mortality [2,39–41], therefore they are contraindicated in this patient population. These reactions are generally acute or subacute, becoming evident within the first few doses or after increase from a previously tolerated dose. When acute deterioration occurs in a confused elderly patient following neuroleptic administration, Lewy body disease should always be considered as part of the differential diagnosis. Following initial positive case reports of the use of newer atypical antipsychotics in DLB, further case studies indicate that neuroleptic sensitivity does occur both with risperidone and olanzapine, especially as the dose is increased [42,43]. Quetiapine did not appear to significantly worsen motor symptoms in a recent, small placebo-controlled trial of 36 patients with DLB [44], but was not associated with significant improvement in psychiatric or cognitive outcome measures. Clozapine may also be useful in treating PD psychosis, but its antimuscarinic properties may increase confusion in patients with dementia [45]. The frequent occurrence of electroencephalogram abnormalities with transient temporal slow waves has prompted the use of carbamazepine and sodium valproate as agents to treat behavioural disturbance, but no systematic reports of efficacy or side-effects are available. The 5HT3 antagonist ondansetron was reported as having antipsychotic effects in hallucinated PD patients, but this has not been independently replicated and the high doses required make the cost prohibitive for routine practice [46]. There is a recent report of the Kampo medicine Yoku-kan-san being effective in treating ChE-I-resistant visual hallucinations and neuropsychiatric symptoms in patients with DLB, and being well-tolerated [47].

Although disorders of affect and depressive features are among the most frequent behavioural symptoms in PD and PD-D, surprisingly there have been no randomized, controlled studies of antidepressants in these populations. A meta-analysis of all studies in PD patients with depression revealed large effect sizes, both under active and placebo. There were, however, no statistically significant differences between them; increasing age and major depression predicted better response [48]. In another systematic review, amitriptyline was reported to be the only compound with evidence of efficacy in PD depression [49]. Amitriptyline, however, is a tricyclic antidepressant which should be avoided in patients with PD-D because of their anticholinergic effects and their potential to worsen cognition. Although evidence from controlled trials is lacking, serotonin-selective reuptake inhibitors (SSRIs) or SNRIs may be preferred. Elevated serotonin 1A receptor density has been reported in temporal cortex of PD-D and DLB patients with a history of depression, suggesting that a serotonin 1A receptor antagonist adjuvant may improve treatment of depression in this group [50].

Disturbances of sleep–wake cycle including excessive daytime sleepiness and rapid-eye-movement (REM) sleep behaviour disorder (RBD) frequently occur in patients with PD-D or DLB [51]. Disturbed sleep with thrashing limb movements, vocalizations and vivid dreams may precede Lewy body disease as an early manifestation, and may persist, sometimes in attenuated form. Treatment of RBD lacks a double-blind, placebo-controlled, evidence base. Clonazepam has been reported as effective and well-tolerated [52] in suppressing the motor features, but does not restore REM-sleep atonia [53]. Melatonin has also proven beneficial, with control of symptoms or significant improvement being noted in 10 of 14 patients who had failed to respond to clonazepam or were unable to tolerate therapeutic doses [54]. Further work is needed to investigate the precise role of these agents in addition to the possible benefits of ChE-Is as treatments for RBD. Excessive daytime sleepiness is also a frequent problem. Although not specifically tested in demented PD patients, modafinil, an agent that promotes wakefulness, might be considered to treat excessive daytime sleepiness. In studies performed in non-demented PD patients, modafinil was found to be significantly better than placebo in two small randomized, placebo-controlled and one open-label study [55–57]; no difference was found in another small, placebo-controlled trial [58]. The drug was well-tolerated in all.

Disease-modifying agents

There are so far no disease-modifying agents available to treat Lewy body disease, and until our understanding of the basic neurobiology of neuronal degeneration improves it is premature to expect their development on a rational basis. Amyloidogenic fibrils of α-synuclein can be instantaneously disintegrated *in vitro* by the antimicrobial agent dequalinium [59], but it is not yet clear whether such disaggregation would be a viable therapeutic strategy. It is also not certain whether early intervention with ChE-Is confers advantage compared with later administration. There is a report that active immunisation of a DLB patient with the amyloid vaccine AN-1792 [60] produced cognitive and behavioural stabilization, associated with a significant clearance of amyloid deposits in the brain at autopsy, with tau and synuclein pathological features remaining. This suggests that trials of successful disease-modifying treatments for AD could also be extended to the Lewy body dementias.

Conclusions

Management of patients with Lewy body-related dementias involves both pharmacological and non-pharmacological measures. The management plan should be developed considering the whole symptom complex and their impact on the family and the patient. Patients with PD-D or DLB should be offered treatment with a ChE-I taking into account expected benefits and potential risks. Some behavioural symptoms such as visual hallucinations may benefit from ChE-I, but treatment with antipsychotics may become necessary in some patients. In such instances classical neuroleptics, as well as risperidone and olanzapine, should be avoided. Quetiapine might be considered, however the strongest evidence for efficacy exists for clozapine. Although evidence from randomized controlled studies is lacking, SSRIs or SNRIs should be given priority to treat depressive features. Clonazepam or melatonin can be tried to treat RBD, and modafinil for the treatment of excessive daytime sleepiness.

References

1 McKeith IG, Galasko D, Wilcock GK, Byrne EJ. Lewy body dementia – diagnosis and treatment. Br J Psychiatry 1995; 167: 709–17.

2 McKeith I, Fairbairn A, Perry R, Thompson P, Perry E. Neuroleptic sensitivity in patients with senile dementia of Lewy body type. Br Med J 1992; 305: 673–8.

3 Aarsland D, Mosimann UP, McKeith IG. Role of cholinesterase inhibitors in Parkinson's disease and dementia with Lewy bodies. J Geriatr Psychiatry Neurol 2004; 17: 164–71.

4 Barber R, Newby J, McKeith IG. Lewy body disease. In: Richter RW, Zoeller Richter B (eds). Current clinical neurology. Alzheimer's disease: a physician's guide to practical management. Totowa, NJ: Humana Press, 2003: pp. 127–35.

5 McKeith I, Dickson D, Emre M, et al. Dementia with Lewy Bodies: Diagnosis and Management: Third Report of the DLB Consortium. Neurology 2005; 65: 1863–72.

6 Emre M, Aarsland D, Brown R, et al. Clinical diagnostic criteria for dementia associated with Parkinson disease. Mov Disord 2007; 22: 1689–1707.

7 Dubois B, Feldman HH, Jacova C, et al. Research criteria for the diagnosis of Alzheimer's disease: revising the NINCDS-ADRDA criteria. Lancet Neurol 2007; 6: 734–46.

8 Cohen-Mansfield J. Non-pharmacological management of DLB. London: Dunitz, 2005.

9 http://www.lbda.org/; http://www.lewybody.org/

10 http://www.mayoclinic.com/health/lewy-body-dementia/DS00795

11 http://www.ninds.nih.gov/disorders/dementiawithlewybodies/dementiawithlewybodies.htm

12 Tiroboschi P, Hansen LA, Alford M, et al. Cholinergic dysfunction in diseases with Lewy bodies. Neurology. 2000; 54: 407–11.

13 Hutchinson M, Fazzini E. Cholinesterase inhibitors in Parkinson's disease. J Neurol Neurosurg Psychiatry 1996; 61: 324–5.

14 McKeith I, Del Ser T, Spano PF, et al. Efficacy of rivastigmine in dementia with Lewy bodies: a randomised, double-blind, placebo-controlled intertaional study. Lancet 2000; 356: 2031–6.

15 Del-Ser T, McKeith I, Anand R, Cicin-Sain A, Ferrara R, Spiegel R. Dementia with Lewy bodies: findings from an international multicentre study. Int J Geriatr Psychiatry 2000; 15: 1034–45.

16 Grace J, Daniel S, Stevens T, et al. Long-term use of rivastigmine in patients with dementia with Lewy bodies: an open-label trial. Int Psychogeriatr 2001; 13: 199–205.

17 Emre M, Aarsland D, Albanese A, et al. Rivastignine for dementia associated with Parkinson's disease. N Engl J Med 2004; 351: 2509–18.

18 Poewe W, Wolters E, Emre M, et al. Long-term benefits of rivastigmine in dementia associated with Parkinson's disease: an active treatment extension study. Mov Disord 2006; 21: 456–61.

19 Oertel W, Poewe W, Wolters E, et al. Effects of rivastigmine on tremor and other motor symptoms in patients with Parkinson's disease dementia – a retrospective analysis of a double-blind trial and an open-label extension. Drug Safety 2008; 31: 79–94.

20 Dubois B, Kulisevsky J, Reichman H, et al. Efficacy and safety of donepezil in the treatment of Parkinson's disease patients with dementia. Neurodegen Dis 2008; 5.

21 Perry EK, McKeith I, Thompson P, *et al.* Topography, extent, and clinical relevance of neurochemical deficits in dementia of Lewy body type, Parkinson's disease and Alzheimer's disease. Ann NY Acad Sci 1991; 640: 197–202.

22 Wesnes KA, McKeith IG, Ferrara R, *et al.* Effects of rivastigmine on cognitive function in dementia with Lewy bodies: a randomised placebo-controlled international study using the Cognitive Drug Research computerised assessment system. Dementia Geriatr Cogn Dis 2002; 13: 183–92.

23 Wesnes KA, McKeith I, Edgar C, Emre M, Lane R. Benefits of rivastigmine on attention in dementia associated with Parkinson disease. Neurology 2005; 65: 1654–6.

24 O'Brien KK, Saxby BK, Ballard CG, *et al.* Regulation of attention and response to therapy in dementia by butyrylcholinesterase. Pharmacogenetics 2003; 13: 231–9.

25 Thomas AJ, Burn DJ, Rowan EN, *et al.* A comparison of the efficacy of donepezil in Parkinson's disease with dementia and dementia with Lewy bodies. Int J Geriatr Psychiatry 2005; 20: 938–44.

26 Minett TSC, Thomas A, Wilkinson LM, *et al.* What happens when donepezil is suddenly withdrawn? An open label trial in dementia with Lewy bodies and Parkinson's disease with dementia. Int J Geriatr Psychiatry 2003; 18: 988–93.

27 Bhanji NH, Gauthier S. Dementia with Lewy bodies: preliminary observations on cholinesterase inhibitor switching. Int Psychogeriatrics 2003; 15: 179.

28 Bhasin M, Rowan E, Edwards K, McKeith I. Cholinesterase inhibitors in dementia with Lewy bodies – a comparative analysis. Int J Geriatr Psychiatry 2007 Jan 30.

29 Ridha BH, Josephs KA, Rossor MN. Delusions and hallucinations in dementia with Lewy bodies: worsening with memantine. Neurology 2005; 65: 481–2.

30 Sabbagh M, Hake A, Ahmed S, Farlow M. The use of memantine in dementia with Lewy bodies. J Alzh Dis 2005; 7: 285–9.

31 Fox C, Umoh G SM, Barbara B, Nil M. Memantine in Parkinson's disease dementia: clinical experience. Mov Disord 2005; 20(Suppl 10): 418.

32 Leroi I, Overshott R, Byrne EJ, Daniel E Burns A. Randomized, controlled trial of memantine in dementia associated with Parkinson's disease. Mov Disord 2009; 24: 1217–21.

33 Aarsland D, Ballard C, Walker Z, *et al.* Memantine in patients with Parkinson's disease dementia or dementia with Lewy bodies: a double-blind, placebo controlled, multicentre trial. Lancet Neurology 2009; 8: 613–8.

34 Emre M and the 11018 Study Investigators. A randomised, double-blind, placebo-controlled, 6-month study of the efficacy and safety of memantine in patients with Parkinson's Disease Dementia (PDD) or Dementia with Lewy Bodies (DLB). Poster No:2009, presented at the 13th Congress of the EFNS, Sept. 12–15, 2009. Florence, Italy.

35 Molloy S, McKeith I, O'Brien JT, Burn D. The role of levodopa in the management of dementia with Lewy bodies. J Neurol Neurosurg Psychiatry 2005; 76: 1200–3.

36 Aarsland D, Larsen JP, Karlsen K, Lim NG, Tandberg E. Mental symptoms in Parkinson's disease are important contributors to caregiver stress. Int J Geriatr Psychiatry 1999; 14: 866–74.

37 Bostrom F, Jonsson L, Minthon L, Londos E. Patients with dementia with Lewy bodies have more impaired quality of life than patients with Alzheimer disease. Alzh Dis Associated Dis 2007; 21: 150–4.

38 Bostrom F, Jonsson L, Minthon L, Londos E. Patients with Lewy body dementia use more resources than those with Alzheimer's disease. Int J Geriatr Psychiatry 2007; 22: 713–9.

39 McKeith I. Why clinical trial design is so important in elderly patients with dementia. Clin Adv Drug Dev 1998; 1: 1–2.

40 Grace J, Ballard C, McKeith IG. Neuroleptic sensitivity in dementia with Lewy bodies (DLB) and Alzheimer's disease (AD). Fifths International Geneva/Springfield Symposium on Advances in Alzheimer Therapy, 1998; p. 144.

41 Aarsland D, Ballard C, Larsen JP, McKeith I, O'Brien J, Perry R. Marked neuroleptic sensitivity in dementia with Lewy bodies and Parkinson's disease. J Clin Psychiatry 2005; 66: 633–7.

42 McKeith IG, Ballard CG, Harrison RWS. Neuroleptic sensitivity to risperidone in Lewy body dementia. Lancet 1995; 346: 699.

43 Walker Z, Grace J, Overshot R, et al. Olanzapine in dementia with Lewy bodies: a clinical study. Int J Geriatr Psychiatry 1999; 14: 459–66.

44 Kurlan R, Cummings J, Raman R, Thal L. Quetiapine for agitation or psychosis in patients with dementia and parkinsonism. Neurology 2007; 68: 1356–63.

45 Burke WJ, Pfeiffer RF, McComb RD. Neuroleptic sensitivity to clozapine in dementia with Lewy bodies. J Neuropsychiatry Clin Neurosci 1998; 10: 227–9.

46 Harrison RH, McKeith IG. Senile dementia of Lewy body type – a review of clinical and pathological features: implications for treatment. Int J Geriatr Psychiatry 1995; 10: 919–26.

47 Iwasaki K, Maruyama M, Tomita N, et al. Effects of the traditional Chinese herbal medicine Yi-Gan San for cholinesterase inhibitor-resistant visual hallucinations and neuropsychiatric symptoms in patients with dementia with Lewy bodies. J Clin Psychiatry 2005; 66: 1612–3.

48 Weintraub D, Morales KH, Moberg PJ, Bilker WB, Balderston C, Duda JE, et al. Antidepressant studies in Parkinson's disease: A review and meta-analysis. Mov Disord 2005; 20: 1161–9.

49 Miyasaki JM, Shannon K, Voon V, et al. Practice Parameter: Evaluation and treatment of depression, psychosis, and dementia in Parkinson disease (an evidence-based review) Report of the Quality Standards Subcommittee of the American Academy of Neurology. Neurology 2006; 66: 996–1002.

50 Sharp SI, Ballard CG, Ziabreva I, et al. Cortical serotonin 1a receptor levels are associated with depression in patients with dementia with Lewy bodies and Parkinson's disease dementia. Dementia Geriatr Cogn Disord 2008; 26: 330–8.

51 Boeve B, Silber M, Ferman T, Lucas J, Parisi J. Association of REM sleep behavior disorder and neuro-degenerative disease may reflect an underlying synucleinopathy. Mov Disord 2001; 16: 622–30.

52 Olson EJ, Boeve BF, Silber MH. Rapid eye movement sleep behaviour disorder: demographic, clinical and laboratory findings in 93 cases. Brain 2000; 123: 331–9.

53 Lapierre O, Montplaisir J. Polysomnographic features of REM-sleep behavior disorder – development of a scoring method. Neurology 1992; 42: 1371–4.

54 Boeve BF, Silber MH, Ferman TJ. Melatonin for treatment of REM sleep behavior disorder in neurologic disorders: results in 14 patients. Sleep Med 2003; 4: 281–4.

55 Adler CH, Caviness JN, Hentz JG, Lind M, Tiede J. Randomized trial of modafinil for treating subjective daytime sleepiness in patients with Parkinson's disease. Mov Disord 2003; 18: 287–93.

56 Hogl B, Saletu M, Brandauer E, et al. Modafinil for the treatment of daytime sleepiness in Parkinson's disease: a double-blind, randomized, crossover, placebo-controlled polygraphic trial. Sleep 2002; 25: 905–9.

57 Nieves AV, Lang AE. Treatment of excessive daytime sleepiness in patients with Parkinson's disease with modafinil. Clin Neuropharmacol 2002; 25: 111–4.

58 Ondo WG, Fayle R, Atassi F, Jankovic J. Modafinil for daytime somnolence in Parkinson's disease: double blind, placebo controlled parallel trial. J Neurol Neurosurg Psychiatry 2005; 76: 1636–9.

59 Park JW, Lee IH, Hahn JS, Kim J, Chung KC, Paik SR. Disintegration of amyloid fibrils of alpha-synuclein by dequalinium. Biochim Biophys Acta 2008; 1780: 1156–61.

60 Bombois S, Maurage CA, Gompel M, et al. Absence of beta-amyloid deposits after immunization in Alzheimer disease with Lewy body dementia. Arch Neurol 2007; 64: 583–7.

Chapter 20

Parkinson's disease: what will the future bring?

John Hardy

Introduction

Predicting the future is notoriously a way to ensure that you appear dimwitted in 20 years' time. However, we are almost exactly 50 years since the discovery of the effects of levodopa in reserpinized (dopamine-depleted) animals and 45 years since the first human levodopa treatment trials [1]. Hence, it is perhaps worth taking stock of progress and thinking about how things might progress from here.

Since the miracle of dopamine replacement therapy, there has been incremental improvement in pharmacological treatment of Parkinson's disease (PD) with first peripheral decarboxylase inhibition and then dopamine agonists [2]. Surgical therapies, too, had initially startling clinical effects, and have subsequently had incremental improvements [3]. Neither current medical nor surgical interventions are believed to have any effects on the progression of neurodegenerative process. In early disease, initial therapy leads to remarkable benefits. Indeed, dopaminergic therapy has more than doubled the life expectancy of patients after their diagnosis [4].

Despite this, I am sure that to patients and caregivers, the current situation leads to great frustration. In nearly all other neurodegenerative diseases, patients get the diagnosis: Alzheimer's disease (AD), motor neuron disease or Huntington's disease, and are told, at diagnosis, that there is no effective treatment to hold disease progression. While this is a cruel outcome, there is no arguing with it. Currently, there are no effective treatments for these diseases and the patients and their families cope with that outcome as best they can. With PD, early treatment really is miraculous and, for a period of a few years, it allows patients and their families to return to a near-normal life. Yet this treatment gradually and frustratingly slips away and the disease gains the upper hand, finally leading to disability and death in a manner no less unpleasant than that caused by the less-teasing diseases which have no treatment at all. It must seem to patients and caregivers that we are close to 'curing' the disease, and yet, of course, we are not.

Since it seems likely that there are only going to be incremental improvements to be made through either further advances in dopaminergic drugs or through surgical treatment, clearly we need to make substantive progress towards either avoiding the disease or in mechanistic therapy. It is in this area that we have to hope we can make progress.

Progress towards understanding disease mechanisms

Over the past 10 years we have made enormous advances in understanding some of the genetic causes of PD (Table 20.1 [5]). A large number of genes have been discovered which, when mutated, lead either to clinically defined Parkinson's disease or to Lewy body disease. Together, mutations in these genes explain a small but significant proportion of the risk of getting PD. This proportion is perhaps 5% in general European populations, but as much as 30% in the Ashkenazi Jews or North African Berber population [6,7].

The general belief is that these genes should map out one or more pathways to disease. This belief is really based on an analogy with AD where the three autosomal dominant genes map onto a pathway of APP metabolism ([8]: see below).

Table 20.1 Parkinsonism and Lewy body disease loci (adapted from Hardy *et al.* [5])

Locus (OMIM)	Gene	Mode of inheritance	Pathology	Comments
PARK1/4 (168601)	α-*synuclein*	Dominant	Lewy bodies	Point mutations and gene duplications
PARK2 (600116)	*parkin*	Recessive	Usually no Lewy bodies	Loss of function variants:
PARK6 (605909)	*PINK1*	Recessive	Not known	Loss of function variants
PARK7 (606324)	*DJ1*	Recessive	Not known	Loss of function variants
PARK8 (607060)	*LRRK2*	Dominant	Usually, but not always Lewy bodies	Variable pathology is a real puzzle
PARK9 (610513)	*ATP13A2*	Recessive	Not known	
Parkinson–pyramidal syndrome	*FBXO7*	Recessive	Not known	
Gaucher's disease	*GBA*	Recessive for Gaucher's, risk locus (OR ~5) for PD	Lewy bodies	PD has Lewy bodies, Gaucher's disease cases also have Lewy bodies
NBIA1 (234200)	*PANK2*	Recessive	Lewy bodies: often brain iron	Variable phenotype: later-onset cases have a dopa-responsive parkinsonian dystonia
INAD1/NBIA2 (256600)	*PLA2G6*	Recessive	Lewy bodies: often brain iron	Identical to above: parkinsonian disorder
Neimann Pick C type 1 (607623)	*NPC1*	Recessive	Lewy bodies and tangles	Neuropathology includes both Lewy bodies and tangles
MAPT (260540)	*MAPT*	Autosomal dominant and complex	Tangles, but contributes to risk of Lewy body disease	Autosomal dominant disease has tangle-like inclusions: haplotype predisposes to PSP and Lewy body PD

PD, Parkinson's disease; PSP, progressive supranuclear palsy.

With 12 genes, it seems remarkable that currently we have no direct biochemical evidence linking any two of them in a pathway to disease, and the question at the moment is to decide whether we are looking at one, two or many pathways to cell death. The best evidence relating to at least one pathway to disease is with *PINK1* and *parkin* [9,10]. It is clear, from work in drosophila, that these two genes are involved in a mitochondrial pathway to disease and that *parkin* is downstream in this pathway. However, *parkin* cases do not have Lewy bodies and we have argued that we should use a pathological, rather than a clinical, definition of disease [5]. On this basis, I would contend that, whereas this work clearly sketched a pathway to parkinsonism, this is unlikely to be the pathway which is operating in that vast majority of cases with disease who have Lewy body pathology [11].

Defining the disease pathologically leads to a different list of genes which we have hypothesized may map onto ceramide metabolism [12], though this remains unproven. Perhaps most importantly, the three genes everyone would agree are important to PD pathogenesis, α-*synuclein*, *LRRK2* and *glucosecerebrosidase*, have not been biochemically linked to each other, which would have allowed an 'amyloid hypothesis' for PD to be developed. This is currently an area of rapid progress and I think it is a fairly safe prediction to suggest that we will know whether there is a link between the *PINK1–parkin/–*mitochondrial pathway and Lewy body disease within the next 5 years, and we should, in the same time frame, be able to sketch a pathway that involves α-*synuclein*, *LRRK2* and *glucosecerebrosidase* and possibly some of the other pathogenic loci. Optimistically, we may then be able to postulate a simple and encompassing hypothesis for disease which will allow a research focus to develop and encourage drug companies to see targets within that framework.

From mechanism to treatment

Let us suppose that by 2015, we have developed a reasonably clear understanding of the biochemical pathways which appear to be dysregulated in typical PD with Lewy bodies: then, our task will be to try to interfere in this pathway and to design clinical trials to test these potential therapies. At that stage, we will want to design small molecules to intervene in these pathways and to start to think about designing clinical trials to slow disease progression. Both of these are formidable tasks. Lining up AD research against PD research (Table 20.2) really shows the magnitude of this task. Mechanistic PD research started 13 years later than mechanistic AD research and we are, optimistically, still 5 years away from the first mechanistic therapies for AD.

Our current problems are clearly both practical: we have no good animal model of the disease yet; and philosophical: there is no generally agreed pathway to disease. Furthermore, we should not forget that AD research has not yet led to disease-modifying treatments, and currently the AD field is worrying about the fact that trials of mechanistic therapies will need to be long and will, therefore, be extremely expensive to run. Additionally therapies need to be tested in individuals who are very early in the disease, possibly even completely asymptomatic. I think, therefore, we are at a rather distressing paradox. It would seem likely that we are more than a decade away from mechanistic therapies. From a practical

Table 20.2 Progress and problems on the road to Alzheimer disease (AD) therapies: comparison with Parkinson's disease (PD) (adapted from Hardy [8])

Year	Progress	Comment	Lesson
1984	Aβ identified	α-Synuclein identified in 1997	PD started 13 years behind
1991	APP mutations identified	α-Synuclein mutations identified in 1993	
1992	Amyloid hypothesis	As yet no PD equivalent	
1995	Presenilin genes discovered	Many other PD genes discovered	Note that AD was defined by pathology
1995	Animal model with some pathology made	AD model was incomplete, but it did at least have plaques	As yet no generally accepted pathological model of PD has been developed
1998	Presenilins shown to be involved in APP metabolism as γ-secretase		No connection between any two parkinsonism genes has yet been found
1998	Delineation of other elements of APP metabolism such as BACE as other targets for intervention		No parkinsonism equivalent as yet
1998	MAPT mutations found in FTD	Led to mice with other pathological elements being developed and eventually to heavily engineered mice with full pathology	
1999	Aβ immunization works in mice	Probably an accidental finding, but depended on having mice with pathology	
2003	First active human vaccination trial halted because of immunogenic side-effects		
2008	Ambivalent phase 2 results reported on passive Aβ antibody trial. Phase 3 trials of this and other agents begin		
2009	Planning stages of next-generation compounds. Drug companies start to plan other approaches such as anti-tau therapies using mice with tangles	The following are the present concerns: Are the AD trials beginning early enough in the disease? Does the amyloid hypothesis relate only to the autosomal dominant form of the disease? How long should a trial be to show disease modification?	We need to be ready with cohorts of high risk, genetically defined individuals so that we can organize trials in defined and characterized individuals
2012	Planned reporting of passive immunization trial: phase 3 trials at least 3 years behind this	28 years from amyloid identification	

perspective this means that we have nothing to offer anyone who currently has the disease except the hope that future generations will not suffer as they are suffering. While to the patient and the caregiver, it seems as if we just need one more push to cure the disease, the truth is that this goal is still beyond the horizon.

References

1 Honykiewicz O. Dopamine miracle, from brain homogenate to dopamine replacement. Mov Disord 2002; 17: 501–8.

2 Schapira AH, Olanow CW. Drug selection and timing of initiation of treatment in early Parkinson's disease. Ann Neurol 2008; 64(Suppl 2): S47–55.

3 Benabid AL, Chabardès S, Seigneuret E, et al. Surgical therapy for Parkinson's disease. J Neural Transm 2006; 70(Suppl): 383–92.

4 Gwinn-Hardy K, Evidente VG, Waters C, Muenter MD, Hardy J. L-dopa slows the progression of familial parkinsonism. Lancet 1999; 353: 1850–1.

5 Hardy J, Lewis P, Revesz, T, Lees, AJ, Paisan Ruiz C. The genetics of Parkinson's syndromes: a critical review. Curr Opin Genet Dev (in press).

6 Clark LN, Wang Y, Karlins E, et al. Frequency of LRRK2 mutations in early- and late-onset Parkinson disease. Neurology 2006; 67: 1786–91.

7 Clark LN, Ross BM, Wang Y, et al. Mutations in the glucocerebrosidase gene are associated with early-onset Parkinson disease. Neurology 2007; 69: 1270–7.

8 Hardy J. A hundred years of Alzheimer's disease research. Neuron 2006; 52: 3–13.

9 Park J, Lee SB, Lee S, et al. Mitochondrial dysfunction in Drosophila PINK1 mutants is complemented by parkin. Nature 2006; 441: 1157–61.

10 Clark IE, Dodson MW, Jiang C, et al. Drosophila pink1 is required for mitochondrial function and interacts genetically with parkin. Nature 2006; 441: 1162–6.

11 Hughes AJ, Daniel SE, Ben-Shlomo Y, Lees AJ. The accuracy of diagnosis of parkinsonian syndromes in a specialist movement disorder service. Brain 2002; 125(Pt 4): 861–70.

12 Bras J, Singleton A, Cookson MR, Hardy J. Emerging pathways in genetic Parkinson's disease: potential role of ceramide metabolism in Lewy body disease. FEBS J 2008; 275: 5767–73.

Index

Please note that page references relating to non-textual content such as Figures or Tables are in *italic* print. PD-D stands for Parkinson's disease with dementia, PD for Parkinson's disease